To Barbara, the perfect companion for the long run.

Fitness and Health

FOURTH EDITION

Brian J. Sharkey, PhD
University of Montana

Human Kinetics

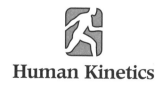

Library of Congress Cataloging-in-Publication Data

Sharkey, Brian J.
    Fitness and health / Brian J. Sharkey. -- 4th ed.
        p.   cm.
    Revision of the 3rd ed. of Physiology of fitness published in 1990
  by Human Kinetics.
    Includes bibliographical references and index.
    ISBN 0-87322-878-2
    1. Sports--Physiological aspects.   2. Physical fitness.
  3. Exercise--Physiological aspects.   I. Sharkey, Brian J.
  Physiology of fitness.   3rd ed.   II. Title.
  RC1235.S52   1997
  613.7--dc20   96-31258
                                                            CIP

ISBN: 0-87322-878-2

This book is a revised edition of *Physiology of Fitness*, published in 1990 by Human Kinetics.

Developmental Editor: Julia Anderson
Assistant Editor: Jacqueline Eaton Blakley
Editorial Assistant: Coree Schutter
Copyeditor: Regina Wells
Proofreader: Jim Burns
Indexer: Diana Witt
Graphic Designer: Judy Henderson
Graphic Artist: Francine Hamerski
Photo Editor: Boyd LaFoon
Cover Designer: Jack Davis
Photographer (cover): John Kelly
Illustrator: M.R. Greenberg
Printer: United Graphics

Printed in the United States of America   10 9 8 7 6 5 4 3 2

Human Kinetics
Web site: http://www.humankinetics.com/

United States: Human Kinetics, P.O. Box 5076, Champaign, IL 61825-5076
1-800-747-4457
e-mail: humank@hkusa.com

Canada: Human Kinetics, Box 24040, Windsor, ON N8Y 4Y9
1-800-465-7301 (in Canada only)
e-mail: humank@hkcanada.com

Europe: Human Kinetics, P.O. Box IW14, Leeds LS16 6TR, United Kingdom
(44) 1132 781708
e-mail: humank@hkeurope.com

Australia: Human Kinetics, 57A Price Avenue, Lower Mitcham, South Australia 5062
(08) 277 1555
e-mail: humank@hkaustralia.com

New Zealand: Human Kinetics, P.O. Box 105-231, Auckland 1
(09) 523 3462
e-mail: humank@hknewz.com

Contents

Preface

I was born in New York, grew up in New Jersey and Pennsylvania, and had just completed work on a doctorate in exercise physiology at the University of Maryland. Neither my wife nor I had ever ventured west of Harrisburg, Pennsylvania, until the summer of 1964. On the first day of September we loaded two kids and some suitcases into our covered wagon, a Volkswagen sedan, and headed west to begin an academic appointment at the University of Montana. I was hired over the phone, sight unseen, without a visit to the campus or the state. But I was happy to have a job, never imagining I would still be in the same place 30 years later. What took place, slowly but surely, was a subtle fusion of my academic interests with the magnificent geography and life of the mountain west. Before long I was hooked on the university, the mountains, and the active life. As our kids grew and we introduced them to the simple pleasures of active living, they responded with a deep sense of belonging in what has been called "The Last Best Place."

After a few years I realized that Montana's long winter nights were ideally suited for writing. In 1968 I began a manuscript that emerged as my first book. Refined by several years of classroom use, *Physiological Fitness and Weight Control* was published in 1974. It provided sound advice for exercise and weight control, advice that could save more than 250,000 lives annually, then and now! That is not to say that we haven't learned a great deal about physical activity, fitness, and health in the past two decades. In fact, exciting research developments led me to author a retitled and expanded version of the original text in 1979, and then follow it with second and third editions in 1984 and 1990. The editions of that book, *Physiology of Fitness*, became a chronicle of new developments and of my journey from fitness enthusiast, to performance advocate, and finally to someone with a healthy respect for the benefits of the active life.

I tell you this to explain why I felt it was important to retitle the fourth (or is it the fifth?) edition to *Fitness and Health*. Epidemiological studies have shown that many of the health benefits of physical activity can be achieved with regular, moderate physical activity. Of course, even greater rewards can be earned by improving your level of fitness, but the greatest gains, for personal and public health, come when individuals move from a sedentary to an active lifestyle. The new title emphasizes the importance of physical activity, highlighting one of the most exciting public health messages of our time.

Written for adults of all ages, this book is especially intended for the individual who wants to develop a deeper understanding, for the enthusiast who wants to know why and how the body responds, for the newcomer who needs more motivation, and for the skeptic who needs more proof. Years ago I set out to write the thinking person's fitness book; I hope you'll find that this edition meets that description.

Part I conveys the importance of regular, moderate physical activity. It describes how the active life contributes to physical and mental health, and the quality of life. The added benefits associated with improved aerobic and muscular fitness are also discussed. Part II covers everything you ever wanted to know about aerobic fitness, and Part III provides information and guidelines for muscular fitness training. Part IV presents new information in the areas of nutrition and weight control, while Part V shows you how to improve your performance in work and sport, and to cope with the environment. Part VI includes an expanded look at the psychology of activity, and a discussion of the role of activity in aging and longevity. The final chapter shows how you can improve your personal life and that of your family and your community. It portrays the importance of the environment to health, fitness, and quality of life, and enlists your aid in the struggle to preserve and expand opportunities for healthful, enjoyable physical activity. Each chapter includes useful information in tables and charts, and some contain testing procedures and proven fitness programs.

So, join me as we enter a new era of physical activity and fitness, in which the benefits are great relative to the effort, guilt and failure are replaced by enjoyment and satisfaction, and physical activity and fitness are recognized as vital to health and the quality of life.

Acknowledgments

Thanks to faculty and graduate students at the University of Montana, to co-workers in the U.S. Forest Service, and to colleagues in the American College of Sports Medicine for inspiration, advice, and review of ideas and interpretations in this book.

Special thanks to Rainer, Julie, and the wonderful folks at Human Kinetics, with extra special thanks to Julia Anderson for her patience, good humor, and attention to detail.

Credits

Figures

Figure 1.1. Reprinted from D.M. Spain, 1966, "Atherosclerosis," *Scientific American* 215: 48-49.

Figure 3.2. Reprinted by special permission from the Canadian Society for Exercise Physiology, Inc., copyright 1994, CSEP.

Figures 5.2 and 9.2. Adapted, by permission, from B.J. Sharkey, 1975, *Physiology and physical activity*, (New York: Harper and Row), 59, 126.

Figure 12.8. This figure is reprinted with permission from the *Research Quarterly for Exercise and Sport*, 1981, p. 382. *RQES* is a publication of the American Alliance for Health, Physical Education, Recreation and Dance, 1900 Association Drive, Reston, VA 22091.

Figures 13.1 and 17.2. Reprinted, by permission, from B.J. Sharkey, 1974, *Physiological fitness and weight control* (Missoula, MT: Mountain Press).

Figure 19.2. Adapted, by permission, from T. Orlick, 1986, *Psyching for sport: Mental training for athletes* (Champaign, IL: Leisure Press), 15.

Tables

Tables 1.1, 1.3, 12.1, 12.2, and 17.2. Reprinted, by permission, from B.J. Sharkey, 1974, *Physiological fitness and weight control* (Missoula, MT: Mountain Press).

Table 3.2. Reprinted, by permission, from J. Stamler, D. Wentworth, and J. Neaton, 1986, "Is relationship between serum cholesterol and risk of premature death from coronary heart disease continuous and graded?" *Journal of the American Medical Association* 256: 2823. Copyright 1986, American Medical Association.

Table 3.5. Reprinted, by permission, from K.H. Cooper, J.G. Purdy, S.R. White, M.L. Pollock, and A.C. Linnerud, 1975, Age-fitness adjusted maximal heart rates. In *The role of exercise in internal medicine* (Medicine and Sport, Vol. 10), edited by D. Brunner and E. Jokl (Switzerland: Karger).

Table 6.2. Reprinted, by permission, from G. Borg, 1985, *An introduction to Borg's RPE scale* (Ithaca, N.Y.: Mouvement Publications), 7.

Table 12.9. Adapted from C.C. Seltzer and J. Mayer, 1965, "A simple criterion of obesity," *Journal of Postgraduate Medicine* 38: A101-A106.

Table 13.1. Reproduced from *The Journal of Clinical Investigation*, 1969, 48:2124-2128 by copyright permission of The American Society for Clinical Investigation.

Table 18.1. Adapted, by permission, from Fries and Crapo, 1981, *Vitality and aging* (San Francisco: W.H. Freeman and Company), 125.

Text

"Principles of Training," pp. 304-309, adapted, by permission, from B.J. Sharkey, 1986, *Coaches guide to sport physiology* (Champaign, IL: Human Kinetics), 10-17.

Introduction

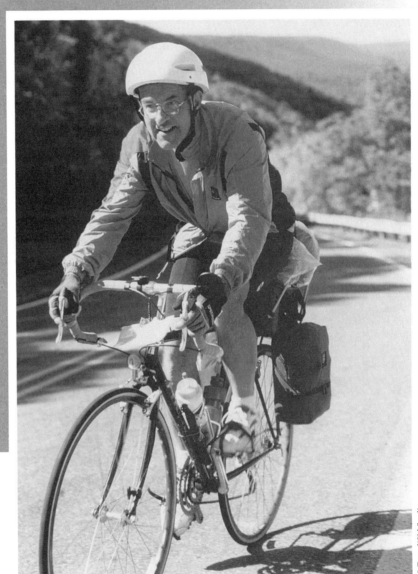

"When you come
to a fork in the
road . . . take it."
Yogi Berra

"Two roads
diverged in a
wood, and I—I
took the one less
traveled by, And
that has made all
the difference."
Robert Frost

You've come to a fork in the road; one path shows evidence of heavy traffic, while the other—the one less traveled—is faintly etched upon the land. One travels downhill, the route of least resistance, while the other rises slowly to distant heights. Will you be seduced by the easy route or motivated by the high road and the view from above? Sadly, many of us have chosen the easy route, and as a consequence we have lost our identity as a vigorous, vital people. Along the way we have become the fattest nation in the world, beset with chronic fatigue, depression, diseases of the heart and lungs, cancer, and diabetes. My goal in writing this book is to convince you to take the road less traveled, knowing it will make all the difference in your life.

What is the one less traveled? Simply stated it is the active life, a way of living based on regular physical activity and a cluster of related behaviors, including healthy food choices, weight control, stress management, abstinence from tobacco and drugs, moderate use of alcohol, attention to safety (seat belts, helmets), and disease prevention. It is the path of individual responsibility that leads not only to health, vigor, and vitality, but also to self-respect and control of your destiny. This family of health-related behaviors has proven to be a profound paradox for our society, simple to comprehend but difficult to adopt.

The active life is the one almost everyone led before people achieved the benefits of industrial modernization, technological developments, the automobile, labor-saving devices, television, and computers. These marvels of ingenuity now make it possible to minimize daily energy expenditure by using buttons, keystrokes, and voice commands to meet survival, work, and entertainment needs. Parallel to the decline in the need for human energy expenditure has been an increase in the consumption of fatty, convenience, and fast foods. Food chemists found it possible to add hydrogen to vegetable oils to prolong shelf (but not human) life, to substitute low-cost palm and coconut oils for other ingredients, and to cater to our demand for tasty food—in a hurry. Individually, the decline in activity and the rise in food consumption may not have been such a problem. However, coming together, as they have in recent years, they create the potential for alarming growth in the epidemic of diseases caused by the way we live, by our lifestyle. Fortunately, these behaviors can be changed.

Healthy Behaviors

The active life is a magnet that attracts a composite of behaviors or habits that, viewed one at a time, seem too simplistic to be of value. Yet collectively they are our greatest hope for personal health and vitality and for the integrity of the nation's health care system. Many of the behaviors remind us of our mother's admonitions. Some years ago researchers at the Human Population Laboratory of the California Department of Health published a list of habits associated with health and longevity (Breslow & Enstrom, 1980).

They included

- regular exercise,
- adequate sleep,
- a good breakfast,
- regular meals,
- weight control,
- abstinence from smoking and drugs, and
- moderate use of (or abstinence from) alcohol.

The study found that men could add 11 years of life and women 7 years just by following six of the seven habits.

Physical Activity

Recently the U.S. Centers for Disease Control and Prevention (CDC) and the American College of Sports Medicine reported that as many as 250,000 lives are lost annually due to the sedentary lifestyle (Pate et al., 1995). If that sounds to you like an enormous number, you are right. Compare it with the lives lost annually in automobile accidents (less than 50,000), with the number of lives lost each year from unprotected sexual intercourse (30,000), or with the number lost in the entire Vietnam War (58,000). Lack of physical activity is now considered as important a risk factor for heart disease as high blood cholesterol, high blood pressure, and cigarette smoking, not because activity is that potent, but because so many of us are inactive or sedentary. Inactivity contributes to a substantial number (34%) of the deaths from heart disease and approaches $5.7 billion in annual medical costs.

As many as 250,000 lives are lost annually due to the sedentary lifestyle.

Healthy Food Choices

Poor food choices contribute directly to overweight, obesity, heart disease, diabetes, and cancer, and indirectly to other problems such as depression and social and economic mistreatment. After years of health education to the contrary, average Americans still get almost 40% of their daily calories from fat. In spite of the books, newspaper and magazine articles, and television programs urging people to reduce fat intake to 30 or even 25%, the public seems surprised or confused about fat and cholesterol, about saturated and unsaturated fat. They seem unable to understand the important nutritional information printed on packages that clearly states the fat and cholesterol content of the food.

Understanding the importance of nutrition and food choices becomes even more critical as greater numbers enter the workforce, work longer hours, and rely more on convenience foods, take-home meals, and eating out. I'm lucky in that I don't eat out that often, so when I do it is a special event. At times I find it difficult to make healthy choices (such as fish versus red meat), to avoid rich sauces, gravies, and desserts, and to eat in moderation. To avoid daily temptation I carry a brown-bag lunch and eat at the desk after a vigorous workout. When I do eat out I ask for skim milk instead of whole, order dry toast, and request dressings on the side. Along with healthy food choices, these changes in eating behavior are survival techniques for modern urban warriors. Poor diet, coupled with lack of exercise, causes at least 300,000 deaths a year, mostly from heart disease, and contributes to an increased risk for cancer and other illnesses.

Weight Control

Dieting for weight loss is the most unsuccessful health intervention in all of medicine. Only 10% of people who have lost 25 pounds or more will remain at their desired weight. Worse yet is the fact that many weight-loss programs have contributed to obesity. The truth that has emerged from the last decade of research is that diet alone won't help you achieve permanent weight loss. What will? The active life, combined with healthy food choices, and behavior therapy if necessary, is the answer to lifelong weight control. Activity maintains or builds the lean tissue (muscle) that has the capability to burn calories. Diet, by itself, leads to the loss of muscle and a reduction in daily caloric expenditure, resulting in an increased storage of fat.

Dieting for weight loss is the most unsuccessful health intervention in all of medicine.

Stress Management

Stress is our emotional response to events in life. What is perceived as stress for one person may be stimulating to another. Stress management implies the learning of effective coping strategies, ways to deal with the many sources of stress in modern life. Stress has been linked to heart disease, cancer, ulcers, immune suppression, and other ills, but the linkage is uncertain due to the difficulty encountered in the measurement of stress. What is certain is that you can learn to cope with minor irritations and most major threats. The best results come when one combines learned behavior changes with an arsenal of coping skills. Regular moderate activity is the ideal way to cope with stress because it is effective, long-lasting, and inexpensive, while providing positive health benefits. As you'll see in chapter 2, activity can be psychologically therapeutic as well as preventive.

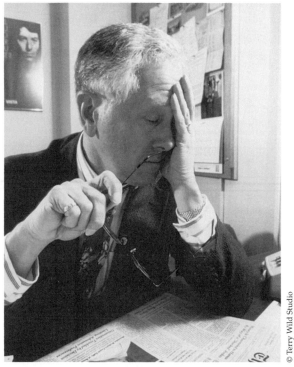

© Terry Wild Studio

Stress has been linked to heart disease, cancer, ulcers, immune suppression, and other ills.

Other Healthy Behaviors

Another important aspect of the active life includes elimination of negative behaviors, such as addiction to tobacco and other drugs, and moderation in the use of alcohol. According to the Public Health Service's Office for Disease Prevention and Health Promotion, tobacco causes 400,000 deaths annually, including 30% of cancer deaths (85% of all lung cancer) and 21% of cardiovascular deaths. Drug deaths total 20,000 per year, including overdose, suicide, homicide, AIDS (HIV infection), and more. Alcohol misuse causes 100,000 deaths a year, including almost half of all deaths from motor vehicle accidents. And yet having one or two drinks of alcohol each day, be they wine, beer, or the hard stuff, is associated with a reduced risk of heart disease. Who says disease pre-

By now you've noticed how many facets of the active life interact and overlap. Activity maintains muscle, which burns calories and fat, helps maintain a healthy weight, and reduces the risk of heart disease, cancer, and diabetes, while it also serves as the centerpiece of a stress management program. Of course, it helps you look better as well. Healthy food choices (sometimes called good nutrition) help maintain or lose weight, lower cholesterol, reduce the risk of heart disease, cancer, and other problems, and make physical activity more enjoyable. The active life is not a hodgepodge of unrelated habits, but rather a highly integrated family of behaviors that become more potent in combination than each is individually.

vention and health promotion have to be boring? One of the enjoyable little moments I experience daily is when I sit down to the evening news, a light beer, and some low-fat pretzels. The beer provides a tasty way to relax, reduce stress, and lower heart disease risk.

The final category of health behaviors I want to mention is the habitual practice of preventive measures appropriate to your age, sex, condition, and family history. These measures include vaccinations and other proven preventive techniques, such as blood pressure and cholesterol checks, mammography, and tests for glaucoma and prostate cancer. The fact is that you, not your doctor, are responsible for your health. Combine personal responsibility and prevention with early-detection tests, and you have a cost-effective strategy for survival. The strategy is cost-effective because prevention is always cheaper than treatment, because you utilize lower-cost health providers, and because you need to see physicians less frequently. If your employer has a comprehensive wellness program, use it. If not, create your own as you take personal responsibility for your health.

The Road Less Traveled?

A recent survey by the Centers for Disease Control and Prevention (Caspersen & Merritt, 1995) estimated the following activity levels for the population:

Physically inactive	30.5%
Irregularly active	28.5%
Regularly active, not intensive	31.9%
Regularly active, intensive	9.1%

Since the active life requires regular activity, only 40% of the population is active enough to ensure the physical and mental benefits of regular physical activity. The rest, a whopping 60%, are deprived of the joys and benefits of the active life and left to burden their families and the health care system. Less than 10% were active at a level known to maintain or promote aerobic fitness. Indeed, the active life is the one less traveled. Isn't it time that you joined the ranks of the few, informed, resolute individuals who have the good sense and conviction needed to take the fork in the road, make the changes, and embark on the active life?

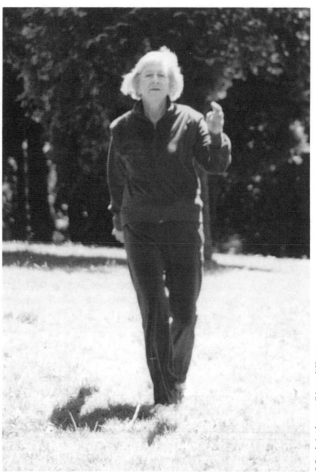

© Stock Art Images/Neena Wilmot

The active life is the road less traveled.

Many people view the active life and its associated behaviors as a medieval torture or religious rite, replete with fasting, denial, and mortification of the flesh. These folks are unwilling to give up the pleasures of rich (fatty) foods and unable to break addictions to cigarettes, drugs, or alcohol. Since behaviors are often interrelated in a dogma of self-indulgence, these same individuals are likely to disdain the pleasures and rewards of the active life. Sadly, they do so at considerable cost to themselves and to society, for while few admit sorrow or repent their indulgences, they are destined to suffer a penance of fatigue, depression, and disease. And the rest of us are expected to pay their bills and pick up the pieces of their lives.

Overly zealous fitness instructors have been heard to say, "No pain, no gain"; "Go for the burn"; or "It has to hurt to be good." Of course, none of these statements are true, unless you are involved in serious training for a highly competitive sport. And then the pain, the burn, and the hurt should be seen as identifiable end points during vigorous exercise. For most of us, pain, burn, and hurt need not be a part of our daily activity. The active life is not one of denial and deprivation, nor is it one of pain and hurt. It is a joyful experience, an affirmation of what we can be physically, mentally, socially, and spiritually. It provides the energy to begin, the vigor to pursue, and the vitality to persist, to go the distance. It replaces overindulgence with moderation, substitutes positive for negative addictions, and yields health, energy, and the capacity to live.

The active life is a joyful experience, an affirmation of what we can be physically, mentally, socially, and spiritually.

How Much Is Enough?

The public and some fitness instructors are confused. For years they thought that exercise had to be intense, as indicated by heavy breathing and a specific percentage of the maximal heart rate, if it was to yield desired benefits. That recommendation still holds true if you are striving to improve your aerobic fitness. But what if your interest is in improving or maintaining health?

In the summer of 1993, the American College of Sports Medicine (ACSM) and the U.S. Centers for Disease Control and Prevention (CDC) brought together a group of world-renowned experts to develop new recommendations for physical activity and health. They reviewed the latest scientific evidence and reached consensus on the following recommendation:

Every American adult should accumulate 30 minutes or more of moderate-intensity physical activity over the course of most days of the week.

- Every American adult should accumulate 30 minutes or more of moderate-intensity physical activity over the course of most days of the week.
- Because most adult Americans fail to meet this recommended level of moderate-intensity physical activity, almost all should strive to increase their participation in moderate or vigorous physical activity.

The recommendation suggests that a wide range of activities can contribute to the 30-minute total, including walking, gardening, and dancing. The 30 minutes (or more) of physical activity may also come from planned exercise or recreation, such as jogging, cycling, and swimming. The recommendation notes that a specific way to meet the standard is to walk 2 miles briskly. The ACSM/CDC recommendation tells those who currently do not engage in regular activity to begin with a few minutes of daily activity, and build gradually to 30 minutes.

These recommendations are based on recent research that shows that adults who engage in regular moderate activity, enough to burn about 200 calories a day (e.g., brisk 2-mile walk or jog), can expect many of the health benefits of exercise (Leon, Connett, Jacobs, and Rauramaa, 1987). From a public health perspective, we'll gain more if millions become active than we will if a few become very fit.

The Activity Index

Before we move on, you may want to gauge your current level of activity using the simple assessment tool called the *activity index*, shown on page 8. Developed in the 1970s, the index has proved to be related to aerobic fitness, as measured in a laboratory procedure that determines the maximal amount of oxygen your muscles are able to utilize. As you increase the intensity, duration, and frequency of exercise, your index score and fitness both go up. How much activity do you need? That is a decision you'll make as you become better acquainted with the pleasures and benefits of activity. A score of 40 or more on the activity index is an indication that you are active enough to earn many of the health benefits associated with physical activity. Increase the amount or intensity of exercise, and you will earn additional health benefits as you increase your aerobic fitness.

If your index score is below 40, you should begin today to increase your daily activity. Then, when we get into a discussion of the extra benefits associated with improved fitness, you will be ready to make a reasoned response to the question: Am I satisfied with my current level of activity and fitness, or do I feel the need to undertake a training program?

The Activity Index

Based on your regular daily activity, calculate your activity index by multiplying your score for each category (Score = Intensity × Duration × Frequency).

	Score	Daily activity
Intensity	5	Sustained heavy breathing and perspiration
	4	Intermittent heavy breathing and perspiration—as in tennis, racquetball
	3	Moderately heavy—as in recreational sports and cycling
	2	Moderate—as in volleyball, softball
	1	Light—as in fishing, walking
Duration	4	Over 30 min
	3	20 to 30 min
	2	10 to 20 min
	1	Under 10 min
Frequency	5	Daily or almost daily
	4	3 to 5 times a week
	3	1 to 2 times a week
	2	Few times a month
	1	Less than once a month

Evaluation and Fitness Category

Score	Evaluation	Fitness category*
100	Very active lifestyle	High
80 to 100	Active and healthy	Very good
40 to 60	Acceptable (could be better)	Fair
20 to 40	Not good enough	Poor
Under 20	Sedentary	Very Poor

*Index score is highly related to aerobic fitness.

From *The Effects of Exercise and Fitness on Serum Lipids in College Women* (p. 46) by D. Kasari, 1976, unpublished master's thesis, University of Montana.

Summary

This introduction began with a description of the road less traveled, the active life; described how the health behaviors of the active life interact; and finished with a simple assessment of your level of activity. Along the way we've documented the fact that only about 20% of the population are active enough to get the physical and mental benefits of regular activity, and we've defined the amount of activity needed to achieve health benefits. What remains is the question: How did we get this way?

We began as a vigorous nation of farmers, miners, loggers, laborers, and merchants; survived a revolution, a civil war, and the Industrial Revolution; migrated across the continent; and continued to thrive in spite of two world wars and the Depression. Yet today, in spite of several decades of unparalleled economic development, we are gaining the reputation of being an overweight, lazy, complacent people, content to while away the hours with fast food, television, and video games. We have become the fattest nation in the world, with one-third of our adult citizens classified as obese. Our educational system is suffering from neglect, and we're the only developed country that has ignored the need for universal health care. We've evolved welfare and unemployment programs that discourage work, and many among us have lost a sense of responsibility for our acts, expecting others to bear the cost of our personal habits and mistakes.

Will the active life change all that? Probably not, but it is a positive way to begin exercising individual responsibility, to lighten our burden on society, and to lead family and friends along the road less traveled. With the active life you'll feel better, look better, and improve your physical and psychological health. Your energy level will increase, along with your productivity. You'll be more attractive, even sexy. And if you stick with the active life, you'll delay chronic illness and prolong the period of adult vigor. You'll be able to romp with your grandchildren and, years later, have the vitality to enjoy your great-grandchildren. You might as well make plans to live for 85 years, give or take a few. Adopt the active life, and you could live with vigor and vitality until the end of your years.

Physical Activity, Fitness, and Health

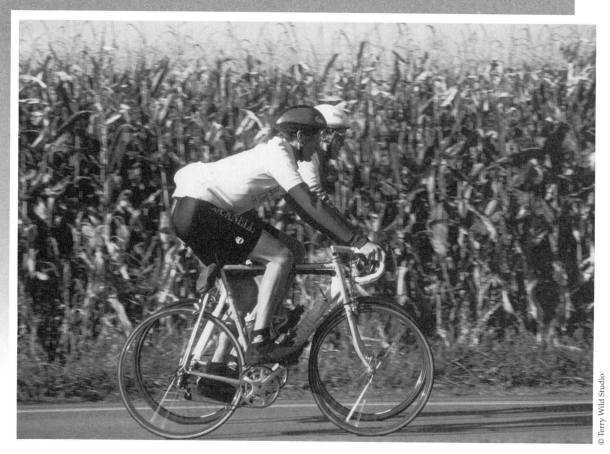

Would you be upset to learn that more than 250,000 lives are lost, every year, for failure to apply a medically proven therapy? It's true; our highly praised health care system has ignored a simple, low-cost health treatment with the capacity to save hundreds of thousands of lives and billions of dollars. This miracle treatment goes unused in favor of expensive drugs, costly operations, even organ transplants. How could this happen? One reason is that physicians have been compensated for performing procedures rather than providing the counseling that leads to improved health habits. With the development of penicillin and other "wonder drugs," we patients have sought a quick fix for problems, and have relinquished personal responsibility for our health. Hospitals, drug and insurance companies, and, yes, even lawyers reaped enormous profits in this so-called health care system, while simple, inexpensive health habits went unused.

Fortunately, the times are changing. As we work to rebuild our ailing health care system, we are searching for ways to reduce costs and the reliance on drugs and medical procedures. At the same time, researchers are questioning the value of operations and drugs, and confirming the contributions of physical activity and related habits to health, longevity, and the quality of life. This section reviews studies that provide the modern foundation for the relationship of physical activity and fitness to physical and psychological health. It discusses the benefits and risks of activity, catalogs the extra benefits of fitness, and provides advice to help you begin your transformation to health, vitality, and the active life.

CHAPTER 1

Health Benefits of Activity and Fitness

"The Surgeon General warns that physical inactivity may be hazardous to your health."

1996 Surgeon General's Report on Physical Activity and Health

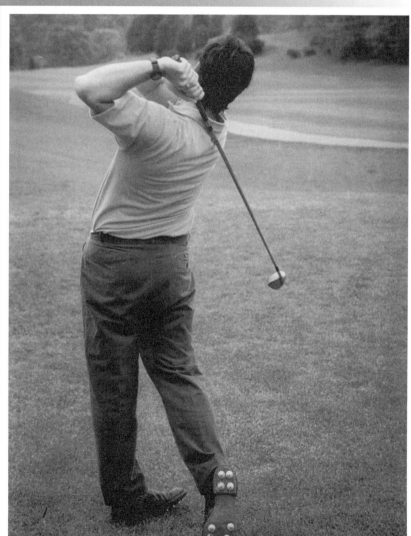

© Terry Wild Studio

The idea that exercise or activity is associated with good health is not a new one. The ancient Chinese practiced a mild form of medical gymnastics to prevent diseases associated with lack of activity. In Rome the physician Galen prescribed exercise for health maintenance more than 1,500 years ago. References to the health values of exercise can be found throughout recorded history, usually with little measurable effect on the populace. Why, then, do I invest time and energy in an effort to provide the latest evidence on the relationships among physical activity, physical fitness, and health? One reason is that I am a devout optimist, the product of more than 30 years of professional experience and many heartwarming success stories. Another reason is that never before in history have we known so much about the health benefits of activity and fitness.

THIS CHAPTER WILL HELP YOU

- understand the relationships among physical activity, fitness, and health;

- see how activity and fitness lower the risk of heart disease, hypertension, and stroke;

- appreciate how activity reduces the risk of chronic diseases such as some cancers and diabetes;

- assess the role of activity in arthritis, osteoporosis, and low back problems; and

- understand how regular moderate physical activity contributes to the length and the quality of life.

The Relationship Among Physical Activity, Fitness, and Health

Epidemiology, which began as the study of epidemics, is a fitting way to study the modern epidemic that is responsible for more than half of all deaths: diseases of lifestyle. The epidemiologist studies populations to determine relationships between behaviors, such as physical activity, and the incidence of certain diseases. Researchers look at morbidity (or sickness) and mortality (or death). Studies can be retrospective, looking back at past behaviors; cross-sectional, looking at chronological slices or age segments of the population; or prospective, following a group into the future. Unfortunately, no type of study is problem-free. Retrospective studies are often troubled by lack of solid information on past activity, fitness, and other health habits, while prospective studies face problems of changing habits and dropouts. Most studies are plagued by issues of access to medical records, or confidentiality, but the major problem is that of self-selection. Critics argue that subjects could be active because they are well, not necessarily well because they are active. Because self-selection confounds the results of retrospective and cross-sectional studies, only carefully controlled prospective studies, involving random assignment of subjects to levels of activity (or inactivity), allow cause-and-effect conclusions. Since these studies are difficult to conduct and probably unethical (inactivity is dangerous to your health), absolute proof of the value of activity and fitness may never be assembled. However, when the preponderance of studies support the health benefits of activity, and when the risks are minimal, it seems reasonable to recommend a prudent—if not proven—course of action.

Since space does not permit a comprehensive review of the role of activity and fitness in health and disease, I will provide a summary of epidemiological findings and review several classic studies. To avoid endless details I will summarize the effects of activity and fitness with reference to the risk ratio (RR), the ratio of morbidity or mortality for the active members of the population to that for the inactive members.

When possible I will indicate reasons why activity may have beneficial effects, and will conclude with a consideration of the risks and benefits of activity, as well as recommendations for prudent behavior.

RISK RATIO

In a study of Harvard alumni, those with the least activity had 78.8 cardiovascular deaths (per 10,000) versus 43 for the most active, yielding a risk ratio of $43 \div 78.8 = .54$ (54%). Stated another way, the risk was 46% lower (100% − 54% = 46%) for the active alumni (Paffenbarger, Hyde, & Wing, 1986).

Activity and the Risk of Coronary Artery Disease

In spite of tremendous progress in the past 25 years, heart disease, or more specifically coronary artery disease (CAD), remains the nation's number one killer. Heart diseases, stroke, and blood vessel diseases kill almost one million people *in one year*, far more than all the lives lost in the four major wars of the 20th century (636,282)! CAD is responsible for more than half of those deaths, often in a sudden dramatic event called a heart attack. But this seemingly sudden event is actually the product of a gradual process called atherosclerosis, which narrows the arteries and restricts the blood flow to the heart.

Atherosclerosis may begin to develop during childhood, and the process is accelerated by a number of primary risk factors. In 1993 the American Heart Association stated that "inactivity is a risk factor for the development of coronary artery disease" and raised lack of physical activity to the level of the big three risk factors—cigarette smoking, elevated blood cholesterol, and high blood pressure (hypertension). Atherosclerosis can be inherited, so a family history is an indicator of personal risk. Table 1.1 presents CAD risk factors and the possible influence of physical activity.

Atherosclerosis may be caused by an injury to the lining of the coronary artery. Thereafter, high levels of circulating fats in the blood infiltrate the region, aided perhaps by high blood pressure and chemicals in cigarette smoke. A scab-like plaque forms and grows until it blocks the flow of blood, or until the artery is clogged by a clot (figure 1.1). Some think viruses may accelerate atherosclerosis, or stimulate immune system responses that contribute to plaque formation and clotting. Gradual narrowing reduces blood flow (ischemia) and often leads to exertional pain (angina) experienced in the chest, left arm, or shoulder. A clot can interrupt blood flow and cause a heart attack (myocardial infarct), which can damage heart muscle if it isn't treated quickly.

Heart diseases, stroke, and blood vessel diseases kill almost one million people in one year, far more than all the lives lost in the four major wars of the 20th century (636,282)!

TABLE 1.1   CAD Risk Factors

Influenced by physical activity	May be influenced by physical activity	Not influenced by physical activity
Endomesomorphic body type	Insulin resistance	Family history of heart disease
Overweight	Electrocardiographic abnormalitites	Gender (male has greater risk until 60s)
Elevated blood lipids	Elevated uric acid	Cigarette smoking
High blood pressure or hypertension	Pulmonary function (lung) abnormalities	Diet (saturated fats, salt)
Physical inactivity	Personality or behavior pattern (hard driving, time conscious, aggressive, competitive)	
	Psychic reactivity (reaction to stress)	

Reprinted from Sharkey 1974.

Autopsy studies show that the process is under way in young adults, and recent surveys have confirmed the presence of CAD risk factors in children of all ages. Thus, a program of risk factor identification and early intervention seems prudent, especially for people with a family history of CAD. The active life can slow or stop the process for all but those with serious genetic disorders, and a demanding intervention program consisting of activity, a very low-fat diet, and medication, if needed, may even reverse the process (Ornish, 1993).

Inactivity and CAD

The famous London bus driver study published in 1954 (Morris & Raffle) focused the world's attention on inactivity as a factor in heart disease. The study compared the incidence of CAD between bus drivers and conductors and found that the conductors, who were more active than the drivers, had a rate 30% below that of the drivers. The disease appeared earlier in drivers, and their mortality rate was more than twice as high following the first heart attack. In

DO YOU KNOW YOUR RISK?

Do you have:
- [ ] high blood pressure (>140 mm Hg)?
- [ ] elevated serum cholesterol (> 240 mg)?
- [ ] excess body weight?

Are you:
- [ ] a cigarette smoker?
- [ ] a bald male with a pot belly?

To calculate your health risk, complete the health risk analysis at the end of chapter 3.

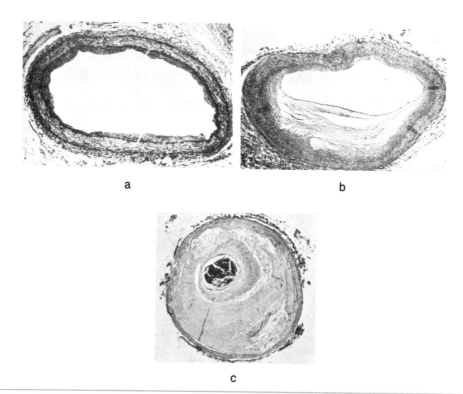

Figure 1.1 The coronary artery: (a) a normal coronary artery; (b) cholesterol deposits that narrow the artery; (c) a blood clot completely blocking a severely occluded coronary artery. Reprinted from Spain 1966.

spite of confounding factors (e.g., the stress of driving; drivers were more likely to be overweight), the study sparked interest in the role of activity.

In a classic epidemiological study cited earlier, Paffenbarger and associates studied thousands of Harvard alumni to determine the influence of activity, vigorous activity, and sports on cardiovascular illness and death (1986). In comparison with less active subjects (those who engaged in less than 1,000 calories of activity per week), moderate and high levels of activity yielded mortality risk ratios of .71 and .54 respectively.

Less than 1,000 calories per week	RR = 1.0
1,000 to 2,500 calories per week	0.71
More than 2,500 calories per week	0.54

Thus, moderate activity yielded a 29% reduction in risk, and high levels of activity yielded a 46% reduction. Those who played light or moderately vigorous sports had mortality ratios of .79 and .63 compared with those who played no sports. Risk ratios for mortality as well as first attacks of coronary artery disease were inversely related to physical activity, as indicated by calories of weekly exercise. The mortality ratio approached .5, which means a 50% reduction in risk, when activity exceeded 2,500 calories per week (see figure 1.2). Paffenbarger and associates (1990) presented data indicating that moderately vigorous activity and sport were more effective than low levels of activity in reducing the risk of CAD. The risk for low-activity alumni who played no vigorous sports was 2.4 times that of active alumni who engaged in vigorous sports.

Most other studies have shown the same results, that heart disease risk is inversely related to the amount of regular physical activity, be it occupational,

Heart disease risk is inversely related to the amount of regular physical activity.

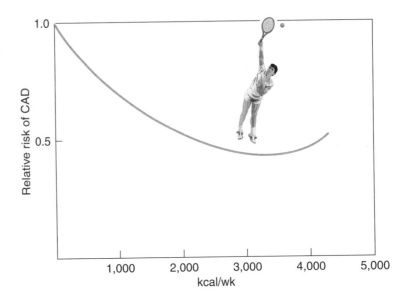

Figure 1.2 Physical activity and the risk of heart disease. The risk declines up to 3,500 kcal/wk and then begins to rise. This unexplained tendency for the risk to go back up may be the result of the small number of cases that report more than 3,500 kcal/wk.

leisure-time, or vigorous sports. They show that the activity must be current or contemporaneous to be beneficial, that participation in high school or college sports did not confer protection later in life. In fact, regularly active adults maintain a lower risk of CAD whether or not they had been physically active during their youth.

Autopsy studies conducted on American soldiers killed in the Korean conflict showed an alarming 77% with evidence of CAD, indicating that the pathology of atherosclerosis is developing by the age of 22 years (Enos, Beyer, & Holmes, 1955). In another study, autopsies of older men (45 to 70 years) found

CALORIES

Throughout this book I use the term *calorie* to refer to the kilocalorie, defined as the amount of heat required to raise 1 kilogram of water (1 liter) 1 degree Celsius. I use calorie because it is the common usage, the one you see when you read food labels. I want you to become very familiar with the calorie cost of activities as well as the calories consumed in food. Then you will be an informed consumer of food and activity, and see how an excess in calorie intake requires an increase in caloric expenditure.

In general you burn about 100 calories when you jog 1 mile. To burn 2,500 calories per week, you would need to jog 25 miles. Or you could combine activities. For example, in one week play singles tennis 3 hours (8 calories per minute × 60 minutes = 480 calories × 3 hours = 1,440 calories), walk 60 minutes (6 calories per minute × 60 minutes = 360 calories), and jog 3.5 miles twice (7 miles × 100 calories per minute = 700 calories), for a total of 2,500 calories of vigorous activity.

that the incidence of scars and obstructions in the arteries and dead tissue was 30% less for those who had been moderately active, and reduced even more for those presumed to be heavily active (Morris & Crawford, 1958).

Animal studies agree that moderate activity is beneficial, but they suggest that exhaustive or stressful effort may somehow accelerate the development of CAD. Exhaustion may be stressful for an animal, and stress provokes a hormonal response that may accelerate the atherosclerotic process, in animals as well as in humans.

Physical Activity Versus Fitness

If activity and sport can lower the risk of CAD, what about fitness? Does one earn extra benefits by raising one's level of fitness? Physical fitness, specifically aerobic fitness, has long been associated with better health. This is surprising, since fitness has only recently been measured in epidemiological studies of physical activity and health. The issue was raised in 1988 at the annual meeting of the American College of Sports Medicine at which Drs. Steven Blair and Harold Kohl reported on their study of more than 10,000 men. They analyzed all-cause death rates for sedentary and active men whose fitness had been assessed in a treadmill test. The surprising results have led to major changes in the way we view activity, fitness, and the prescription of exercise.

The all-cause death rate was almost three times higher for the sedentary men. And within the sedentary classification, aerobic fitness level made a difference only at the lowest level, where the least fit had twice the risk of other sedentary subjects (five times the risk for active men). Among the active subjects, the death rates were not significantly different, regardless of the level of aerobic fitness! These findings suggested that, for the male subjects in this study, activity conferred most of the health benefits of exercise, and that higher levels of aerobic fitness didn't provide greater protection from all-cause mortality (heart disease contributes more than one-half of all-cause mortality) (see table 1.2).

Does this mean that physical fitness is not associated with better health? No, it certainly does not. In fact, when the sedentary and active subjects are analyzed together, there is a trend toward a reduced death rate with increasing fitness (Blair, Kohl, Paffenbarger, et al., 1989).

Fitness Level		Death Rate*
1	Lowest	64
2		25.5
3	Medium	27.1
4		21.7
5	Highest	18.6

*All-cause deaths per 10,000.

TABLE 1.2   Physical Activity Versus Fitness

	Fitness level				
	Low	2	3	4	High
Sedentary	74*	31	35	28	33
Active	13	8	14	16	13

*Age-adjusted death rate per 10,000; Blair & Kohl, 1988.

Although the higher levels of fitness are associated with only minor reductions in all-cause death rate, they are correlated with fewer risk factors and probably do provide added protection, especially for those with an elevated risk (elevated cholesterol, triglycerides, hypertension, diabetes, obesity).

Are you wondering why some sedentary subjects are more fit than others? Physical fitness is a product of heredity and training. With good heredity a sedentary individual could have a higher level of fitness than an active friend. The good news is that moving from sedentary to active living imparts a sizable drop in health risk and all-cause mortality. When an already active individual improves his or her fitness, the decrease in risk is more subtle but still important, especially for someone with inherited risks.

Further proof of the extra benefits of fitness can be found in a recent study conducted in Finland. The authors concluded that higher levels of both leisure-time physical activity and fitness had a strong inverse relationship with the risk of heart attack. The study supports the conclusion that lower levels of physical activity and lower levels of fitness are independent risk factors for coronary artery disease in men (Lakka, Venalainen, Rauramaa, et al., 1994).

> For now let me emphasize one of the most important public health messages of our time: Regular moderate physical activity conveys many if not most of the important health benefits associated with exercise. From a public health standpoint, an increase in physical activity will provide millions of Americans with some level of protection from heart disease, hypertension, adult-onset diabetes, certain cancers, osteoporosis, depression, premature aging, and more. Improved aerobic fitness provides some added benefits. However, in both the Blair and Lakka studies, the level of fitness associated with extra benefits was not extremely high.

Cardioprotective Mechanisms

Numerous studies have shown that physical activity and fitness are associated with a lower risk of CAD. Yet, due to self-selection, most of the studies do not allow cause-and-effect statements and the level of assurance desired in scientific and medical research. To further investigate the influence of activity on cardiovascular health, researchers have explored a number of hypotheses concerning cardioprotective mechanisms (see table 1.3).

Among the many possible ways in which activity may prevent or help minimize the process of atherosclerosis, few are directly related to the heart itself. In my opinion, the major benefit of activity is its ability to mobilize and metabolize fat, and to lower circulating levels of fat in the blood (triglycerides and cholesterol). Let's explore some of these mechanisms to help explain why something as simple as regular moderate activity is so good for your health.

Activity's Effect on the Heart

Physical activity does have some direct effects on the heart, but not as many as you have been led to believe. Indeed, studies on the therapy called cardiac rehabilitation have been surprising in that they show little visible effect of exer-

TABLE 1.3   Cardioprotective Mechanisms

Physical activity may	
Increase	Decrease
Oxidation of fat	Serum cholesterol and triglycerides
Number of coronary blood vessels	Glucose intolerance
Vessel size	Obesity, adiposity
Efficiency of heart	Platelet stickiness
Efficiency of peripheral blood distribution and return	Arterial blood pressure
Electron transport capacity	Heart rate
Fibrinolytic (clot-dissolving) capability	Vulnerability to dysrhythmias
Arterial oxygen content	Overreaction to hormones
Red blood cells and blood volume	Psychic stress
Thyroid function	
Growth hormone production	
Tolerance to stress	
Prudent living habits	
Joy of living	

Reprinted from Sharkey 1974.

cise or training on the heart. Only when the training is prolonged and strenuous do we see measurable effects on the heart, and strenuous training may not reduce the risk of heart disease much more than moderate activity.

• **Efficiency of the heart:**   Regular activity reduces the workload of the heart. Changes in skeletal muscle, including improved oxygen-using (aerobic) enzymes and enhanced fat metabolism, allow the heart to meet exercise demands with a lower heart rate. The lower rate means a lower level of oxygen utilization in the heart muscle and a more efficient heart. Drugs are sometimes prescribed to lower the workload of the heart, but activity and fitness are a more natural approach to the problem, without undesirable side effects.

Some of the improved efficiency of the heart is due to improved contractility of the cardiac muscle, to diminished myocardial response to the hormone epinephrine (adrenaline), and to an increase in blood volume with training. If the heart pumps more blood each time it beats, it doesn't have to beat as often. Regularly active and fit individuals have lower resting and exercise heart rates, and a higher stroke volume (amount of blood pumped each beat).

• **Heart size:**   Since skeletal muscle gets larger with training, some people have wondered if the same holds true for the heart. Studies of endurance training suggest that the trained heart is larger, but the increase is in the volume of the left ventricle, allowing a greater stroke volume. Little change has been noted in the concentration of aerobic enzymes in heart muscle, which is not surprising, since the heart is already the ultimate endurance muscle. People who do serious long-term resistance training may experience some increase in the thickness of the heart muscle as it strains to pump blood against the resistance of contracting muscles. Cardiac hypertrophy, or an enlarged heart, is a natural consequence of exercise training. There is no suggestion that it is associated with more or less risk of CAD.

• **Blood supply:** Studies show that activity improves the circulation within the heart. Animal and human studies suggest that in some subjects, moderate activity enhances the development of coronary collaterals, alternative circulatory routes that help distribute blood and minimize the effects of narrowed coronary arteries. A fascinating effect of regular activity, first suggested after the autopsy on marathon runner Clarence DeMar, is an increase in the diameter of the coronary arteries, perhaps minimizing the effect of plaque formation. Kramsch and associates (1981) studied the effect of moderate exercise and an atherosclerotic diet on the development of CAD in monkeys. ECG changes and sudden death occurred only in the sedentary animals, whereas the exercise group had larger hearts and larger-diameter coronary arteries.

Activity's Effect on the Vascular System

The following discussion suggests ways that activity may lower the risk of CAD via changes in or within the blood vessels. They include beneficial changes in blood clotting, blood pressure, and blood distribution.

• **Blood clotting:** Blood is designed to form a clot and stem the flow of blood when we are injured. But a clot (called a thrombus) that forms within an uninjured vessel is dangerous, and a clot in a narrowed coronary artery could be disastrous. Clots form when the soluble protein fibrinogen is converted to insoluble threads of fibrin. Normally we have some ability to dissolve unwanted clots by dissolving the fibrin that keeps the clot together (fibrinolysis). Exercise enhances this process, but the effect lasts only for a day or two. Moreover, the stress of exhaustive or highly competitive exercise seems to inhibit this system, allowing a more rapid clotting time. Regular, moderate, or even vigorous activity is the way to enhance the body's ability to dissolve unwanted clots (Molz, Heyduck, Lill, et al., 1993). In fact, a recent review of the literature concluded that regular exercise is the most practicable approach known to date to lower plasma fibrinogen levels (Ernst, 1993).

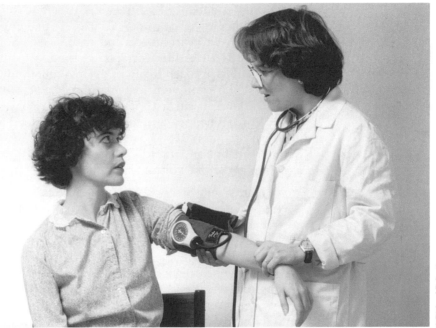

© Richard B. Levine

Regular, moderate physical activity has been shown to reduce blood pressure.

ASPIRIN

Studies have shown that one aspirin a day (or one every other day) reduces the risk of clots associated with heart disease and stroke. The aspirin reduces the stickiness of platelets, small particles in the blood that get caught in the fibrin threads of a developing clot. One aspirin a day, taken with a meal, is tolerated by most folks. It is an inexpensive way to reduce the risk of CAD and stroke, and it may help reduce the risk of colon cancer.

• **Blood pressure:**   High blood pressure, or hypertension, increases the workload of the heart by forcing it to contract against greater resistance. Anything that lowers blood pressure also reduces the workload of the heart. Regular moderate physical activity has been shown to reduce blood pressure in middle-aged or older individuals. And walking but not weight lifting has been shown to reduce systolic blood pressure in elderly individuals (Rejeski, Neal, Wurst, et al., 1995). Recent studies suggest that regular activity may help maintain the elasticity of blood vessels in aging subjects. Of course, changes in blood pressure could also be the consequence of weight loss or reduced stress, both known outcomes of regular activity.

• **Blood distribution:**   Regular physical activity teaches the body to better distribute the blood to muscles during exercise, further reducing the workload of the heart. Constricting vessels leading to digestive and other organs and dilating vessels that serve working muscles allow the blood to flow where it is needed. Of course, the 10-to-15% increase in blood volume that comes with endurance training further enhances the performance of both the heart and skeletal muscles. These changes serve to lower the heart rate and blood pressure during physical activity. Since the oxygen needs of heart muscle are directly related to the product of heart rate and blood pressure, these improvements reduce the likelihood that you'll exceed the ability to supply oxygen to cardiac muscle. As with most other effects of activity and training, the benefits depend on regular, not occasional, activity.

Metabolic Changes Due to Activity

The package of metabolic mechanisms may be the most important in the fight against CAD, as well as several other disorders.

• **Fat metabolism:**   Eat too much, and you gain weight in the form of stored fat. Excess fat is a health risk for heart disease, hypertension, diabetes, and some forms of cancer. You can diet (starve) to get rid of fat, but there is a hitch: the starving breaks down muscle tissue for energy, so you lose the only tissue that is capable of burning large amounts of fat. Muscular activity is the proven way to mobilize fat from adipose tissue storage, and then to burn it for energy in skeletal muscles. Exercise burns fat and avoids loss of muscle protein; in fact, regular activity can build additional muscle, thereby enhancing your ability to burn additional fat.

Regular activity burns calories, helping you to maintain a desirable body weight and percent body fat, and a leaner, healthier figure. Fitness training leads to an enhanced ability to mobilize and metabolize fat. The physically fit

The physically fit individual is the owner of an efficient fat-burning furnace.

individual is the owner of an efficient fat-burning furnace. This enhanced ability to utilize fat as an energy source leads to even greater benefits that are closely tied to prevention of atherosclerosis and CAD.

• **Blood lipids:**   Lipid is another word for fat; the blood lipids include cholesterol and triglycerides, and each is related to the risk of heart disease. The level of cholesterol in the blood is an important predictor of the risk of heart disease. Total cholesterol includes two main forms, low-density lipoprotein cholesterol (LDL) and high-density lipoprotein cholesterol (HDL). Regular activity can lead to a modest decline in total cholesterol, but that is only part of the story. LDL is the dangerous form of cholesterol found in the plaques that clog coronary arteries. Activity, diet, and weight loss all contribute to a drop in LDL. Regular activity, particularly vigorous activity, and weight loss both contribute to a rise in HDL cholesterol, the beneficial form of cholesterol that collects cholesterol from the arteries and transports it to the liver for removal from the body. So, exercise reduces total cholesterol (especially the LDL portion), raises HDL, and greatly improves your total cholesterol/HDL ratio, one of the best predictors of heart disease risk.

Interestingly, it has been shown that a high fat diet inhibits formation of the liver's LDL receptors that are needed to clear LDL cholesterol from the circulation (Brown & Goldstein, 1984). We'll say much more about dietary fat in chapters 11, 12, and 13.

Triglycerides, consisting of three fatty acids and a molecule of glycerol, constitute a transport and storage form of fat. High levels are associated with heart disease, obesity, and hypertension. Regular activity is a proven way to lower circulating levels of triglycerides. Levels are reduced several hours after exercise, and the effect persists for 1 or 2 days. Several days of exercise lead to a progressive reduction of triglyceride levels. The final plateau depends on the diet, body weight, intensity and duration of exercise, and one's genetic tendency. It is clear that regular moderate activity leads to a significant reduction in triglycerides.

• **Other metabolic mechanisms:**   A number of additional metabolic mechanisms support the value of activity as a cardioprotective therapy. Regular activity and training have been shown to increase insulin sensitivity and glucose tolerance. This effect of exercise is particularly important for obese people and people with adult-onset diabetes (also called type II diabetes, or non-insulin-dependent diabetes mellitus—NIDDM). High levels of circulating fat inhibit insulin's ability to help transport glucose into muscles. Exercise enhances the transport, even in the absence of insulin. Thus, regular activity helps by reducing body weight and fat levels, and by increasing insulin sensitivity and glucose transport. All these improvements reduce the risk of heart disease and NIDDM.

TOTAL CHOLESTEROL/HDL RATIO

Before training and weight loss, Bill had a cholesterol level of 240 and an HDL of 40, for a ratio of 240/40 = 6, and a moderately high risk of CAD. Training and weight loss reduced the cholesterol to 200 and raised the HDL to 50, yielding a much improved ratio of 4. He could continue to improve his lipid profile and further reduce his risk of CAD by continuing the fitness training, maintaining his body weight, and reducing his consumption of total and saturated fat.

- **Electrolytes:**   Electrolytes, including potassium, sodium, and calcium, are essential to the function of muscles, such as the heart. During exertion the untrained heart may experience a diminished oxygen supply, which can trigger an imbalance of electrolytes, electrical instability, and disturbances in heart rhythms. Death can result from lethal rhythm disorders, such as tachycardia (rapid beating) or fibrillation (irregular, uncontrolled, unsynchronized beating). Fitness training minimizes this likelihood by reducing the heart's workload, improving oxygen supply and efficiency, and correcting electrolyte imbalance.

Psychological Stress

Most folks and some researchers are convinced that stress, or our reaction to it, is a major factor in the development of atherosclerosis and CAD. Years ago Friedman and Rosenman (1973) identified the Type A personality, characterized by competitiveness, ambition, and a profound sense of time urgency, as a risk factor. They claimed that among the subjects in their studies, Type As had a greater incidence of CAD. However, analysis of the Framingham study (Wilson, Castelli, & Kannel, 1987), a long-term (longitudinal) study of an entire community, failed to find a link between stress and heart disease. This could be due to the fact that stress is hard to measure with a paper-and-pencil test. Recent work in this area suggests that anger and repressed hostility are related to heart disease, and that Type A behavior by itself does not pose a problem. Others are searching for "hot reactors," individuals who have exaggerated increases in blood pressure and stress hormones when faced with daily events.

I do know that regular activity is a coping mechanism that serves to improve tolerance to psychological stress. It is my opinion that regular moderate activity is the best form of stress management. Why? Simply because it provides the benefits of meditation and relaxation while it delivers added health-related benefits, including weight loss; reduced risk of CAD, hypertension, cancer, diabetes, and other ills; and control of anxiety and depression; as well as improved appearance, vitality, even longevity. I'll say more about stress in chapter 2.

Physical Activity Reduces the Risk of Chronic Diseases

I've taken a lot of time and space to establish the role of activity and fitness in reducing the risks and risk factors of heart disease. Now I will briefly sketch how activity can protect you from an impressive list of chronic diseases and disorders.

Hypertension and Stroke

Individuals with high blood pressure (greater than 160/95) are three times more likely to experience CAD and four times more likely to get congestive heart failure than others. Hypertension also increases the risk of stroke and kidney failure. The causes of hypertension are still under investigation, but we do know that inactivity increases the risk of developing hypertension by 35%, and that unfit subjects have a 52% greater risk than the fit. Regular endurance exercise lowers systolic and diastolic pressures about 10 mm Hg. Active hypertensive patients have half the risk of death from all causes compared with inactive hypertensives (Paffenbarger, 1994). A stroke, due to a clot or hemorrhage of a blood vessel in the brain, can result in loss of speech or muscle control, or even death. The risk factors are similar to those for CAD. In most studies the risk of stroke decreases as activity increases. However, with more vigorous activity, and possibly heavy lifting, the trend may reverse. Transient ischemic attacks (TIAs) are sudden, brief periods of weakness, vertigo, loss of vision, slurred speech, headache, or other symptoms that sometimes precede a stroke. Similar symptoms have been associated with heavy weight-lifting exercises. Thus, time and again we find compelling arguments for moderation.

Cancer and Immunity

The active lifestyle is associated with a lower risk of certain types of cancers.

In recent years, evidence that the active lifestyle is associated with a lower risk of certain types of cancers has been accumulating. Most often studied is the link between activity and a lower risk of colon cancer. Some researchers hypothesize that regular activity shortens intestinal transit time for potential carcinogens in the fecal material. If that is the mechanism, it is hard to understand why the incidence of rectal cancer in active individuals isn't lower as well.

Women who were active in their youth have fewer cancers of the breast and the reproductive system, according to Frisch, Wyshak, Albright, et al. (1985). These authors noted that body fat was lower in the previously active women. The role of dietary fat and obesity in the development of cancer continues to interest researchers. A few studies suggest that activity may help reduce the risk of prostate cancer.

Cancers may be initiated by a substance that causes genetic damage (e.g., by carcinogens in meat or cigarette smoke), then promoters (such as estrogen in the case of breast cancer) stimulate cell proliferation. The healthy immune system may play a role in the control of initiators or in the suppression of transformed cells or their by-products. On the other hand, a compromised immune system may allow initiation and promotion to go unchecked. Regular moderate physical activity enhances the function of the immune system, while high levels of stress or exhaustive exercise seem to suppress the system.

Diabetes and Obesity

Researchers have begun to suspect a link between non-insulin-dependent diabetes (NIDDM), CAD, and hypertension, specifically that all three share insulin resistance, and that obesity and lack of activity are part of the problem. Insulin-resistant cells can't take in glucose, so glucose levels rise and the body secretes more insulin, which tends to increase blood pressure (via increased blood volume and constriction of small blood vessels). Obesity and high levels of blood lipids seem to foster a resistance to insulin, while exercise increases insulin sensitivity and the movement of glucose into working muscles. Regular activity has returned to a place of prominence in the treatment of NIDDM, and for some it removes the need for insulin substitutes. In general, regularly active adults have a 42% lower risk of NIDDM (RR, or risk ratio, = .58).

Arthritis, Osteoporosis, and Back Problems

This group of musculoskeletal problems accounts for significant pain and suffering, as well as billions of dollars for often inadequate treatments. All of these problems can be treated or prevented with activity. Arthritis isn't caused by exercise unless there is a previous injury. Regular moderate activity is an essential part of the treatment for arthritis. Osteoporosis is the progressive loss of bone mineral that occurs faster in women, especially after menopause. It is accelerated by cigarette smoking, low body weight—especially from dieting—and lack of activity. With age the condition can lead to brittle bones, hip fractures, and the characteristic dowager's hump caused by the collapse of vertebrae. The bone mineral loss can be slowed with adequate calcium intake, regular weight-bearing exercises, and, if necessary, hormonal therapy after menopause.

Back problems result from the acute or chronic assault to underused and undertrained bodies. The risk can be minimized or rehabilitated with regular attention to abdominal and flexibility exercises. Among the many therapies used on back problems—including surgery, injections, and drugs—none has been proven more effective than a rapid return to activity. I'll provide specific suggestions for back health in chapter 10.

Physical Activity Increases Longevity

By decreasing the risk of CAD, cancer, and other diseases of lifestyle, regular activity extends the period of adult vigor and compresses the period of sickness that often precedes death. In a real sense, activity adds life to your years, and now there is evidence that it can also add years to your life. When Paffenbarger (1994) analyzed the effects of changing to more favorable health habits, moderate activity (1,500 calories per week) conferred an average of 1.57 years above less active living, and vigorous sports provided 1.54 years over no sports participation.

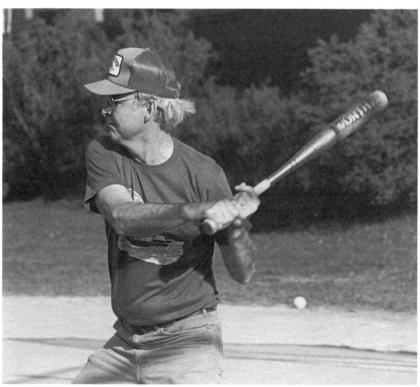

© CLEO Freelance Photo

Activity adds life to your years.

Data on Harvard alumni indicated that vigorous activity (defined as more than 6 times resting metabolism, or 6 METs, or about 6.5 to 7.5 calories per minute, the equivalent of a brisk walk) was associated with reduced mortality. Mortality declined with increasing levels of vigorous activity up to about 3,500 calories per week, but not for nonvigorous activity (Lee, Hsieh, & Paffenbarger, 1995).

A recent report from the Institute for Aerobics Research (Blair, Kohl, Barlow, et al., 1995) confirmed that fit folks live longer. Based on 9,777 men aged 20 to 82, the data showed that men who were unfit when they entered the study were 44% less likely to die over the 18-year period of the study if they improved their fitness. Those who were fit at the start of the study and remained fit were 67% less likely to die than those who remained unfit. The benefits were found across all age groups, and the individuals who were the most fit had the lowest risk of premature death. I'll say more about aging and how to live better and longer in chapter 18.

Summary

For 40 years epidemiologists have studied the relationships of occupational and leisure-time activity to health, and an impressive list of benefits has emerged. The studies clearly show how activity enhances health while it reduces the risk of CAD, hypertension, and stroke as well as some cancers, diabetes, osteoporosis, obesity, and other chronic disorders. I've presented evidence of additional health benefits associated with vigorous activity and fitness, and shown how regular moderate physical activity extends the length and quality of life. Now we will turn our attention to the topic of psychological health, to see how the active life contributes to mental health and the joy of living.

CHAPTER 2

Activity and Mental Health

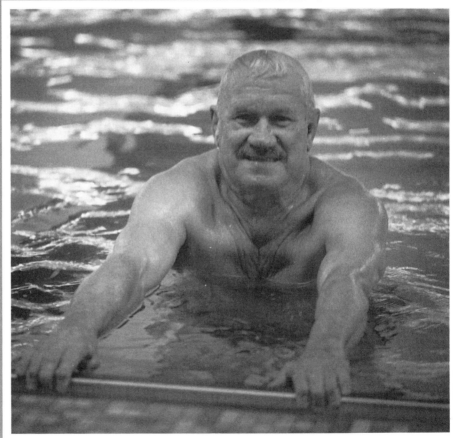

"A sound mind in a sound body, is a short but full description of a happy state in this world."

John Locke

Everyone has heard of psychosomatic illness, a physical ailment caused or exacerbated by the state of mind. But few have heard the term somatopsychic, which suggests the effect of the body (soma) on the mind. This chapter describes how use of the body, specifically with regular moderate physical activity, has a beneficial effect on the mind and mental health. While the research in this area is still in its infancy and many questions remain, it is important to review the case for what may be the most important role for activity and fitness.

As with activity and physical health, we must wonder about self-selection: Does activity promote mental health, or does mental health promote activity? Do happy, less anxious, and nondepressed individuals have the interest, vigor, and energy to be active? Evidence from epidemiological studies indicates that the level of physical activity is positively associated with good mental health, when mental health is defined as positive mood, general well-being, and relatively infrequent symptoms of anxiety and depression (Stephens, 1988). And as you will see, in intervention studies, activity has been associated with reduced levels of anxiety and depression. If it is true, as some have estimated, that at any given time as many as 25% of the population suffer from mild to moderate anxiety, depression, and other emotional disorders, we should not ignore the potential of this safe, low-cost therapy.

THIS CHAPTER WILL HELP YOU

- understand how activity reduces anxiety and depression,
- appreciate how activity helps us deal with stress, and
- recognize positive aspects of an addiction to activity.

Activity Reduces Anxiety and Depression

If activity were a drug, and it could be proven effective in the prevention and treatment of anxiety and depression, it would be hailed as a modern miracle, worth billions to the company with legal rights to the formula. Well, activity isn't a drug, but rather a learned behavior that requires the motivation to begin and the persistence to adhere to a program. This chapter deals with mental health problems, while chapter 19 provides the psychological support you'll need to begin and continue the active life.

Anxiety

Anxiety has been defined as a diffuse apprehension of some vague threat, characterized by feelings of uncertainty and helplessness. It is more than ordinary worry, since it can be perceived as a threat to one's self-esteem. *State anxiety* is a transitory emotional phase characterized by feelings of tension, apprehension, and nervousness. *Trait anxiety* is considered a relatively stable level of anxiety proneness, a predisposition to respond to threats with elevated anxiety. Studies have investigated the effects of acute and chronic activity on state and trait anxiety.

Activity such as walking has been shown to reduce state anxiety, as have meditation, biofeedback, and some other forms of mental diversion. So, if you are tense and apprehensive about an upcoming responsibility, meeting, or presentation, go for a walk. It certainly can't hurt, and it probably will help. If your state anxiety is associated with an immediate physical threat such as a steep ski slope or white-water rapids, then lessons, practice, and improved skill will help diminish future anxiety. Of greater importance is the question: Will regular (chronic) activity or training reduce trait anxiety? Studies of police, firefighters, athletes, and even patients indicate that training and improved fitness are associated with reductions in trait anxiety. Most medical, psychological, and exercise scientists agree that long-term exercise is usually associated with reductions in trait anxiety (Morgan & Goldston, 1987).

Depression

Depression is characterized by sadness, low self-esteem, pessimism, hopelessness, and despair. Symptoms range from fatigue, irritability, lack of direction, and withdrawal to thoughts of suicide. While mild depression may resolve without treatment, and moderate depression may go away in 6 months, severe cases, in which suicide is a real risk, are usually treated with drugs. Most activity studies have been conducted on mild to moderate cases or nonclinical subjects.

A comprehensive statistical review of studies related to activity and depression concluded that activity significantly decreased depression for all age groups and fitness levels, and that larger decreases were associated with more sessions and longer exercise programs (North, McCullagh, & Tran, 1990). While some researchers have hypothesized that exercise had to lead to improvements in aerobic fitness in order to decrease depression, results have not supported that theory. It seems safe to say that those with mild to moderate depression may experience at least as much relief from activity and training as they may from conventional forms of therapy. Let's consider some reasons why this may be so.

These statements, suggested by the National Institute of Mental Health, can help determine if you may be suffering from depression. Indicate whether you agree or disagree with the following:

- ☐ I feel downhearted, blue, and sad.
- ☐ I don't enjoy the things I used to.
- ☐ I feel that others would be better off without me.
- ☐ I feel that I am not useful or needed.
- ☐ I notice that I am losing weight.
- ☐ I have trouble sleeping at night.
- ☐ I am restless and can't keep still.
- ☐ My mind isn't as clear as it used to be.
- ☐ I get tired for no reason.
- ☐ I feel hopeless about the future.

Total the number of statements with which you agreed. If you agreed with at least five, including one of the first two, and if you have had the symptoms for at least 2 weeks, professional help is recommended. If you agreed with the third statement, seek help immediately.

How Activity Affects Anxiety and Depression

A number of hypotheses have been advanced to explain the effect of activity and training on mental health. They range from simple behavioral strategies to complex biochemical theories.

Coping Strategies

Regular activity serves as a positive coping strategy, a diversion from the stress of everyday life. It occupies the mind, allowing the passage of time during difficult periods. It allows the substitution of good habits for bad ones, positive addictions for negative ones. It is a form of meditation, providing the benefits of other approaches along with improvements in health and fitness. It provides a sense of control over one's life and environment. People can be separated into two groups: "internals" who believe they can control outcomes in their lives, and "externals" who believe their lives are controlled by chance or by others. Internal controllers are more likely to adhere to healthy behaviors. Can this locus of control be changed? Can one become an internal and improve adherence to healthy behavior?

Coping behavior is influenced by the perception of acquiring mastery in a particular area, skill, or sport. Perception of mastery influences performance, and it is theorized that experience alters perception. Thus, successful experience may reinforce a coping behavior, thereby ensuring continuation of the behavior. It has even been suggested that this enhanced *self-efficacy*, defined as a sense of one's ability to organize and execute actions required to achieve designated outcomes, may generalize to other areas of performance. Much remains to be learned concerning these theories. We can say that regular activity provides a sense of control and mastery over one dimension of life, and it may improve control and mastery over others.

> *Regular activity serves as a positive coping strategy, a diversion from the stress of everyday life.*

I DON'T DO LUNCH

Years ago I decided that midday was the best time for my personal exercise program. I've continued to enjoy a noon-hour workout, with or without the company of friends, followed by a shower and a brown-bag lunch at the desk. Sometimes I head out with a problem and come back with a solution. Exercise before work, on the other hand, is a struggle, and after work I am more inclined to crash in front of the nightly news, with low-fat pretzels and a light beer (for medicinal purposes). I look forward to my daily activity and do all I can to keep the noon hour open. On weekends we often start early for extended workouts, but during the week the noon hour is my time. In this era of power lunches you don't influence people or enhance your career when you announce, "I don't do lunch," and, of course, there are times when I must make exceptions, but this resolve to keep the exercise time sacred is an indication of how important regular activity is for my physical and mental health. Regular activity is my primary coping mechanism.

Self-Esteem, Self-Concept, and Body Image

Can regular activity or improved fitness have a beneficial effect on self-esteem and self-concept, and could that reduce or prevent anxiety or depression? One widely used test of self-concept employs 100 statements and a five-point answering scale to determine five components of self-concept: personal self, social self, family self, moral/ethical self, and physical self (body image). You might not expect activity and fitness to alter all the scales, but changes in physical, social, and personal self seem possible.

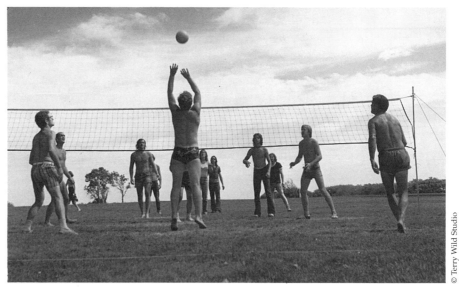

Social contact is only one of the benefits of activity.

An extensive review of research on children indicated that activity was associated with a positive self-concept, that participation in activity programs contributed to self-esteem, and that fitness activities were more effective than other components of the physical education program in developing self-concept (Gruber, 1986). Research on adults agrees that activity and fitness improve self-concept. When you take control of your life, lose weight, and improve strength, endurance, and your appearance, you feel better about yourself and your body. This new confidence may alter your outlook on life, even your personality. When middle-aged male subjects in a fitness study discussed the influence of their participation in a fitness program, many claimed an improvement in their sex lives. As activity and fitness alter the body image, this renewed confidence in the body can be an important step toward improved personal relations.

Self-esteem can be enhanced through participation in physical activity, perhaps by enhancing physical ability and self-estimation. Runners and other athletes identify with other participants. We define ourselves as runners, cyclists, swimmers, and so on, and derive social acceptance from the group. One fear associated with injury is the loss of identity and social acceptance.

Biochemical Mechanisms

Activity and training can influence metabolism and a number of hormones. Regular participation provides biofeedback that leads to changes in heart rate,

ENDORPHINS AND LACTIC ACID

A recent study correlated a number of measures to beta endorphin release during exertion. The level of lactic acid in the blood was found to be one of the measures most associated with endorphins, suggesting that strenuous effort that produces lactic acid is more likely to lead to their release. When the acid was buffered during exertion, endorphin release was suppressed (Taylor, Boyajian, James, et al., 1994).

blood pressure, and other measures. Activity temporarily raises the body temperature and induces relaxation and mild fatigue, factors related to the tranquilizing effect of exercise. A study by deVries and Adams (1972) showed that a single bout of exercise (walking) was as effective in reducing tension as a tranquilizer, and that the effect of the exercise lasted longer. Fitness training leads to profound metabolic effects that include increased efficiency and responsiveness to hormones such as insulin. Training also favorably influences hormones and neurotransmitters associated with depression.

Some researchers believe that activity increases levels of mood-altering substances called endorphins. Studies show that endorphins, morphine-like compounds produced in the brain, can reduce pain and induce a sense of euphoria. When beta endorphins were reported to increase in runners after a marathon run, runners were quick to speculate that these opiates were responsible for the euphoric sensation known as the runner's high. Subsequent research cast doubt on that hypothesis. Although the blood endorphin levels are elevated during and after an endurance effort, findings have indicated that the levels do not correspond with mood states (Markoff, Ryan, & Young, 1982). It isn't surprising, though, that blood levels and moods might not correlate, because a barrier prevents easy transport between the general circulation and the brain. Hence, blood levels of endorphins do not tell us what is happening to endorphin levels in the brain, where moods are formed. The increased levels in the blood are probably a reflection of endorphins' role as a narcotic. Running feels easier after about 20 minutes, which is when increased levels of beta endorphin have been detected. So, if you have tried running and found it uncomfortable, try to continue beyond 20 minutes; you may find it becomes easier with the help of your natural painkillers.

It is clear that activity and fitness have the potential to improve mild to moderate cases of anxiety and depression. But why wait until you are anxious or depressed to begin? Start now and you may be able to prevent or minimize these assaults on your mental health.

Activity and Stress

Many people believe that stress has become one of the modern age's major health problems. Physiological fight-or-flight responses that were necessary for the survival of primitive peoples may be unhealthy in highly complex societies. Stress, tension, and reactive behavior patterns have been associated with heart disease, hypertension, suppression of the immune system, and a variety of other ills. The emotional response to life events is mediated by structures in the brain, including the hypothalamus. When something excites or threatens us, the hypothalamus tells the anterior pituitary gland to secrete adrenocorticotropic hormone (ACTH), a chemical messenger that travels to the adrenal cortex and orders release of hormones called glucocorticoids (e.g., cortisol). These hormones are necessary for the body's response to stressful situations. Without them the body cannot deal with stress; it collapses and dies. Stress has been defined as anything that increases the release of ACTH or glucocorticoids.

Stressful situations also elicit a response in the sympathetic nervous system that leads to secretion of hormones from the adrenal medulla, including adrenaline (epinephrine) and norepinephrine. These hormones mobilize energy and support the cardiovascular response to the stressor. This aspect of the stress response is called the fight-or-flight mechanism. The hormones prepare the body to battle or run, but they have other effects that can be bad for the health. Epinephrine makes the blood clot faster, an advantage in a fight but a disadvantage in the workplace, where it can precipitate a heart attack or a stroke.

Prolonged exposure to stress hormones eventually suppresses the immune system.

The stress response is necessary to prepare an athlete for a maximal effort in a race or physical challenge, but it can be unhealthy if it occurs too often in the wrong setting. If you become stressed on the job, when a natural physical catharsis is impossible or improper, the circulating hormones can be a problem. As mentioned in chapter 1, recent research suggests that some of us are hot reactors, exhibiting exaggerated responses to everyday stressors. Hot reactors become enraged when the driver in front goes too slowly, or when they are forced to stand in line at the supermarket. This hostility elicits a flood of hormones designed for combat. Blood pressure and heart rate increase, energy is mobilized, and clotting time shortens. And the hot reactors are forced to stew in their own juices, setting the stage for future health problems. We do know that prolonged exposure to stress hormones eventually suppresses the immune system. Reduced resistance to infection is a sign of stress.

TYPE A

The Type A behavior pattern is characterized by extreme competitiveness, ambition, and a profound sense of time urgency. The Type B personality, the opposite of the Type A, is relaxed, calm, even phlegmatic. In studies by cardiologists Friedman and Rosenman (1973), Type A subjects had higher cholesterol levels, faster blood clotting times, higher adrenaline levels, more sudden deaths, and a sevenfold greater risk of heart disease. However, subsequent studies, including the massive Framingham study, failed to find a link between the Type A behavior pattern, stress, and heart disease. They did find a link between anger, repressed hostility, and heart disease risk (Wilson, Castelli, & Kannel, 1987).

While most of us accept the idea that excess stress may be a risk factor for heart disease, the Type A personality, in the absence of anger and hostility, does not seem to be related to heart disease risk. Studies of the corporate structure suggest that it is the employees, not the hard-driving executives, who face the most stress. Executives live fast-paced lives but retain a sense of control. Employees are also busy but they often feel they have no control over their lives, and that sense of lack of control is stressful.

Some early rat studies suggested that exercise itself was a stressor (Selye, 1956). However, those results must be considered in light of the fact that the animals were forced to run on a treadmill and were given shocks when they tried to rest, or forced to swim to exhaustion in a deep tank with a weight tied around the tail. Electroshock and fear of drowning are stressful for most of us. And for humans, exercise is stressful when it is highly competitive, exhausting, or threatening. For example, rock climbing is stressful for the neophyte and exhilarating for the veteran. Stress is in the eye of the beholder. Regular moderate activity minimizes the effects of stress. It is relaxing and tranquilizing, and has been shown to counter the tendency to form blood clots. Regular activity enhances the function of the immune system, while the exhaustion of a marathon is immunosuppressive. Occasional exposure to stressful activity is fine if you have trained for the event. Regular moderate activity and fitness contribute to your health.

Psychoneuroimmunology

A relatively new area, psychoneuroimmunology (PNI) studies links among the brain, the nervous system, and the immune system. PNI focuses on how thoughts, emotions, and personality traits interact with the immune system and become manifest in sickness or health. Thoughts or emotions can enhance or suppress the immune system, via neurotransmitters secreted by the sympathetic nervous system, or via hormones released upon command of the brain

---

Certain life events, both positive and negative, have been proven to be stressful. Here are some of the events and their relative stressfulness. A score of more than 300 points covering events in the past year has been associated with emergence of a serious illness, such as heart disease or cancer, within 2 years.

Death of spouse	100 points
Divorce	73
Separation	65
Jail term	63
Death of family member	63
Personal injury or illness	53
Marriage	50
Fired from job	47
Marital reconciliation	45
Retirement	45
Pregnancy	40
Death of friend	37
Mortgage	31
Personal achievement	28
Spouse starts/stops work	26
Trouble with boss	23
Change residence	20
Vacation	13

If life is getting too stressful, slow the pace of change. (Roth & Holmes, 1985)

(e.g., ACTH). The immune system is immensely complicated, consisting of lymphocytes, T cells, natural killer cells, antibodies, immunoglobulins, and more. It serves to protect the body from foreign assaults. However, when exposed to prolonged stress, the system tends to break down, allowing invading microorganisms to proliferate. PNI suggests that by altering your perception of the supposed threat, by reprogramming your thinking and your outlook on life, you can reduce exposure to stress and spare the immune system.

Another way to bolster the immune system is with regular activity. Recent studies confirm the beneficial effect of activity and training on components of the immune system. The studies agree that regular, moderate activity and training are the answer to a healthy immune system (Mackinnon, 1992). Excessive intensity, duration, or frequency of training risks overstraining, a condition characterized by fatigue, poor performance, and suppression of the immune system. Activity, relaxation, imagery, and other coping strategies help you deal in a rational way with difficult problems, freeing the immune system to function on your behalf.

Activity and Addiction

Substance abuse with nicotine, alcohol, prescription or recreational drugs, or cocaine and heroin presents a health and social dilemma of such dimensions it threatens to tear our society apart. Each presents a staggering cost in health care, rehabilitation, and social services, not to mention the loss of human potential. I don't pretend to have answers to this national problem, but I do have some suggestions for prevention and individual responsibility.

In his book *Positive Addiction*, Dr. William Glasser contrasts positive and negative addictions (1976). Negative addictions such as drugs or alcohol relieve the pain of failure and provide temporary pleasure but at a terrible cost in terms of family, social, and professional life. Positive addictions lead to psychological strength, imagination, and creativity. Dr. Glasser suggests that as a person participates in meditation, yoga, or running, he or she eventually achieves the state of positive addiction. When this state is reached the mind is free to become more imaginative or creative. The mind conceives more options in solving difficult or frustrating problems; it has more strength. Proof of addiction comes when you are forced to neglect your habit, or when guilt and anxiety accompany the early stages of withdrawal.

In the chapter entitled "Running—The Hardest but Surest Way," Dr. Glasser suggests that running, perhaps because it is our most basic solitary survival activity, produces the non–self-critical state more effectively than any other practice. He recommends running to all, from the weakest to the strongest. He feels that once one can run an hour without fatigue, it is almost certain that the positive addiction state will be achieved on a regular basis. If competition is avoided and the runner runs alone in a pleasant setting, addiction should occur within the year.

I knew I was addicted to running long before Dr. Glasser wrote his book; it took far less than an hour per day of running or a year to achieve. Over the years the addiction to running has evolved into an addiction to activity. It works with walking, cycling, cross-country skiing, swimming, even weight training, so long as I keep it noncompetitive and uncritical. As interests change or injuries occur, I've been able to transfer the addiction to new activities. And the addiction ensures that I am hooked and will remain active for the rest of my life.

Is it possible to be too dedicated to activity, fitness, or training, to be negatively addicted or dependent? Probably so. An old friend, the eminent and venerable sport psychologist Dr. William Morgan, first called attention to the possibility, noting runners who were so addicted that they neglected family and work. Some continued to train in spite of an illness or injury (Morgan, 1979). I too have seen runners with an obsessive compulsion for their sport. On closer inspection it seemed that some lives were confounded with other problems, that these people had turned to running as therapy. Several studies have linked compulsive running with the eating disorder anorexia nervosa. However, others found that addicted runners fell within the normal range of behavior while anorexics did not.

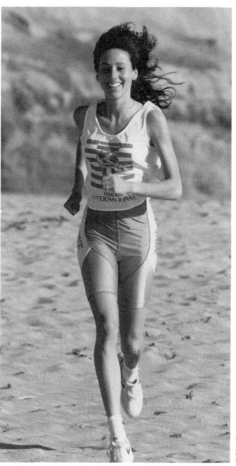

Is it possible to be too dedicated to activity, fitness, or training?

For my part I'd prefer a negative addiction to running over an addiction to alcohol or drugs. The compulsive activity may alter family relationships and work performance, but so does alcohol or drug abuse, and running won't destroy the body and the mind. The obsession with running may serve as a therapy, just as activity has served to reduce anxiety and depression. I've long thought that it might be possible to substitute a positive for a negative behavior, that a commitment to exercise might help a smoker give up the habit. While this clearly works for some individuals, its application is limited by the sizable dropout rates common to exercise and smoking cessation programs.

Positive addiction can be achieved from almost any activity you choose, so long as it meets the following criteria:

- ☐ It is not competitive
- ☐ You do it for approximately 1 hour daily
- ☐ It is easy to do and doesn't take much mental effort
- ☐ You can do it alone or occasionally with others, but you don't rely on others to do it
- ☐ You believe it has some physical, mental, and spiritual value
- ☐ You believe that if you persist you will improve
- ☐ You can do it without criticizing yourself

Summary

Health has been called "the first of all liberties." What some call optimal health or wellness implies a vitality and zest for living that is much more than the absence of disease. Our definition of health also embraces psychological, emotional, or mental health. Thus, healthy people are free from disease, anxiety, and depression; their physical condition, nutritional state, and emotional outlook enable them to carry out daily tasks with vigor and alertness, without undue fatigue, and with ample energy to enjoy leisure-time pursuits and meet unforeseen emergencies.

The International Society of Sport Psychology (Tenebaum & Singer, 1992) believes that the benefits of regular vigorous activity include

- reduced state anxiety,
- decreased level of mild to moderate depression,
- reductions in neuroticism and anxiety,
- an adjunct to professional treatment of severe depression,
- reduction of stress indices, and
- beneficial emotional effects for all ages and both sexes.

We have seen how regular moderate activity serves to enhance both physical and mental health. Now let's explore the role of health care in the active life.

CHAPTER 3

Activity and Personal Health

"Better to hunt in fields, for health unbought, Than fee the doctor for a nauseous draught. The wise, for cure, on exercise depend: God never made his work for man to mend."

John Dryden

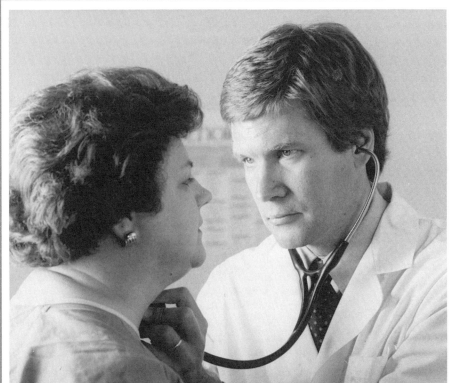

© Mark Anderman

The so-called American health care system is not about health, nor is it a system; instead it is a complex, chaotic, expensive arrangement of doctors, hospitals, drug and insurance companies, lawyers, and—oh, yes—patients, held together by mutual dependence, economic necessity, and self-interest. It isn't focused on prevention or health, but on the treatment of illness, disease, and disabling injury. It isn't a system because it wasn't planned; it just grew. It defies economic theory; if demand goes down, prices go up. Worst of all, it has fostered an unhealthy attitude: If I ignore common-sense health habits and become sick or injured, the health care system will perform a miracle cure, and the insurance will pay the enormous costs. Insurance programs have insulated individuals from the real costs of treatment, thereby reducing incentives for good habits and cost containment. At the same time, this so-called health care system leaves a staggering 40 million citizens without health insurance! Meaningful reform will require changes in all parts of the system.

- Doctors who gravitated toward specialization to enhance stature, income, and lifestyle, and to fit a reimbursement system that paid for procedures, will return to primary care.
- Hospitals that became highly competitive corporate profit centers will return to cooperation and community service.
- Pharmaceutical corporations that invested millions to develop and billions to market new drugs will settle for a bit less on the bottom line.
- Insurance companies that practiced cherry picking, insuring only the healthy, will cover everyone, with fair rates and simplified forms.
- Lawyers who filed questionable malpractice cases for huge contingency fees will adjust to reasonable fees and tort reform.
- Patients who impatiently expected instant cures will assume greater responsibility for their health.

Prevention is inexpensive; crisis medicine is not. The active life is the enlightened, cost-effective way to individual responsibility and prevention. It should be the keystone of a real health care system.

Many Americans have come to rely on their doctors to take care of their health. Of course, it doesn't work; your doctor can't make you stop smoking, lose weight, eat less fat, fasten your seat belt, or get some exercise. These simple habits have more to do with health and disease than all the influences of medicine. More than half of all disease and death can be attributed to diseases of lifestyle. Granted, there are medical tests and treatments that prevent or minimize disease and disability, but not all of the procedures require a physician. Let's review features and limitations of health screening, early diagnosis, and the medical examination.

More than half of all disease and death can be attributed to diseases of lifestyle.

This CHAPTER WILL HELP YOU

- recognize the values and limitations of health screening and early detection,
- develop a schedule for periodic medical examinations,
- determine the need for a pre-exercise medical exam, and
- understand the risks and benefits of regular, moderate physical activity.

Health Screening

I have the pleasure of working in two bureaucracies, a university and a federal agency. While they are different in many respects, they share an interest in the health of their employees: Both have employee wellness programs. Most wellness programs utilize a computerized health risk analysis as the start of a comprehensive health screening program. The analysis uses answers to questions about health habits, and some basic information (age, sex, weight, blood pressure, cholesterol) to calculate health risks and to compute one's risk age. An overweight smoker with a family history of heart disease may have a risk age years above his or her chronological age. The health risk analysis is a simple, low-cost way to focus future health habits. A sample health risk analysis and longevity estimate is included in figures 3.6 and 3.7 at the end of this chapter.

Results from a cholesterol test could lead to a class on healthy food choices, an activity program, or even a doctor's visit and a prescription for cholesterol-lowering medication. The principle is simple: Use low-cost approaches to identify health habits and risks, apply more expensive tests but only for those at risk, and reserve high-cost tests and treatments for those in real need. Years ago, testing advocates thought health screening tests should be applied broadly. Now we realize that many tests should be reserved for those who, by virtue of age, risk factors, family history, or symptoms, are most in need of the procedure. Generalized testing is costly, wastes time and effort of medical personnel, and risks false positive results (indication of a problem when none exists).

Various factors, including age, sex, health risks, family history, and occupation, influence the need for health screening. Young, apparently healthy individuals do well with infrequent tests, unless of course they have a family history or symptoms, or they change habits. It is regrettable that age alone increases the need for certain onerous tests, such as a proctoscope (for rectal and colon cancer) and digital prostate examination. A family history of glaucoma raises the need for a regular glaucoma test, and occupational exposure to noise or toxic chemicals calls for evaluation of hearing or lung function, respectively. A comprehensive worksite wellness program provides a wide range of health screening procedures (see figure 3.1), along with appropriate immunizations (e.g., flu shots for retired employees) and booster shots.

Early Detection

For a period of time there was great interest in the development of tests to detect problems, such as cancer. The idea was that early detection would improve the prognosis for recovery. Indeed, some studies showed that early detection was associated with extended survival. Fine, so long as the extension of life exceeds the improvement in detection time. However, early detection is meaningless if there is no effective treatment for the disease. Of course, if the disease can be transmitted and one can effectively limit its spread, early detection makes sense from a public health standpoint.

In recent years medical opinion has changed concerning the course of treatment for several problems. For example, in older men, aggressive treatment of prostate cancer (surgery, radiation) has not proven superior to benign neglect.

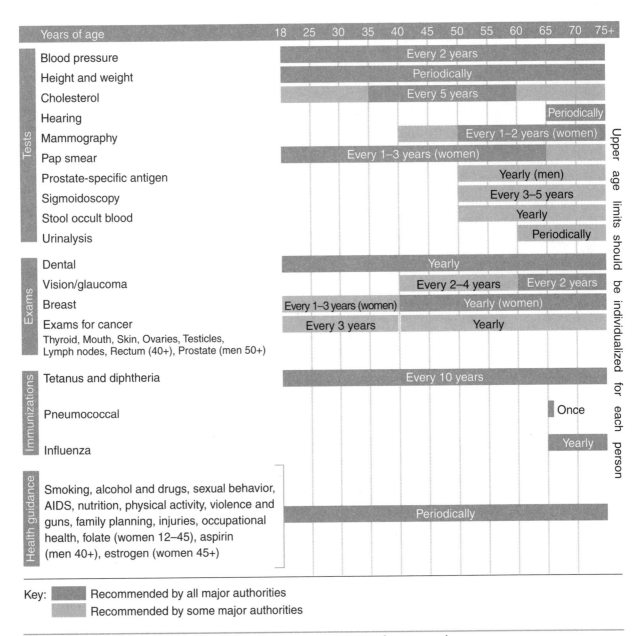

Figure 3.1 Adult preventive care timeline: recommendations of major authorities.
Reprinted from U.S. Public Health Service.

Survival time doesn't improve, and the quality of life is often impaired. Similarly, back operations and heart surgery, even for patients with obvious symptoms, have been performed more often than necessary, leading one to question the accuracy of detection and diagnosis. But many tests are warranted, especially when they lead to changes in behaviors. Low-cost blood pressure and cholesterol tests can identify problems while there is still time to slow, stop, or even reverse the disease process. So, if your age, sex, race, family history, health habits, or exposures put you at risk for a disease, by all means utilize an early detection test, if the proposed test meets the following criteria:

- The disease has a significant effect on the quality of life
- Acceptable methods of treatment are available
- Treatment during the asymptomatic (no symptom) period significantly reduces disability or death
- Early treatment yields a superior result
- Detection tests are available at a reasonable cost
- The incidence of the disease in the population is sufficient to justify the cost of screening

Few tests meet these criteria; blood pressure, breast examinations, and Pap smears do, while exercise stress tests, diabetes screening, and X-rays for lung cancer do not. You may be surprised to know that the routine (annual) medical examination also fails to meet the criteria.

BLOOD PRESSURE

High blood pressure, or hypertension, a silent killer with no obvious symptoms, is easy and inexpensive to test. Moreover, several acceptable methods of treatment are available, and successful control extends the quantity and quality of life. So periodic blood pressure checks are both prudent and cost effective. You can even purchase a cuff and stethoscope for home use.

Systolic pressure is the pressure exerted against arterial walls when the heart contracts to send blood into the system. Diastolic pressure is the pressure against arterial walls between beats, when the heart is relaxed. Both measures contribute to the mean arterial pressure, the average pressure exerted on arterial walls, and both have consequences for your health. Use the information in table 3.1 to evaluate your blood pressure. Borderline and stage 1 cases often respond to diet, weight loss, and exercise. Stage 2 cases that remain elevated with diet, weight loss, exercise, and stress reduction will also require medication, as will most stage 3 and stage 4 cases. Studies clearly show the value of controlling blood pressure. High blood pressure can damage arterial walls and contribute to atherosclerosis, and excess pressure increases the risk of strokes. While salt intake, being overweight, and stress may exacerbate the problem, the cause is poorly understood, and more than 90% of all cases are of unknown origin. Modern molecular biology will someday unlock the cause of these constricted arteries, but you can't wait for someday. Check your pressure regularly, and never rely on a single measure. If the pressure is elevated in several checks, see your physician, who will advise you to restrict salt and fat, lose weight, engage in regular moderate activity, and learn how to manage stress. If all that isn't enough, new medications are available to provide control of blood pressure with fewer side effects. But don't rely on medications for control; continue with diet, exercise, weight loss, and stress management.

TABLE 3.1   Blood Pressure Evaluation

	Systolic BP	Diastolic BP	Action
Normal BP	<130 mm Hg	<85 mm Hg	Retest annually
Borderline	130-139	85-89	Retest in 6 mo
Hypertension			
Stage 1	140-159	90-99	Recheck
Stage 2	160-179	100-109	See doctor soon*
Stage 3	180-210	110-120	See doctor very soon
Stage 4	>210	>120	See doctor now!

*For recheck, diet, weight loss, activity, stress reduction, and possible medication.

Medical Examination

The typical medical examination includes a history, physical examination, and tests dictated by the patient's age and sex and the outcome of the exam. In the past, we all assumed that the annual medical examination would help us stay healthy and reduce the likelihood of illness or premature death. But when researchers compared those who had annual exams with those who did not, they found an equal number of chronic diseases and deaths in both groups. Today most doctors agree that for persons with no symptoms or chronic disease, the annual medical exam is a waste of time and money. A past president of the American Medical Association has said he hasn't had a routine physical since he joined the army decades ago, and he asks patients who request a checkup: What do you want one for? Let's consider a typical scenario to see why the annual medical pays off for the doctor and the laboratory but not for the patient.

Joe is a typical patient; he is 45, somewhat overweight and out of shape, still smokes a pack a day, and indulges his love for meat and potatoes. His company pays for his annual medical exam, so the physician schedules a battery of tests, including a blood lipid panel, chest X-ray, electrocardiogram (ECG), pulmonary function tests, and other procedures. Aside from somewhat elevated blood pressure and cholesterol, and a low level of HDL cholesterol, Joe's tests appear normal. So, Joe goes out and celebrates his "clean bill of health" with a prime rib, a baked potato with butter, sour cream, and bacon bits, a salad with lots of dressing, and a slice of cheesecake. The next morning he experiences a crushing pain in his chest and is rushed to the hospital with a heart attack.

This all-too-common scenario illustrates the fact that many tests lack the sensitivity to provide early detection. A resting ECG seldom predicts an impending myocardial infarction (heart attack). While an exercise electrocardiogram (stress test) may have indicated Joe's problem, this test occasionally indicates heart disease when none is present. Pulmonary function tests and chest X-rays seldom detect lung cancer early enough to improve the prognosis (and the X-ray increases the risk of cancer). And some tests increase the likelihood of surgery when it may not be needed. If Joe had complained of a back problem and the doctor had ordered an MRI (magnetic resonance imaging) that revealed a bulging disk, he might have been scheduled for an operation that could make things worse (Jensen, Brant-Zawadzki, Obuchowski, et al., 1994). Does this mean that all tests and medical exams are a waste of time? Of course not; there are many valid reasons for a medical examination.

If you have symptoms or are in doubt about the condition of your health, by all means see your physician. If you have a history of hypertension, or if a member of your family has, check your pressure regularly. Buy a stethoscope and a blood pressure cuff (sphygmomanometer) and do it at home, at the drugstore, or at your worksite wellness program. Check elevated cholesterol regularly at worksite screenings, health fairs, or walk-in clinics. Check your kids to see if they need to use diet and exercise to minimize a family problem. Use screening programs to check blood sugar, and if problems arise see your physician. Of course, women should be checked regularly throughout pregnancy. For adults, the National Conference on Preventive Medicine recommends periodic medical exams according to this schedule:

If you have symptoms or are in doubt about the condition of your health, by all means see your physician.

- At around 18 and 25 years of age
- Every 5 years between ages 35 and 65
- Every 2 years after age 65

In my view, this schedule could be too intensive for the apparently healthy adult who is willing to take charge of his or her health. My last medical exam, more than 15 years ago, was an inconclusive search for a problem I later diagnosed with the aid of the *Merck Manual*, the book doctors use when they are stumped. I have a wellness program blood panel twice a year to keep track of an inherited tendency for elevated cholesterol, and I take advantage of other worksite wellness and community health screening programs that fit my needs. I see the dentist often enough and have periodic eye exams to adjust my prescription and to test for glaucoma. Otherwise, my visits to the doctor's office are for specifics, such as a trip to the dermatologist to check on a suspicious growth. But, as I said, if you have symptoms or are in doubt about the condition of your health, by all means see your physician.

Cholesterol Screening

Cholesterol is a serious heart disease risk factor, and the risk rises with the level of cholesterol (see table 3.2). Why some people with relatively low cholesterol experience problems with atherosclerosis is beginning to be understood. Cholesterol is a fat-like substance found in all human and animal tissues, but not in plants. It is ingested in foods from animals (e.g., meat, eggs, fish, poultry, dairy products) or can be synthesized in the body. If you don't eat much cholesterol, the body will make all it needs from other fats. It is transported in the blood in low- or high-density lipoprotein packages.

TABLE 3.2   Cholesterol and CAD Death Rate

Cholesterol (mg/100 ml)	Risk ratio
Under 181	1.00
182-202	1.29
203-220	1.73
221-244	2.21
Over 245	3.42

Reprinted from Stamler, Wentworth, and Neaton 1986.

Cholesterol values from 200 to 220 milligrams should respond to a moderate reduction of dietary fat (saturated fat, hydrogenated fat). Levels above 220 milligrams call for a concerted effort to reduce dietary fat and cholesterol. Oat bran, niacin, and other natural foods may also help reduce serum cholesterol. Values that remain above 240 after dietary and exercise intervention may require drug therapy, especially if other risk factors exist. Fortunately, several new drugs have successfully reduced cholesterol and the incidence of heart disease. See your physician for details.

Low-density lipoprotein cholesterol (LDL) is the dangerous version that finds its way into the lining of the coronary arteries. It can combine with oxygen and enhance the development of plaques in arteries. *High-density lipoprotein cholesterol* (HDL) acts like a transport system that picks up cholesterol and delivers it to the liver for reprocessing or removal. Thus, higher HDL levels are protective, with a 1-milligram increase associated with a 2 to 3% reduction in CAD. Conversely, low values are an independent risk factor. So, you can have a low cholesterol level and still be at risk if your HDL level is low. You should know all three numbers (total cholesterol, LDL, and HDL), as well as your total cholesterol/HDL ratio. Table 3.3 shows the risk associated with LDL cholesterol, and table 3.4 displays how the risk declines as HDL levels rise.

TABLE 3.3   LDL Cholesterol and CAD Risk

Risk	LDL (mg/dl)
Low	<100
Desirable	100-129
Borderline	130-159
High	>160

TABLE 3.4   HDL Cholesterol and CAD Risk

Risk	HDL (mg/dl)*
Very low	75
Average (1.0 risk ratio)	45 (55 for women)
High	25

*dl = one-tenth of a liter, or 100 ml.

Another way to assess your risk is to calculate your total cholesterol/HDL ratio. A ratio under 4 (e.g., 200/50) is associated with a low risk of heart disease, while one over 6 (e.g., 240/40) is not. All adults should be tested every 5 years unless values are borderline or high, which calls for annual testing and treatment, including weight loss, dieting (reduced intake of saturated fats and cholesterol; increased soluble fiber and vitamins C and E), increased exercise duration, some alcohol (one to two drinks a day), no smoking, and if all that isn't enough, cholesterol-lowering drugs. I'll say more about cholesterol as well as triglycerides, another blood lipid (fat), in later chapters.

Pre-Exercise Medical Examination

A medical examination is more urgent for those who plan to remain inactive than for those who intend to get into good physical shape.

Should you see your doctor before you embark on an increase in your physical activity? Here is the opinion of the eminent Swedish physician and exercise scientist Dr. Per-Olof Åstrand (Åstrand & Rodahl, 1970):

> There is less risk in activity than in continuous inactivity . . . . It is more advisable to pass a careful medical examination if one intends to be sedentary.

The active life is certain to enhance—not threaten—your health if you are free of symptoms, if you make a gradual transition to a more active life, and if you follow a sensible program. On the other hand, you should consider a pre-participation medical examination if you have been sedentary, you are concerned about your health, you have one or several of the primary heart disease risk factors (hypertension, elevated cholesterol, cigarette smoking, or inactivity), or you are over 40 years of age (50 for women) and plan to engage in a vigorous exercise program. The American College of Sports Medicine (1995) recommends a pre-participation exam including a progressive, ECG-monitored exercise test (stress test) for everyone with known cardiac, pulmonary, or metabolic disease, and for patients with symptoms, before participation, and for those over 40 (50 for women) before participation in vigorous exercise.

Inexpensive pre-participation health screening can substantially reduce the risk of participation in activity and fitness programs. Canadian researchers have developed a simple questionnaire to identify the small number of adults for whom physical activity might be inappropriate or those who should have medical advice prior to participation (see figure 3.2).

Answer no to all the questions, and you are ready to increase your level of physical activity. If you answer yes to any question, you should postpone vigorous exercise until you consult with your physician.

The Exercise Stress Test

Severe chest pain (angina pectoris) or even a heart attack can sometimes be the first sign of coronary artery problems. Indications of previously undiagnosed heart disease can be detected in a gradually increased exercise challenge known as a stress test. Narrowed coronary arteries may be able to supply the blood you need for sedentary pursuits, but during exercise the oxygen needs of heart

The *coronary bypass* is an operation to repair one or more of a body's narrowed coronary arteries. A small blood vessel is taken from the leg or chest and used to bypass the section of severely narrowed artery. *Coronary angioplasty* involves insertion of a catheter tipped with a balloon into the artery. Inflation of the balloon opens the artery and improves blood flow. Neither procedure is always successful, and neither usually lasts as long as the patient would like, so prevention seems a far wiser course of action. Some day lasers, which are being tested on animals, may be used to clear arteries blocked by atherosclerosis. In the meantime, prevention would appear to be prudent.

Physical Activity Readiness
Questionnaire - PAR-Q
(revised 1994)

PAR - Q & YOU

(A Questionnaire for People Aged 15 to 69)

Regular physical activity is fun and healthy, and increasingly more people are starting to become more active every day. Being more active is very safe for most people. However, some people should check with their doctor before they start becoming much more physically active.

If you are planning to become much more physically active than you are now, start by answering the seven questions in the box below. If you are between the ages of 15 and 69, the PAR-Q will tell you if you should check with your doctor before you start. If you are over 69 years of age, and you are not used to being very active, check with your doctor.

Common sense is your best guide when you answer these questions. Please read the questions carefully and answer each one honestly: check YES or NO.

YES	NO		
☐	☐	1.	Has your doctor ever said that you have a heart condition <u>and</u> that you should only do physical activity recommended by a doctor?
☐	☐	2.	Do you feel pain in your chest when you do physical activity?
☐	☐	3.	In the past month, have you had chest pain when you were not doing physical activity?
☐	☐	4.	Do you lose your balance because of dizziness or do you ever lose consciousness?
☐	☐	5.	Do you have a bone or joint problem that could be made worse by a change in your physical activity?
☐	☐	6.	Is your doctor currently prescribing drugs (for example, water pills) for your blood pressure or heart condition?
☐	☐	7.	Do you know of <u>any other reason</u> why you should not do physical activity?

If

you

answered

YES to one or more questions

Talk with your doctor by phone or in person BEFORE you start becoming much more physically active or BEFORE you have a fitness appraisal. Tell your doctor about the PAR-Q and which questions you answered YES.

- You may be able to do any activity you want — as long as you start slowly and build up gradually. Or, you may need to restrict your activities to those which are safe for you. Talk with your doctor about the kinds of activities you wish to participate in and follow his/her advice.
- Find out which community programs are safe and helpful for you.

NO to all questions

If you answered NO honestly to <u>all</u> PAR-Q questions, you can be reasonably sure that you can:

- start becoming much more physically active — begin slowly and build up gradually. This is the safest and easiest way to go.
- take part in a fitness appraisal — this is an excellent way to determine your basic fitness so that you can plan the best way for you to live actively.

DELAY BECOMING MUCH MORE ACTIVE:

- if you are not feeling well because of a temporary illness such as a cold or a fever — wait until you feel better; or
- if you are or may be pregnant — talk to your doctor before you start becoming more active.

Please note: If your health changes so that you then answer YES to any of the above questions, tell your fitness or health professional. Ask whether you should change your physical activity plan.

<u>Informed Use of the PAR-Q</u>: The Canadian Society for Exercise Physiology, Health Canada, and their agents assume no liability for persons who undertake physical activity, and if in doubt after completing this questionnaire, consult your doctor prior to physical activity.

You are encouraged to copy the PAR-Q but only if you use the entire form

NOTE: If the PAR-Q is being given to a person before he or she participates in a physical activity program or a fitness appraisal, this section may be used for legal or administrative purposes.

I have read, understood and completed this questionnaire. Any questions I had were answered to my full satisfaction.

NAME _____

SIGNATURE _____   DATE _____

SIGNATURE OF PARENT _____   WITNESS _____
or GUARDIAN (for participants under the age of majority)

© *Canadian Society for Exercise Physiology*
  Société canadienne de physiologie de l'exercice

Supported by: Health   Santé
                           Canada   Canada

Figure 3.2 PAR-Q pre-exercise screening test.

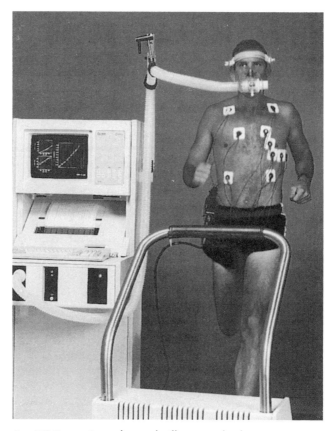

An ECG-monitored treadmill test with direct measurement of oxygen intake.

muscle go up, and electrocardiographic abnormalities or physical symptoms may indicate a problem.

A physician uses a progressive ECG-monitored exercise test as a diagnostic tool to identify the problem early, to avoid a heart attack, and to initiate effective treatment. The stress test has been used to diagnose or verify the presence of heart disease, as a pre-exercise test to reduce risks or set limits, as a post-coronary test to indicate the extent of damage and subsequent progress in therapeutic programs, or after a coronary bypass or angioplasty procedure to establish the extent of recovery as well as work and activity limits. Although most stress tests are conducted on the treadmill, arm testing (cranking) may be required for individuals returning to jobs that require strenuous use of the arms or upper body. Maximal or near-maximal workloads may be needed to elicit the symptoms of previously undiagnosed heart disease. However, many physicians terminate the stress test when the heart rate reaches some percentage of the age-adjusted maximal heart rate, reasoning that it is unnecessary to risk a maximal test. Unfortunately, there is such variability in maximal heart rates that the test may be too strenuous for some and too easy for others (see table 3.5).

One reason for maximal testing is to evaluate individuals' functional capacity, their maximal attainable workload. The stress test can be used to clear a patient for hard work and to establish his or her work capacity. However, when treadmill tests are used to predict aerobic fitness, the subject should not support his or her weight by holding the railing of the treadmill. This all-too-common practice lowers the actual workload and invalidates the prediction of fitness and work capacity.

TABLE 3.5   Age- and Fitness-Adjusted Maximal Heart Rates

Age	Predicted maximal heart rates*		
	Below-average fitness	Average fitness	Above-average fitness
20	201	201	196
25	195	197	194
30	190	193	191
35	184	190	188
40	179	186	186
45	174	183	183
50	168	179	180
55	163	176	178
60	158	172	175
65	152	169	173
70	147	165	170

*Maximal heart rate (MHR) declines with age. The rate of decline is related to activity and fitness. The decline is slower among active and fit individuals. These age- and fitness-adjusted MHRs are based on a sample of more than 2,500 men, but are averages—there is considerable variability in this measure.

Reprinted from Cooper et al. 1975.

The stress test should be terminated when the subject cannot continue or has symptoms of exertional intolerance (chest pain, intolerable fatigue) or distress (staggering, dizziness, confusion, pallor, labored breathing, or nausea), when there are significant electrocardiographic changes, or when blood pressure drops in spite of an increasing workload. Termination of the test at some predetermined percentage of the assumed maximal heart rate, on the other hand, as discussed earlier, risks missing important signs or symptoms. As I have noted, the maximal heart rate is highly variable. Using an age-related maximal heart rate (e.g., 220 beats per minute minus age equals the predicted maximal heart rate) can lead to substantial errors. For example, the maximal heart rate for 40-year-old patients may average 180 beats per minute (bpm) (220 – 40 = 180), but the range goes from below 144 bpm to above 216. So, a test terminated at 85% of the predicted maximal heart rate (.85 × 180 = 153 bpm) may be too strenuous for a few and too easy for others.

MAXIMAL HEART RATE

The variability in maximal heart rate, as defined by a statistic called the standard deviation (SD), is ± 12 bpm: 68% of all cases fall within ± one SD, 95% within ± two SD, and 99% within ± three SD. For 40-year-olds (220 – 40 = 180), it is possible that one in 100 may have a max HR below 144 or above 216. Incidentally, as you'll see in chapter 4, this variability in max HR complicates the use of the heart rate for the prescription of exercise. And to make matters more confusing, the standard deviation in max HR goes up to 15 bpm for older individuals!

The Exercise Electrocardiogram

The electrocardiogram (ECG) is a strip of paper with a record of the electrical activity of the heart. Each complete ECG cycle (see figure 3.3) represents one beat of the heart. The P wave shows the electrical activity that immediately precedes the contraction of the upper chambers, or atria. The QRS complex represents the electrical discharge of the lower chambers or ventricles, and the T wave results when the depolarized ventricles are recharged. Under normal conditions the heart receives excitation at the sinoatrial node, located near the right atrium, via the sympathetic nervous system. The impulse spreads across both atria, causing contraction of the upper chambers as the impulse flows, and finally arrives at the atrioventricular node, which is located between the atria and ventricles. Here the impulse finds its way down specialized fibers to the muscle of the ventricles, causing them to contract and pump blood to the body.

The ECG is wired to indicate a positive deflection when the depolarization wave is flowing toward the positive electrode. The P wave and QRS complex normally yield positive deflections. If the stimulus to contract originates from the wrong direction (e.g., from the ventricles) the QRS could deflect downward. Because the recording paper moves at a specified speed (usually 25 millimeters per second) the width of the wave can provide information about the rate of conduction. For example, if conduction is slow or blocked, the width of the QRS will be broad. The physician, nurse, or exercise test technologist administering a stress test pays careful attention to the ECG waveform as it travels across the screen of the oscilloscope. Changes of sufficient importance to terminate the test include:

- S-T segment depression in excess of 0.2 millivolts (mv) (2 millimeters below baseline)
- Irregular rhythms (e.g., premature ventricular contractions), particularly when they originate in the ventricles and come in volleys of 3 or more or as many as 10 per minute
- Left ventricular conduction disturbances

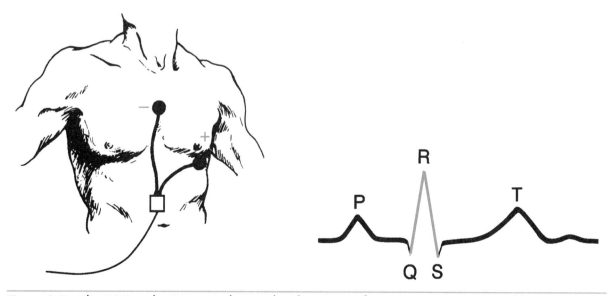

Figure 3.3   The ECG cycle. *P* wave indicates depolarization of atria. *QRS* wave is caused by spread of excitation through ventricles. *T* wave indicates repolarization of ventricles.

Exercise-induced premature ventricular contractions (PVCs) may lead to ventricular tachycardia (extremely rapid rate) and occasionally to fibrillation, an uncontrolled and uncoordinated action of heart muscle fibers that is incapable of pumping blood. Fibrillation requires immediate emergency action: The defibrillator provides a strong direct current that depolarizes the entire heart muscle, thereby allowing return to the normal pattern of stimulation. Conduction disturbances occasionally occur during stress tests, so it is important that emergency equipment and trained personnel are available when high-risk patients are being evaluated. Fortunately, most patients recover and are able to return to supervised activity after defibrillation. Tests conducted on apparently healthy individuals are not considered unsafe, but test administrators should be thoroughly trained in CPR and other emergency techniques.

Test Results

When the exercise stress test results are suggestive of heart problems (e.g., ECG abnormalities, chest pain, or abnormal blood pressure response) the test is called positive. Interestingly, a problem-free test is called negative, indicating a lack of significant findings. Stress test findings are verified when they are confirmed with cardiac catheterization, an invasive imaging technique. In this procedure a catheter is inserted into a blood vessel in the leg and worked into position in the aorta. An opaque dye is injected into each coronary artery to allow X-ray detection of narrowing due to atherosclerosis. Results of a positive stress test are called false when the catheter test reveals normal coronary arteries (i.e., a false positive stress test), thereby disproving the results of the stress test. On the other hand, if narrowed arteries are found after a normal, or negative, stress test, indicating the presence of disease, it is called a false negative test.

False Negative Test.   False negative results are disturbing because they indicate a failure to diagnose the presence of existing coronary artery disease. A small number of cases fall into this category, and most of them do not go on for further evaluation. In such cases, the first indication of a problem may be the last, a myocardial infarction or heart attack. Because of this, the physician cannot rely on the stress test alone, but must employ clinical judgment, the medical history, and other diagnostic tools. For example, patient reports of indigestion or chest pain during exertion may be useful, because the gradual warm-up of the stress test may allow patients with narrowed arteries to adjust to the increased workload, thus disguising the problem.

False Positive Test.   False positive tests are disturbing because they may cause otherwise healthy individuals to become cardiac neurotics, morbidly obsessed with a heart condition that may not exist. Estimates of the frequency of false positive results range from more than 50% to as little as 8%, depending on the group studied. False positive results are more prevalent in highly active subjects and women (who may be more likely to hyperventilate during the test). Endurance athletes often exhibit ECG abnormalities during the stress test, and doctors have learned to disregard the findings in the absence of other signs or symptoms. But what about the active nonathlete who receives word that the stress test indicates possible coronary artery disease? What does he or she do next?

Until recently the coronary angiogram was the only way to confirm or deny the existence of coronary artery disease. If the stress test indicated possible disease, the patient had two choices: Have the invasive catheter test, or ignore the findings and fret about the possibilities, even giving up an active lifestyle for a heart condition that might not exist. Today the patient has other choices. Myocardial scintigraphy involves a less invasive assessment of myocardial blood flow during rest and exercise. In this procedure, radioactive thallium is injected into the circulation, and its uptake in cardiac muscle is observed with a scintillation camera. Cold spots indicate areas where blood flow is inadequate during exercise, allowing confirmation of stress test results (Froelicher, 1984). Recently, drugs have been used to stress the heart and simulate the stress test, and computerized tomography scans (CT scans) are being used successfully as well to detect plaques in coronary arteries. I'm waiting for simple, noninvasive, low-cost alternatives, such as a comparison of blood pressure readings taken from the arm and leg. In such a case, a leg reading lower than that taken on the arm may indicate the presence of atherosclerosis. These developments may someday make the stress test obsolete.

Actually, some experts think there may be few false positive tests. They reason that a coronary artery spasm may occur during the vigorous effort of the stress test. Because the catheterization test is routinely performed at rest, the spasm may not show up. The thallium scan mentioned earlier helps solve this problem, and drugs can indicate the tendency for spasms during catheterization. (For more on exercise testing consult *ACSM's Guidelines for Exercise Testing and Prescription [5th ed.]*, 1995.)

The Risk of Activity

When Jim Fixx, author of a popular book on running, died during a run, millions became concerned about the risks of vigorous activity. Subsequent research has confirmed the fact that activity reduces but doesn't eliminate the risks associated with inherited or lifestyle diseases. The risk of heart attack for habitually active individuals rises during exercise to a level slightly above that of sedentary living, but only during the period of exercise. Throughout the rest of the day, the active individual has a much lower risk than a sedentary counterpart (Siscovick, LaPorte, & Newman, 1985).

The risks of activity and fitness range from minor musculoskeletal problems to major coronary events. The risks are low for low-intensity and moderate-duration activity. Overuse injuries are more common when distance is increased rapidly, with more miles per week, with high-intensity (e.g., interval) training, and with eccentric exercise (e.g., downhill running). The risk of a coronary event is low for an asymptomatic adult, in either training or testing. And the risk can be cut in half by taking the pre-exercise screening test (see figure 3.2).

When patients take a stress test in a medical setting, the risks are fewer than one death, four heart attacks, and five hospital admissions per 10,000 tests. But when presumably healthy (asymptomatic) individuals are tested, the risks are much lower. The risk of death while jogging for middle-aged men has been estimated at one death per year for every 7,620 joggers. When those with known heart disease are excluded, the rate falls to one death per year for every 15,200 joggers (Siscovick et al., 1985).

Figure 3.4 provides a graphic view of the relationships between the benefits and risks of activity. The figure shows that benefits increase rapidly at first but eventually plateau, with little additional reward at higher levels of activity. Risks, on the other hand, rise slowly at first, then more rapidly at higher levels of activity. It seems prudent to maximize benefits while minimizing risks and to engage in a level of activity associated with enhanced health, regular moderate activity.

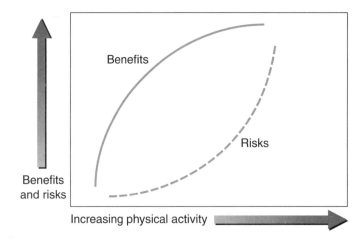

Figure 3.4   Relationships of benefits and risks with level of physical activity.
Reprinted from K. Powel and R. Paffenbarger, 1985, "Workshop on epidemiologic and public health aspects of physical activity and exercise: A summary," *Public Health Reports* 100: 123.

Special Considerations

This section provides a brief summary for those with special exercise needs. Consult specific references, community services, or your physician for additional information.

Senior Citizens

With age comes an increasing need for muscular fitness. Seniors should undertake exercises to develop and maintain muscular endurance and—if needed—strength. It would be wise to increase strength to required levels before loss of strength limits self-sufficiency.

Women

The exercise prescriptions in this book work for both men and women. However, women should consider a few specifics. Young women need to know that vigorous prepubertal training may delay the onset of the menstrual cycle, but on the positive side, early training also seems to reduce the incidence of sex-related cancers in later years. Excess endurance training in young women could reduce mineralization of bones, cause stress fractures, and pose future problems. Strength training strengthens bones and leads to improved strength *and* to increases in muscle mass (hypertrophy). During pregnancy, exercise habits can be continued with physician approval. Most doctors recommend eliminating high-impact aerobics and keeping the heart rate below 140 beats during exercise. Postmenopausal women should be certain to include exercises that put a moderate degree of stress on the muscles and bones of the upper body as well as the legs, to minimize the threat of osteoporosis. Women of all ages need to be aware of their special nutritional needs (e.g., iron and calcium) and make sure they get adequate amounts.

African Americans

A series of articles on blacks and exercise (Lubell, 1988) documented the greater prevalence of hypertension among African Americans. One in every three black adults has hypertension, compared with one in four nonblacks, and blacks are two times more likely to have moderate hypertension and three times more likely to have severe hypertension than whites. Although black people will benefit from aerobic and other activities, those with hypertension should avoid exercises with an isometric component, such as heavy weight lifting. Aerobic exercise and weight loss will help lower blood pressure, but people with hypertension should undergo a thorough pre-exercise medical evaluation and be certain to take prescribed medication.

People With Disabilities

Each disability carries its own special restrictions, but each has potential as well. People with diabetes compete in international competition, but only after establishing control over their condition. Individuals with multiple sclerosis find that moderate activity, such as swimming, expands their potential. Wheelchair athletes compete in marathons and play basketball, and now they can fish at handicapped access sites. Individuals with disabilities have learned to ski, to kayak, to do just about anything, and more opportunities are becoming available. For more information contact your recreation department or community service organizations.

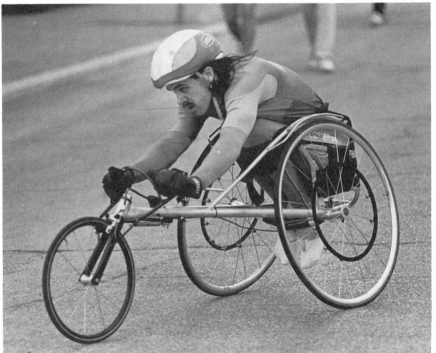

Courtesy of *The Daily Illini*

A disability needn't prevent you from living the active life.

Children

Children are not miniature adults; their bones are still being formed, and their capacity for exercise in certain circumstances is different from that of adults. Moreover, the value of prepubertal strength or endurance training is still far from established. Therefore, it is wise to encourage but not force children's participation. Avoid heavy training, prolonged hard work in hot environments, and excess competition (if only to prevent later burnout). Give children the freedom to develop their own games, to play, to explore, and to be kids. Don't impose an adult model or adult goals and objectives on children.

Warning Signs

As you train, be aware of these warning signs.

Group 1

If any of these occur, *even once*, stop exercising, and consult your physician before resuming exercise.

- *Abnormal heart action.* This may include irregular pulse; fluttering, pumping, or palpitations in the chest or throat; a sudden burst of rapid heartbeats; or a very slow pulse that a moment earlier had been beating at a moderate rate (this may occur during exercise, or it may be a delayed reaction).
- *Pain or pressure in the middle of the chest or in the arm or throat.* This can occur during or after exercise.
- *Dizziness, lightheadedness, sudden loss of coordination, confusion, cold sweat, glassy stare, pallor, blueness, or fainting.* In this case, stop the exercise—don't try to cool down—and lie with feet elevated or sit and put your head down between your legs until the symptoms pass.

Group 2

Try the suggested remedy briefly; if no help results, consult a doctor.

- *Persistent rapid heart action.* This can occur when you're near the training zone and 5 to 10 minutes after exercise. To correct the condition, keep the heart rate at the lower end of the zone or below, and increase very slowly. Consult a physician if the action is persistent.
- *Flare-up of arthritic conditions.* Rest, and don't resume exercise until the condition subsides. If you have no relief with usual remedies, consult a physician.

Group 3

These usually can be remedied without medical consultation, though you may wish to report them to your doctor.

- *Nausea or vomiting after exercise.* Exercise less vigorously, and take a more gradual cool-down period.

- *Extreme breathlessness lasting more than 10 minutes after stopping exercise.* Stay at the lower end of the training zone or below. Be sure you're not too breathless to speak during exercise; if you are, stop exercising. Consult a doctor.
- *Prolonged fatigue.* If you are tired 24 hours after exercising or have insomnia not present before starting your exercise program, stay at the lower end of the training zone or below, and increase the level gradually.
- *Side stitch* (diaphragm spasm). Lean forward while sitting, attempting to push the abdominal organs up against the diaphragm.

Health and Wellness

In the past, health was defined as the absence of disease, and that is how many individuals still think of the term. Recently the definition of health has been expanded to include a state of complete physical, mental, and emotional well-being, not merely the absence of disease or infirmity. In that context the relationship of activity to health becomes more clear. The relationship of health and wellness is equally clear. Ardell (1984) defined wellness as "a conscious and deliberate approach to an advanced state of physical and psychological/spiritual health." So, wellness defines movement toward an advanced state of health, which is also called optimal or high-level health (figure 3.5).

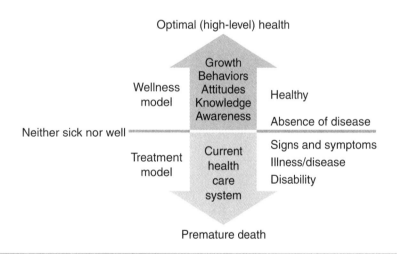

Figure 3.5 The health continuum.

The old view of health placed illness on one side of a line and health on the other, with doctors and the treatment-oriented health care system defending the line. Wellness, on the other hand, is viewed as a dynamic process in which you—the individual—are responsible for your health. The health care system is treatment-oriented: Workers in the system focus on correcting problems brought on by illness, disease, injury, or disability. Wellness involves disease prevention and promoting behaviors that lower the risk of illness or injury. The treatment system employs an army of high-priced professionals and costs billions of dollars. Wellness relies on individual responsibility and low-cost helpers, and reduces reliance on costly specialists and procedures. The active life is the keystone of health and wellness.

Health Risk Analysis

Utilize the health risk analysis in figure 3.6 as a learning tool to identify positive and negative aspects of your health behavior. While many of the effects are based on real findings from large epidemiological investigations, the estimates are generalized and should not be taken too seriously. It is impossible to predict with accuracy how long you will live or when you will die. A more accurate estimate can be achieved by calculating risk according to age, sex, and race, using computerized analyses.

Plus one (+1) represents a positive effect that could add a year to your life or life to your years, and minus one (-1) indicates a loss in the quality or quantity of life. Complete each section and record the totals in figure 3.7.

Summary

Until recently the medical community had been cautious concerning exercise, suggesting a visit to the physician and even a stress test prior to participation. This is understandable, since few medical schools offer more than one or two lectures on exercise physiology. Unless your doctor is active or has special training in physiology or sports medicine, he or she may know very little about the benefits of activity and how to prescribe exercise to achieve those benefits. But as the benefits and risks become better understood, physicians are turning to exercise physiologists to design and conduct preventive and rehabilitative exercise programs.

Of course, you don't have to see your physician in order to participate in moderate activity such as walking. If you feel good and answer no to all the questions in the pre-exercise screening test (figure 3.2), you don't have to spend hundreds of dollars to confirm what you already know. Start slowly, increase intensity and duration gradually, and read the next section of this book. And use health screening, early detection, and periodic medical examinations to help you maintain your health.

Coronary Heart Disease (CHD) Risk Factors

Cholesterol, total cholesterol/HDL ratio

under 160	160-200	200-220	220-240	over 240	
< 3	3-4	4-5	5-6	> 6	
+2	+1	−1	−2	−4	_____

Blood pressure $\left(\dfrac{systolic}{diastolic} \right)$

110	110-130	130-150	150-170	170	
60-80	60-80	80-90	90-100	> 100	
+1	0	−1	−2	−4	_____

Smoking

never	quit	smoke cigar or pipe or close family member smokes	1 pack cigarettes daily	2 or more packs daily	
+1	0	−1	−3	−5	_____

Heredity

no family history of CHD	1 close relative over 60 with CHD	2 close relatives over 60 with CHD	1 close relative under 60 with CHD	2 or more close relatives under 60 with CHD	
+2	0	−1	−2	−4	_____

Body weight (or fat)

5 lb below desirable weight (< 10% fat—M; < 16% fat—F)	5 lb below to 4 lb above desirable weight (10-15% fat—M; 16-22% fat—F)	5-20 lb overweight (15-20% fat—M; 22-30% fat—F)	20-35 lb overweight (20-25% fat—M; 30-35% fat—F)	35 lb overweight (> 25% fat—M; > 35% fat—F)	
+2	+1	0	−2	−3	_____

Sex

female under 45 years	female over 45 years	male	stocky male	bald, stocky male	
0	−1	−1	−2	−4	_____

Stress

phlegmatic, unhurried, generally happy	ambitious but generally relaxed	sometimes hard-driving, time-competitive	hard-driving, time-conscious, competitive (Type A)	Type A with repressed hostility	
+1	0	0	−1	−3	_____

Physical activity

high-intensity, over 30 minutes daily	intermittent, 20-30 minutes 3-5 times/week	moderate, 10-20 minutes 3-5 times/week	light, 10-20 minutes 1-2 times/week	little or none	
+2	+2	+1	0	−2	_____

Total: I CHD Risk Factors _____

Enter on figure 3.7

(continued)

Figure 3.6   Health risk analysis.

II Health Habits (associated with good health and longevity)

Breakfast

daily	sometimes	none	coffee	coffee and doughnut	
+1	0	–1	–2	–3	_____

Regular meals

3 or more	2 daily	not regular	fad diets	starve and stuff	
+1	0	–1	–2	–3	_____

Sleep

7-8 hr	8-9 hr	6-7 hr	9 hr	6 hr	
+1	0	0	–1	–2	_____

Alcohol

none	women 3/wk	men 1-2 daily	2-6 daily	6 daily	
+1	+1	+1	–2	–4	_____

Total: II Health Habits   _____

Enter on figure 3.7

III Medical Factors

Medical exam and screening tests (blood pressure, diabetes, glaucoma)

regular tests, see doctor when necessary	periodic medical exam and selected tests	periodic medical exam	sometimes get tests	no tests or medical exams	
+1	+1	0	0	–1	_____

Heart

no history of problems self or family	some history	rheumatic fever as child, no murmur now	rheumatic fever as child, have murmur	have ECG abnormality and/or angina pectoris	
+1	0	–1	–2	–3	_____

Lung (including pneumonia and tuberculosis)

no problem	some past problem	mild asthma or bronchitis	emphysema severe asthma, or bronchitis	severe lung problems	
+1	0	–1	–2	–3	_____

Digestive tract

no problem	occasional diarrhea, loss of appetite	frequent diarrhea or stomach upset	ulcers, colitis, gall bladder, or liver problems	severe gastrointestinal disorders	
+1	0	–1	–2	–3	_____

Figure 3.6 *(continued)*

III Medical Factors (continued)

Diabetes

no problem or family history	controlled hypoglycemia (low blood sugar)	hypoglycemia and family history	mild diabetes (diet and exercise)	diabetes (insulin)	
+1	0	−1	−2	−3	_____

Drugs

seldom take	minimal but regular use of aspirin or other drugs	heavy use of aspirin or other drugs	regular use of amphetamines, barbiturates, or psychogenic drugs	heavy use of amphetamines, barbiturates, or psychogenic drugs	
+1	0	−1	−2	−3	_____

Total: II Medical Factors _____
Enter on figure 3.7

IV Safety Factors

Driving in car

4,000 mi/ year, mostly local	4,000-6,000 mi/ year, local and some highway	6,000-8,000 mi/ year, local and highway	8,000-10,000 mi/ year, highway and some local	10,000 mi/ year, mostly highway	
+1	0	0	−1	−2	_____

Using seat belts

always	most of time (75%)	on highway only	seldom (25%)	never	
+1	0	−1	−2	−3	_____

Risk-taking behavior
(motorcycle, skydive, mountain climb, fly small plane, etc.)

some with careful preparation	never	occasional	often	try anything for thrills	
+1	0	−1	−1	−2	_____

Total: IV Safety Factors _____
Enter on figure 3.7
(continued)

Figure 3.6 *(continued)*

V Personal Factors

Diet

low-fat, high-complex carbohydrates	balanced, moderate fat	balanced, typical fat	fad diets	starve and stuff	
+2	+1	0	−1	−2	_____

Longevity

grandparents lived past 90, parents past 80	grandparents lived past 80, parents past 70	grandparents lived past 70, parents past 60	few relatives lived past 60	few relatives lived past 50	
+2	+1	0	−1	−3	_____

Love and marriage

happily married	married	unmarried	divorced	extramarital relationship	
+2	+1	0	−1	−3	_____

Education

postgraduate or master craftsman	college graduate or skilled craftsman	some college or trade school	high school graduate	grade school graduate	
+1	+1	0	−1	−2	_____

Job satisfaction

enjoy job, see results, room for advancement	enjoy job, see some results, able to advance	job OK, no results, nowhere to go	dislike job	hate job	
+1	+1	0	−1	−2	_____

Social

have some close friends	have some friends	have no good friends	stuck with people I don't enjoy	have no friends at all	
+1	0	−1	−2	−3	_____

Race

white or Asian	black or Hispanic	American Indian	
0	−1	−2	_____

Total: V Personal Factors _____

Enter on figure 3.7

Figure 3.6   *(continued)*

VI Psychological Factors

Outlook

feel good about present and future	satisfied	unsure about present or future	unhappy in present, don't look forward to future	miserable, rather not get out of bed	
+1	0	−1	−2	−3	_____

Depression

no family history of depression	some family history—I feel OK	family history and I am mildly depressed	sometimes feel life isn't worth living	thoughts of suicide	
+1	0	−1	−2	−3	_____

Anxiety

seldom anxious	occasionally anxious	often anxious	always anxious	panic attacks	
+1	0	−1	−2	−3	_____

Relaxation

relax or meditate daily	relax often	seldom relax	usually tense	always tense	
+1	0	−1	−2	−3	_____

Total: VI Psychological Factors _____

Enter on figure 3.7

VII For Women Only

Health care

regular breast and Pap exam	occasional breast and Pap exam	never have exam	treated disorder	untreated cancer	
+1	0	−1	−2	−4	_____

Birth control pill

never used	quit 5 years ago	still use, under 30 years of age	use pill and smoke	use pill, smoke, over 35	
+1	0	0	−2	−3	_____

Total: VII For Women Only _____

Enter on figure 3.7

Figure 3.6 *(continued)*

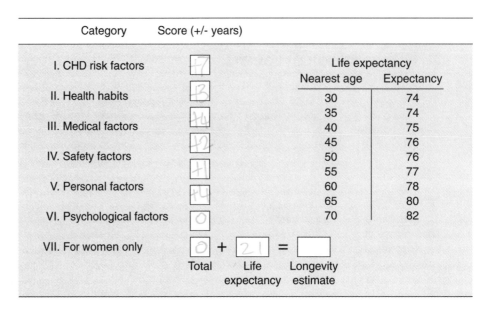

Category	Score (+/- years)		
I. CHD risk factors	+7		
II. Health habits	13	Life expectancy	
		Nearest age	Expectancy
III. Medical factors	+4	30	74
		35	74
IV. Safety factors	+2	40	75
		45	76
V. Personal factors	+1	50	76
		55	77
VI. Psychological factors	+4	60	78
	0	65	80
VII. For women only		70	82

0 + 21 = ☐

Total   Life   Longevity
        expectancy   estimate

Figure 3.7 Health risk summary. Now go back and see how you can add years to your life by improving behaviors and lifestyle. Check each category for possible changes you would like to make in your current lifestyle.

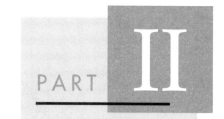

Aerobic Fitness

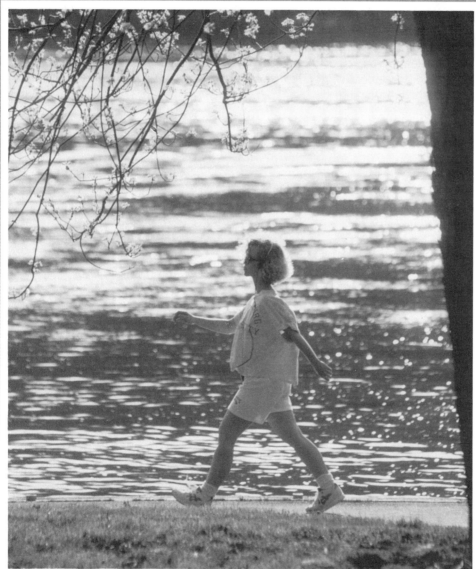

Somewhere above the pace of your normal daily activities but well below maximal effort you will find aerobic exercise. If you do aerobic exercise often enough you will improve your aerobic fitness, and as fitness improves you'll further enhance your health, appearance, vitality, and quality of life. Aerobic fitness describes how well you are able to take oxygen from the atmosphere into the lungs and then the blood, and pump it via the heart to working muscles where it is utilized to oxidize carbohydrate and fat to produce energy. No other measure says more about the health and capacity of your respiratory system, heart, blood and blood vessels, and skeletal muscles. Rhythmic large-muscle activities such as brisk walking, jogging, cycling, swimming, cross-country skiing, and rowing are aerobic exercises. They demand sustained increases in respiration, circulation, and muscle metabolism, and lead to adaptations in the systems and muscles involved. Participation in aerobic exercise is associated with health benefits and longevity, and regular participation leads to improved aerobic fitness. In many physical, psychological, and social ways, aerobic fitness is good for health and the quality of life. It improves appearance, boosts self-confidence and body image, and opens the door to a challenging new world filled with new experiences and interesting people. Let's see how you can integrate fitness into your busy schedule so you can reap the many extra benefits.

CHAPTER 4

Understanding Aerobic Fitness

"The firm, the enduring, the simple, and the modest are near to virtue."

Confucius

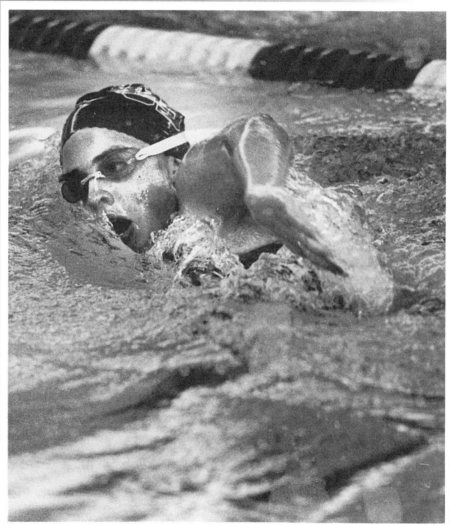

© Mary Langenfeld

To me, *aerobic fitness* stands for "endurance" or "stamina." It describes the ability, part inherited and part trained, to persevere or persist in strenuous or prolonged endeavors. People who pursue fitness earn far more than enhanced health and performance. For many the process becomes more important than the goal, providing discipline, challenge, and time for reflection. For the moment we'll consider the physiology of fitness; later we'll ponder its other dimensions.

THIS CHAPTER WILL HELP YOU

- understand the terms *aerobic* and *anaerobic*,
- determine the meaning of aerobic exercise and aerobic fitness,
- identify and experience the concept of anaerobic threshold, and
- understand the factors that influence aerobic fitness.

Aerobic Exercise

Dress for exercise, warm up, and head out at a walking pace. Increase the pace a little as each minute passes, going from a slow to a fast walk. At about 5 miles per hour (12 minutes per mile) you'll begin to jog. Continue to gradually increase your speed until the effort becomes uncomfortable, breathing becomes labored, and you doubt your ability to continue. Up to this point the exercise has been aerobic, which means "in the presence of oxygen." Energy has come from the oxidation of fat and carbohydrate. If you continued to increase the intensity of exercise, the muscles would shift to anaerobic, or non-oxidative, energy production, which involves intense effort of necessarily short duration and the accumulation of lactic acid in the muscles and blood.

Lactic acid is both an energy carrier and a metabolic by-product of intense effort. Its accumulation is a sign that you are using energy faster than it can be produced aerobically. Too much lactic acid interferes with the muscle's contractile and metabolic capabilities. Lactic acid and the high levels of carbon dioxide produced in vigorous effort are associated with labored breathing, fatigue, and discomfort. Aerobic exercise can be defined as exercise below the point at which blood lactic acid levels rise rapidly, below the lactate threshold (see figure 4.1).

FIBER TYPES

Humans have three main types of muscle fibers: slow twitch (slow oxidative, or SO) fibers that are efficient in the use of oxygen; a faster-contracting type that can work with oxygen or without (fast oxidative glycolytic, or FOG); and a fast twitch fiber that uses muscle glycogen for short, intense contractions (fast glycolytic, or FG). As we go from a walk to a jog to a run we recruit SO, FOG, then FG fibers to help us go faster. Recruit too many FG fibers and the effort becomes anaerobic; the fibers produce lactic acid, and we are forced to slow down or stop.

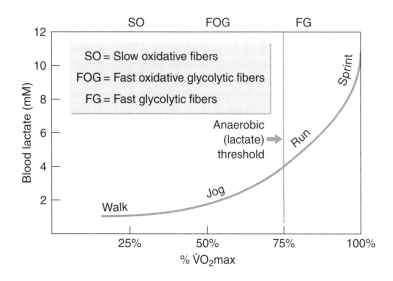

Figure 4.1 Anaerobic (lactate) threshold. As exercise intensity (% $\dot{V}O_2$max) increases we recruit FOG fibers, then FG fibers. More blood lactate accumulates because FG fibers produce more lactic acid and because most muscle fibers are active and therefore unable to remove (take up) lactate.

Aerobic metabolism is far more efficient than anaerobic, yielding 38 molecules of adenosine triphosphate (ATP—the compound that fuels muscular contractions) per molecule of glucose, versus only 2 molecules via the anaerobic route. Since it produces little lactic acid, aerobic exercise is relatively pleasant and relaxing. And the oxidation of abundant fat reserves ensures an adequate supply of energy for extended periods of effort. Aerobic exercise can be sustained for several minutes to many hours. You can even carry on a conversation during moderate aerobic exercise.

Aerobic and anaerobic exercises differ in intensity; light to moderate activity is aerobic, while extremely vigorous or intense effort is anaerobic. Table 4.1 illustrates how heart rate and breathing increase with exercise intensity, and how we switch from burning fat to burning carbohydrate as exercise becomes more vigorous. The table also shows how the nervous system recruits different muscle fiber types as the intensity of the effort increases.

TABLE 4.1   Levels of Exercise Intensity

| | Exercise intensity | | |
	Light	Moderate	Intense
Example exercise	Walking	Jogging	Running
Metabolism	Aerobic	Aerobic	Aerobic/anaerobic
Energy source	Fat and CHO	CHO and fat	CHO and fat
Heart rate	<120	120-150	>150
Breathing	Easy	Can talk easily	Hard to talk
Muscle fiber recruited	SO	FOG	FG

CHO = carbohydrate

Aerobic Fitness

Aerobic fitness is the maximal capacity to take in, transport, and utilize oxygen.

Aerobic fitness, defined as the maximal capacity to take in, transport, and utilize oxygen, is best measured in a laboratory test called the maximal oxygen intake (or $\dot{V}O_2$max). The test, which defines the highest sustainable intensity of effort, requires a treadmill or other exercise device; a metabolic measurement system to measure oxygen, carbon dioxide, and the volume of expired air; and a computer to do the calculations. After a health risk assessment, the subject signs an informed consent form and is fitted with ECG electrodes to keep track of the heart and measure heart rate.

Following a brief warm-up, the subject begins the test wearing a mask or mouthpiece to direct the expired air into the analyzer. The test involves a walk (or run, for the more fit) on the treadmill, which is programmed to increase grade every minute or two. Oxygen intake is computed each minute as the test proceeds toward maximal effort. The test is terminated when the oxygen intake levels off in spite of increased treadmill grade, or when the subject can no longer keep up with the treadmill. The highest level of oxygen attained is called the maximal oxygen intake or aerobic fitness.

$\dot{V}O_2$max Test

The $\dot{V}O_2$max test protocol, the result of many years of experience, is suitable for a wide range of subjects, from the sedentary to elite athletes. The test, which takes from 8 to 12 minutes, can utilize either metabolic measurements (oxygen and carbon dioxide concentrations and volume of expired air) to measure oxygen intake or a table to estimate the value. The protocol allows the test to be tailored to the subject's level of fitness and previous training. Figure 4.2 describes the protocol, and table 4.2 provides information for the estimation of the $\dot{V}O_2$max. (Note that the subject should not be allowed to hold on to the railing of the treadmill if the intention is to estimate the max value. Holding on to the railing reduces the workload and overestimates the estimation of oxygen intake.)

Use the final rate and grade on the treadmill to estimate the $\dot{V}O_2$max (see table 4.2). For example, if the last minute of the test was at 6 miles per hour and 10% grade, the aerobic fitness estimate is 50 ml/kg · min, or 50 milliliters of oxygen per kilogram of body weight per minute.

Scores in the range of 3 to 4 liters of oxygen per minute (L/min) are common, and values of 5 to 6 liters have been reported for endurance athletes. When reported in L/min (called *aerobic capacity*) the score provides information about the total capacity of the cardiorespiratory systems and is a good predictor of endurance performance in non–weight-bearing sports (e.g., cycling). However, since this value is related to body size, larger individuals tend to have higher scores. To eliminate the influence of body size, the maximal oxygen intake score in liters is divided by the body weight in kilograms (1 kg = 2.2 lbs). In this example, maximal oxygen intake score is 3 liters, and body weight is 60 kilograms:

$$3 \text{ L/min} \div 60 \text{ kg} = 50 \text{ ml/kg} \cdot \text{min}$$

The resulting value, expressed in milliliters of oxygen per kilogram of body weight per minute, allows direct comparison of individuals, regardless of body size. This measure, also known as aerobic power, is more related to endurance

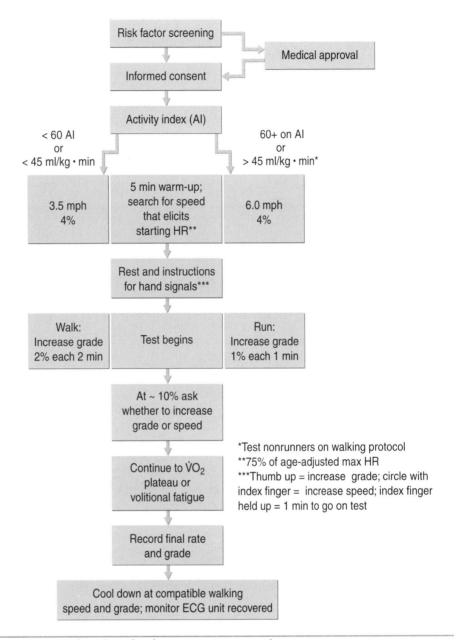

Figure 4.2 Flowchart for $\dot{V}O_2$max test protocol.

performance in running and other weight-bearing sports, and it is the preferred way to express aerobic fitness. If two individuals of different weight have the same score in liters, which one is more fit? If one weighs 60 kilograms as in the preceding example and the other weighs 100 kilograms (220 pounds), likewise divide the score for the latter by the respective body weight:

$$3 \text{ L/min} \div 100 \text{ kg} = 30 \text{ ml/kg} \cdot \text{min}$$

In a footrace, the one with a score of 50 would be better able to take in, transport, and utilize oxygen in the working muscles than the one with the score of 30. The average young male (18 to 25 years old) scores 45 to 48 ml/kg · min, while the average female scores 39 to 41. Active men score in the 50s and 60s, with similarly active women in the 40s and 50s. Male endurance athletes have

TABLE 4.2   Estimating $\dot{V}O_2$max:
Approximate Oxygen Intake Requirements for Final Rate/Grade Combinations*

Miles per hour	Grade				
	8%	10%	12%	14%	15%
Walk					
3.0		26	30	34	
3.5		29	34	39	
4.0		32	38	44	(48)
Run					
6.0	(47)	50	53	56	
7.0		58	61	65	
8.0		66	70	74	

*Ml/kg · min; varies with efficiency. (Numbers in parentheses represent $\dot{V}O_2$max in ml/kg · min.)

Maximal oxygen intake is a test of exercise intensity, while lactate threshold is an indicator of exercise duration.

been measured in the 80s, and top female athletes are not far behind with scores in the 70s (see table 4.3). While average values decline with age, as much as 10% per decade in sedentary populations, regular activity cuts the rate in half (5% per decade), and aerobic training can cut that rate in half (2 to 3% per decade).

Until recently, the aerobic fitness score ($\dot{V}O_2$max) was viewed as the best measure of fitness, and was believed to be correlated to health and related to performance in work and sport. While all this is still true, other ways to measure fitness have begun to emerge, and some seem better correlated to endurance and to performance. The maximal oxygen intake or $\dot{V}O_2$max test, which uses the highest score attained, is a test of exercise *intensity*, best correlated to events lasting 12-15 minutes. Measures that reflect the oxidative capacity of muscle (e.g., the lactate threshold) reflect exercise *duration*, or how long an effort can be sustained. So, the lactate threshold is a better indicator of performance in activities lasting 30 minutes or more (Sharkey, 1991).

TABLE 4.3   Fitness Comparison

Subjects	Age	Men (ml/ kg · min)	Women (ml/kg · min)
Untrained	18-22	45	39
Active	18-22	50	43
Trained	18-22	57	53
Elite	18-22	70	63
World class	18-22	80+	70+
Untrained	40-50	36	27
Active	40-50	46	39
Trained	40-50	52	44
Elite	40-50	60+	50+

Lactate Threshold

When exercise becomes very intense, more energy is produced anaerobically, lactic acid begins to accumulate in the blood, and carbon dioxide production increases along with the rate and depth of breathing. The discomfort caused by lactic acid and the labored breathing are sure signs that you have stepped across the anaerobic threshold. The threshold defines the upper limit of sustainable aerobic exercise, and it is a good indicator of endurance performance. Note, however, that physiologists discourage use of the term anaerobic threshold, since not all fibers may be anaerobic; lactate may be produced in one muscle fiber and used as an energy source in another. So, I'll use the more specific terms *lactate threshold* (LT) and *ventilatory threshold* (VT) to define the upper limit of aerobic metabolism and transition to anaerobic metabolism.

Threshold measurements can be made during the $\dot{V}O_2$max test. For this, blood is drawn after each stage (% grade) of the treadmill test and analyzed in a lactate analyzer. The lactate threshold may be defined as the point at which lactate production increases dramatically or at a particular level (e.g., 4 millimoles [mM]), and reported as a percent of the $\dot{V}O_2$max or the velocity at LT (e.g., 85% $\dot{V}O_2$max

ESTIMATING THE THRESHOLD

The lactate threshold is a better indicator of endurance performance than aerobic fitness ($\dot{V}O_2$max) in events such as a 10-kilometer road race. The lactate threshold indicates the oxygen utilization capabilities of the muscles. You can predict your threshold using equations developed by Dr. Art Weltman (1989) at the University of Virginia.

The prediction equation uses the time for a 3,200-meter run to predict the lactate threshold, expressed as the $\dot{V}O_2$ (oxygen uptake) at the threshold (4 millimoles [mM] lactate). You can use this value and the results of your aerobic capacity test to determine the percentage of the maximum that you can sustain.

For men:

$$\dot{V}O_2 \text{ (ml/[kg} \cdot \text{min])} = 122.0 - (5.31 \times [3,200\text{-m time in min*}])$$

  *In minutes and decimal fractions; e.g., 30 s = .5 min.

For women:

$$\dot{V}O_2 = (-1.12\ 3\ [3,200\text{-m time}]) + 61.57$$
(note negative in equation)

Example:

A 40-year-old male with 3,200-meter time of 14 minutes:

$$\dot{V}O_2 = 122 - (5.31 \times 14)$$
$$= 122 - 74.34$$
$$= 47.66$$

Divide the result (47.66) by the max (56) to get the lactate threshold as a percentage of the max, 47.6 ÷ 56 = 85% of the $\dot{V}O_2$max. Use the aerobic fitness and threshold tests to gauge the progress of your training.

or 10 miles per hour respectively). A less invasive way to estimate the threshold involves measuring and plotting the rise in ventilation during the progressive treadmill test. The ventilatory threshold is defined as the point at which the ventilation (in liters of air per minute) rises disproportionally, a point that has been called breakaway ventilation. This rise in ventilation provides a perceptible signal that indicates you are flirting with exhaustion and had better ease off. Perceptive athletes learn to listen to the information provided by their bodies.

While the thresholds are often similar, they can be disassociated, indicating that they are measuring different aspects of the exercise response. Taken together, the $\dot{V}O_2max$ and the lactate threshold tell a lot about aerobic fitness and performance potential, with the $\dot{V}O_2max$ indicating the capacity for intensity, and the threshold defining the capacity for duration or endurance. Now let us explore the factors that influence aerobic fitness.

Factors Influencing Aerobic Fitness

Is a high aerobic fitness score the product of heredity or training, and how do other factors such as sex, age, and body fat influence your attainable level of fitness?

Heredity

It takes tremendous natural endowment and years of systematic training to achieve high-level endurance performances. Canadian researchers have studied differences in aerobic fitness among fraternal (dizygotic) and identical (monozygotic) twins, and found that intrapair differences were far greater

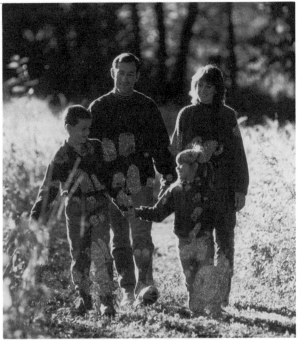

Heredity and environment influence aerobic fitness.

among fraternal than identical twins. The largest difference between identical twins was smaller than the smallest difference between fraternal pairs (Klissouras, 1976). More recently, Malina and Bouchard (1991) have estimated that heredity accounts for 25 to 40% of the variance in $\dot{V}O_2$max values, and Sundet, Magnus, and Tambs (1994) contend that more than half of the variance in maximal aerobic power is due to genotypic differences, with the remainder accounted for by environmental factors (nutrition, training). This supports the notion that the way to become a world-class endurance athlete is to pick your parents carefully!

We inherit many factors that contribute to aerobic fitness, including the maximal capacity of the respiratory and cardiovascular systems, a larger heart, more red cells and hemoglobin, and a high percentage of slow oxidative and fast oxidative-glycolytic muscle fibers. Mitochondria, the energy-producing units of muscle and other cells, are inherited from the maternal side. Recent evidence indicates that the capacity of muscle to respond to training may also be inherited. Other inherited factors such as physique and body composition will also influence fitness and the potential to perform at a high level.

Training

The potential to improve aerobic fitness with training is limited; while most studies confirm the potential to improve 15 to 25% (more with loss of body fat), only adolescents can hope to improve much more than 30%. Consider

ENDURANCE

A biologist friend who has studied locomotion throughout the animal kingdom has noted that humans are inferior to other species at short distances. The cheetah, gazelle, antelope, horse, camel, and even grizzly bear are much faster than humans. But as the distance increases, the human becomes more competitive, and at long distances human endurance qualities stand out. Unfortunately, this superiority emerges only at distances that few are willing to negotiate.

When a proud Montana horseman bragged about the endurance and speed of his Arabian, a local physician wagered he could outrun the horse over a mountainous marathon course (26.2 miles). Perhaps the distance wasn't long enough because the horse finished 16 minutes ahead of the human. Of course, it is also possible that the fit but 49-year-old physician was slightly past his prime and the horse was not.

We have ample evidence that humans are able to cover 100 miles or more in one day. The Tarahumara Indians of Mexico run more than 100 miles while kicking a small ball, and runners throughout the world compete in 100-mile races, sometimes over difficult mountainous terrain. Years ago, crowds flocked to watch 6-day races, where athletes attempted to run as far as possible. Today the 6-day record is well over 635 miles, for an average of 106 miles per day! In spite of the publicity given short races and sports that emphasize bursts of speed, the human body has evolved with the capacity to accomplish prodigious feats of endurance.

two untrained women, one with a $\dot{V}O_2$max of 40 ml/kg · min, the other with a score of 60. Let us assume that heredity accounts for the difference in scores. What happens if each trains and gains a 25% improvement in oxygen intake?

    a. $40 \times 25\% = 10 + 40 = 50$ ml/kg · min
    b. $60 \times 25\% = 15 + 60 = 75$ ml/kg · min

Training raises "a" above the average for young men, while "b" is elevated to a level of elite endurance athletes. Even in the untrained state, "b" has a higher $\dot{V}O_2$max than "a" does when trained. Who ever said life was fair?

Training improves the function and capacity of the respiratory and cardiovascular systems and boosts blood volume, but the most important changes take place in the muscle fibers that are used in the training. Aerobic training improves muscles' ability to produce energy aerobically and shifts metabolism from carbohydrate to fat. This outcome makes muscle an efficient furnace for the combustion of fat, which may produce the single most important health effect of exercise. Burning fat reduces fat storage, blood fat levels, and cardiovascular risk; it also improves insulin sensitivity and reduces the risk of diabetes. This fat metabolism may also contribute to a lower risk of some cancers. Of course, training enhances the ability to perform, but the improvement is limited to the activity used in training. I'll say more about the effects and specificity of training in later chapters.

Gender

Before puberty, boys and girls differ little in aerobic fitness, but from then on girls fall behind. Young women average 15 to 25% less than young men in aerobic fitness, depending on their level of activity. But highly trained young female endurance athletes are but 10% below male endurance athletes of the same

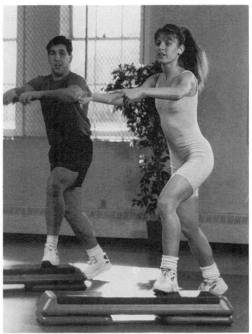

Aerobic training makes muscle an efficient furnace for burning fat.

age in $V\cdot O_2$max and performance times. One reason for the difference between sexes may be hemoglobin, the oxygen-carrying compound found in red blood cells. Men average about 2 grams more per 100 milliliters of blood (15 versus 13 grams per deciliter [g/dl]), and total hemoglobin is correlated to $V\cdot O_2$ and endurance. On the other hand, some females have higher values than male endurance athletes.

Other reasons may be that women are smaller and have less muscle mass, or that women average more body fat than men (25% versus 12.5% for college-age women and men, respectively). Because aerobic fitness is usually reported per unit of body weight, those women with more fat and less lean tissue (muscle) will have some disadvantage. Of course, a portion of the difference is sex-specific fat that is essential for reproductive function and health. For these and other reasons (e.g., osteoporosis) women shouldn't try to become too thin. I raise the issue only to explain why the average male has some advantage over the average female in aerobic fitness.

Until the 1970s women were prohibited from competing in races longer than one-half mile. Overprotective or prejudiced officials worried that frail females couldn't stand the strain. Today women run marathons and 100-mile races, compete in the Iron "Man" triathlon, and swim, ski, and cycle prodigious distances. A woman led for three-quarters of the 1994 high-altitude Leadville 100 until she was passed by a male Tarahumara Indian from Mexico. We've learned that women are well suited for fat-burning endurance events, and that some tolerate heat, cold, and other indignities as well as or better than men. Yet, at the highest level, women's endurance performances remain about 10% behind the best males.

Age

Earlier I alluded to the effects of age on aerobic fitness, with a decline approaching 8 to 10% per decade for inactive individuals, regardless of their initial level of fitness (see figure 4.3). Those who decide to remain active can cut the decline in half (4 to 5% per decade), and those who engage in fitness training can cut that rate in half (2.5% per decade).

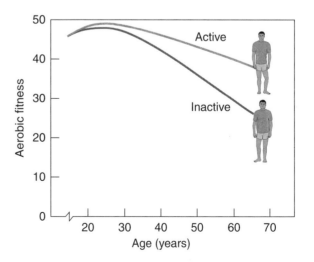

Figure 4.3   Age and aerobic fitness.
Adapted from Sharkey 1977.

A colleague of mine, who served as a subject in many studies, had a $\dot{V}O_2$max of 46 ml/kg · min when he started aerobic training at the age of 30. His score rose to 54 in a few months, then declined slowly as he continued his active lifestyle. Now at age 60 and retired, he has time for even more activity, and his fitness tests out at 52, well above his starting point at age 30. While trainability may decline somewhat with age, exercise gerontologist Dr. Herb deVries has shown that fitness can be improved, even after the age of 70 (deVries, 1986). And it is never too late to start. At 81 years Eula Weaver had a heart attack to add to her problems of congestive heart failure and poor circulation. Unable to walk 100 feet at first, she worked up to jogging a mile each day, and riding her stationary bicycle for several more. She even lifted weights several days a week. At 85 she won the gold medal for the mile run in her age group at the Senior Olympics. I'll say more about age and performance in chapter 18.

Body Fat

Remember that fitness is calculated per unit of body weight, so if fat increases, your fitness declines. About one-half of the decline in fitness with age can be attributed to an increase in body fat. So, the easiest way to maintain or even improve fitness is to rid yourself of excess fat. For example, if Bob (at 100 kilograms, or 220 pounds, and 20% fat) loses 10 kilograms (22 pounds), or half of his body fat, his aerobic fitness score will go from

$$4 \text{ L} / 100 \text{ kg} = 40 \text{ ml/kg} \cdot \text{min}$$
$$\text{to}$$
$$4 \text{ L} / 90 \text{ kg} = 44.4 \text{ ml/kg} \cdot \text{min}$$

About one-half of the decline in fitness with age can be attributed to an increase in body fat.

Without any exercise, just weight loss, his fitness has improved 10%! Now if he earns an additional 20% improvement from training, his fitness could rise above 53 ml/kg · min ($44.4 \times 20\% = 8.88$ ml/kg · min + 44.4 = 53.3). Unlikely? Not at all. My old friend Ernie at one time smoked two packs a day, weighed more than 250 pounds, and bragged about his sedentary lifestyle. When he took a fitness test it was all he could do to finish with a score in the low 30s. Then Ernie got the message: He stopped smoking, started training, and paid attention to his diet. Now, 10 years later, you wouldn't recognize him. Under the fat he discovered a trim, handsome body. He weighs around 170, his fitness score is 58, and he enjoys the active life.

Activity

Finally, let me comment on the most obvious influence on fitness: your regular level of activity. Remember that it is what you do day by day, year after year, that shapes your health, vitality, and quality of life. The effect of years of training can be lost in a mere 12 weeks with the cessation of activity (Coyle, Hemmert, & Coggan, 1986). Three weeks of complete bed rest, for example, may cause a fitness decline of 29%, or almost 10% per week, but the good news is that the loss can easily be restored with regular activity (Saltin et al., 1968). Moderate activity leads to above-average fitness and substantial health benefits, training leads to higher levels of fitness and extra health benefits, and prolonged, systematic training helps you achieve your potential. The choice is yours, but bear in mind: Health has more to do with regular moderate activity than with your level of fitness.

Aerobic Fitness Field Tests

Another way to estimate your aerobic fitness is with a simple, inexpensive field test. If you are a walker use the 1-mile walking test to estimate your $\dot{V}O_2$max. If you are a runner you can use the 1.5-mile run test. Be sure to take the pre-exercise screening test (figure 3.2, page 50) before engaging in either test.

Walking Test

The 1-mile walking test utilizes the time for a 1-mile walk and some personal information to estimate the $\dot{V}O_2$max. Walk the measured course as quickly as possible, then substitute the time (to the nearest hundredth of a minute), posttest heart rate, and other information in the equation.

$$\dot{V}O_2\text{max} = 132.853 - (0.0769 \times \text{weight in pounds})$$
$$- (0.3877 \times \text{age in years}) + (6.315 \times 1 \text{ for male, } 0 \text{ for female})$$
$$- (3.2649 \times \text{time}) - (0.1565 \times \text{HR at end of test})$$

The result in $ml/kg \cdot min$ is highly correlated to a laboratory measure of aerobic fitness (Kline, Pocari, Hintermeister, et al., 1987).

Running Test

The 1.5-mile running test requires a near-maximal effort. If you've been inactive, precede the test with 6 to 8 weeks of training. People over the age of 40 should consider a medical examination. Be sure to stretch and warm up before the test. The time for the 1.5-mile run is used to predict aerobic fitness and is based on the oxygen cost of running (figure 4.4).

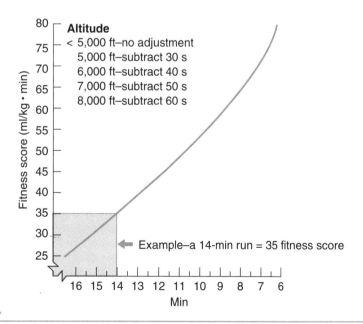

Figure 4.4   1.5-mile aerobic fitness test.

Note: Subtract altitude adjustment from 1.5-mi run time. Then use the graph to find your score.

Montana Bicycle Test

Because some individuals don't like running tests, several people set out to develop a bicycle test to predict aerobic fitness. The result, the Montana Bicycle Test, was developed by Jim Tobin, Kathy Miller, Ted Coladarci, and me. This version was developed on male subjects. I include it to see how you like it and so others can evaluate and improve on the procedure.

The test involves a 5-mile bike ride over a level out-and-back or loop course. Wind speed should be under 10 miles per hour. The test is taken on a 27-inch road bike. The gear remains constant throughout, with the chain on the large chainwheel in front and smallest rear sprocket. Use the drop position on the handlebars throughout the test.

After a warm-up, rest and prepare for the 5-mile ride. Then ride the course as fast as possible. Use the time for the ride and your percent body fat to predict your aerobic fitness (see table 4.4). (Use figure 12.8, page 246, to estimate your body fat.) When the test is conducted above 5,000 feet, use the altitude adjustments found on the 1.5-mile run test (see figure 4.4).

When conducted properly this test correlates highly with treadmill or bicycle ergometer tests of the maximal oxygen intake (aerobic fitness). Remember, the test has been validated only for young men; however, I encourage women to use it as a reference point for bicycle training.

Bicycle Ergometer Test

The bicycle ergometer test is a submaximal test that predicts fitness ($\dot{V}O_2max$). It uses several workloads to determine the relationship between HR and workload, then extrapolates to the maximum HR to predict the maximal working capacity and $\dot{V}O_2max$. The test requires a bicycle ergometer, a stationary bicycle that allows precise measurement of the workload. The Monark or Tuntari ergometers are found at most health clubs.

TABLE 4.4   The Montana Bicycle Test

	Time for the 5-mile bicycle test (min*)										
% Fat	12.0	12.4	12.8	13.2	13.6	14.0	14.4	14.8	15.2	15.6	16.0
4	65.2	64.1	63.2	61.0	60.7	59.6	58.5	57.3	56.2	55.1	54.0
6	63.9	62.8	61.7	60.6	59.4	58.3	57.2	56.0	54.9	53.8	52.7
8	62.6	61.5	60.4	59.3	58.1	57.0	55.9	54.7	53.6	52.5	51.4
10	61.4	60.2	59.1	58.0	56.8	55.7	54.6	53.4	52.3	51.2	50.1
12	60.1	58.9	57.2	56.7	55.5	54.4	53.3	52.1	51.0	49.9	48.8
14	58.8	57.6	56.5	55.4	54.2	53.1	52.0	50.8	49.7	48.6	47.5
16	57.5	56.3	55.2	54.1	52.9	51.8	50.7	49.5	48.4	47.3	46.2
18	56.2	55.0	53.9	52.8	51.6	50.5	49.4	48.2	47.1	46.0	44.9
20	54.9	53.7	52.6	51.5	50.3	49.2	48.1	47.0	45.8	44.7	43.6
22	53.6	52.4	51.3	50.2	49.0	47.9	46.8	45.7	44.5	43.4	42.3

*Minutes and decimal fractions: 12.4 = 12 min 24 s; 12.8 = 12:48, etc.

The workload per minute (power in kilogram meters per minute—kgm/min) is calculated using the following measures:

- Pedal revolutions per minute (rpm)—this test uses 60 rpm
- Force—the resistance to pedaling (from 1 to 7 kg)
- Distance—a combination of mechanical advantage and wheel circumference (totals 6 on the Monark bicycle)

Thus, the workload is

$$60 \text{ rpm} \times 1 \text{ kg} \times 6 = 360 \text{ kgm/min}$$
$$60 \text{ rpm} \times 2 \text{ kg} \times 6 = 720 \text{ kgm/min}$$
$$60 \text{ rpm} \times 3 \text{ kg} \times 6 = 1{,}080 \text{ kgm/min}$$

Adjust the seat height so your leg is *almost* extended when the pedal is in its lowest position (the ball of your foot is on the pedal). Warm up for 2 minutes with easy pedaling at a low resistance. Become familiar with the cadence—use a metronome set at 60 to pace your cadence, or watch a clock and push down with your right foot every second. After a brief rest begin the test.

Stage 1: Begin the first of three 2-minute stages with a setting of 1 kilogram. Maintain the cadence; in the last 30 seconds of the first stage, carefully take a 15-second HR reading at the throat (use gentle contact at the throat to avoid pressure on the carotid artery, which causes a reflex lowering of the heart rate). Multiply that number by 4, and record the HR and setting (1 kg). Stage 2: Increase the resistance (see the following guide to selection), and take the HR as in Stage 1. Record the HR and setting. Stage 3: Increase the resistance, and take your HR as in Stage 1. Record the HR and setting. Cool down with easy cycling.

Use this guide to select workloads:

Men:

Stage 1   Begin at 1 kg (360 kgm/min)

Stage 2   HR below 95, set at 3 kg
           HR 95 to 110, set at 2.5 kg
           HR over 110, set at 2 kg

Stage 3   Increase 1 kg for Stage 3

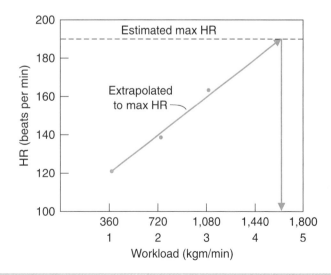

Figure 4.5   Heart-rate–workload relationship. In this example, the subject is 30 years old and thus has an estimated max HR of 190 (220 – 30).

TABLE 4.5   Predicting Aerobic Fitness From Max Workload on Bicycle Test

Weight (kg)	Workload (kgm/min)								
	600	750	900	1,050	1,200	1,350	1,500	1,650	1,800*
50	30**	36	42	48	54	60	66	72	
60	25	30	35	40	45	50	55	60	65
70		26	30	34	39	43	48	52	57
80		22	26	30	34	38	42	46	50
90			23	27	31	35	39	43	46
100				24	27	31	34	38	42

*Extrapolate for values above 1,800 kg/m.

**Values for aerobic fitness scores are in ml/kg · min.

Women:

Stage 1   Begin at 0.5 kg (180 kgm/min)*

Stage 2   HR below 110, set at 1.5 kg
          HR above 110, set at 1 kg

Stage 3   Increase 1 kg for Stage 3

*Active women can follow the men's protocol.

Plot the HR and corresponding workloads on graph paper (see figure 4.5). Then draw a line that comes closest to all three points and extrapolate the line to the estimated maximal heart rate (220 minus age). Now draw a vertical line down to the baseline to read the maximal working capacity (in kilogram meters per minute).

Example: For a 30-year-old individual

- 120 HR = 360 kgm/m
- 138 HR = 720 kgm/m
- 162 HR = 1,080 kgm/m

Then enter the correct value from table 4.5 to predict aerobic fitness ($\dot{V}O_2max$) in milliliters per kilogram of body weight per minute, or ml/kg · min.

Summary

Aerobic fitness, defined as the ability to take in, transport, and utilize oxygen, is a measure of exercise intensity. The anaerobic (lactate) threshold, which defines the upper limit of sustainable aerobic exercise, is a measure of exercise duration and an excellent predictor of performance. Aerobic fitness is influenced by heredity and training, as well as other factors such as age, gender, and body fat. Your ability to perform an endurance event will also be influenced by your current health, diet, hydration, level of rest, and acclimatization to heat and altitude. Few of us ever reach our potential for fitness and endurance, and there is no laboratory test to pinpoint this potential. World-class athletes train daily for years in order to be the best they can be. Most of us must be content to do the best we can within constraints of family, profession, community, and other responsibilities. The best time to start training is as you approach puberty. The second best time to start is now. Chapter 6 provides a prescription to get you started, and chapter 16 provides additional guidance to help you reach your potential.

CHAPTER 5

Benefits of
Aerobic Fitness

"Nothing in the
world can take the
place of persis-
tence."
Calvin Coolidge

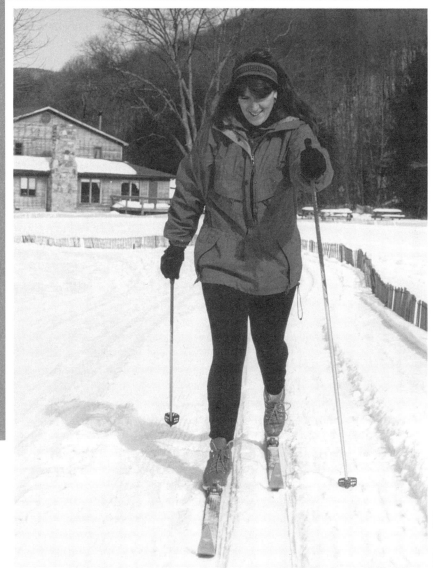

© W. Lynn Seldon

Years ago, as I began my career in exercise physiology, we used the term *cardio-vascular* to define fitness. Next came the term *cardiorespiratory*, and today we speak of *aerobic* fitness. The changes in terminology reflect insights derived from several decades of research, based on a clearer view of the effects of training. We used cardiovascular when the best documented effects were on the heart and circulation. Cardiorespiratory became popular when we began to understand the importance of oxygen intake as well as transport. And aerobic was adopted to indicate that oxygen intake, transport, and utilization were all improved with training. Since 1967, when research first documented the effects of endurance training on the muscles' ability to use oxygen, there has been a growing awareness that some of the major effects of training are on skeletal muscles themselves and their ability to carry out oxidative, or aerobic, energy production. To emphasize that point I like to say that skeletal muscle is the target of training.

Skeletal muscle is the target of training.

You've been told that fitness is good for the heart and the lungs, and that is true. But training requires the use of muscles, and major changes take place in the muscles used in training. Of course, important secondary adaptations take place in the respiratory, cardiovascular, and neuroendocrine systems and other tissues (fat, bone, ligaments, tendons). But it is impossible to improve the health or function of organs such as the heart without utilizing the muscles. All the beneficial changes begin with muscular activity. Train the muscles properly, and the secondary benefits follow: Fail to train the muscles, and the other changes are unlikely to occur.

THIS CHAPTER WILL HELP YOU

■ understand how systematic exercise (training) stimulates changes in:

- muscle fibers
- respiration and oxygen transport
- blood volume
- the heart and circulation
- the endocrine system
- fat metabolism and body composition
- bones, ligaments, tendons, and

■ understand the specificity of training and its importance for the design of effective programs.

The Training Effect

When you engage in an exercise such as walking or jogging at a level above your normal daily activity (load), you *overload* the muscles and other systems. Repeat the exercise regularly (e.g., every other day) and your body begins to adapt to the overload imposed by the exercise. We call the many adaptations *the training effect*. The exercise somehow signals muscle fibers to undergo changes that will permit more exercise in the future.

In this analysis of the effects of training, I try to rely on studies conducted on humans. A typical study involves pretesting of volunteer subjects for aerobic fitness, lactate threshold, and other measures; random assignment to experimental or control groups; weeks or even months of systematic and progressive training; and posttesting to measure the adaptations due to training. Studies have ranged from low to high intensity, using low- to high-fit subjects.

A variation of the training study involves *detraining* of already fit subjects. Researchers ask habitual exercisers to forgo training for a period while they observe the decline of important measures and performance. Although this approach has limits, it eliminates the need for prolonged training. We'll look at both types of studies as well as animal research to help you understand the training effect.

THE TRAINING STIMULUS

Figure 5.1 illustrates the basic structure of a muscle fiber. The functional unit of muscle, the sarcomere, consists of contractile proteins—the thin actin and thicker myosin. Contraction takes place when myosin heads attach to actin, swivel, and cause the protein filaments to slide past each other. Energy from stored fat and carbohydrate (glycogen) fuels contractions. Something associated with training (metabolic by-products, chemical messenger, hormone) tells the DNA in the muscle fiber's nuclei to produce specific messengers in the form of RNA. The messenger RNA (mRNA) travels to structures within the fiber called ribosomes to direct the synthesis of specific proteins, such as aerobic enzymes. Transfer RNA (tRNA) reads the mRNA blueprint and then goes forth to capture appropriate amino acids for use in the synthesis of the desired protein. Endurance training leads to an increase in the concentration of oxidative enzymes and to a rise in the size and number of mitochondria, the cellular power plants in which all oxidative metabolism takes place. These particular adaptations are specific to endurance training, and they take place only in the muscles used in training.

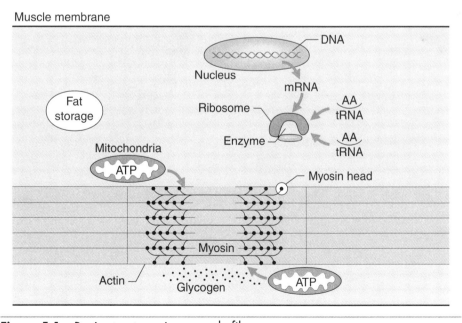

Figure 5.1   Basic structures in a muscle fiber.

Muscle: The Target of Training

Muscle is the primary target of training. The effects of aerobic training on muscle relate to the utilization of oxygen. Oxidative metabolism, the enzymatic breakdown of carbohydrate and fat to produce energy for muscular contractions, takes place in cellular powerhouses called mitochondria. Training has the following effects on muscle:

- It increases the concentration of aerobic enzymes (protein compounds that catalyze metabolic reactions) needed for the metabolic breakdown of carbohydrate and fat to produce energy in the form of ATP (adenosine triphosphate, the cellular energy supply).
- It increases the size and number (volume) of mitochondria, the cellular powerhouses that produce energy aerobically (with oxygen).
- It increases the muscle's ability to use fat as a source of energy.
- It increases the size of the fibers used in training: Long-slow training improves the oxidative capabilities of slow oxidative fibers, while high-intensity training enhances the capabilities of fast oxidative glycolytic fibers.
- It increases the myoglobin (a compound that carries oxygen from the cell membrane to the mitochondria) content in muscle fibers.
- It increases the number of capillaries serving muscle fibers.

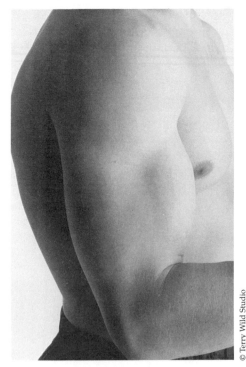

© Terry Wild Studio

Skeletal muscle is the target of training.

Today we know that the increase in mitochondrial mass is due to branching of existing mitochondria, and that the increase provides greater capacity for oxidation of energy sources, especially our abundant supply of fat (we store 50 times more fat energy than carbohydrate, and training makes that supply more available).

CELLULAR EFFECTS

Prior to 1967, research had failed to demonstrate the effects of training on muscle fibers. Dr. John Holloszy reasoned that previous studies failed to overload aerobic pathways, so he subjected rats to a strenuous treadmill program. Trained rats eventually were able to continue exercise for 4 to 8 hours, while untrained animals were exhausted within 30 minutes. Following the 12-week program, the animals were sacrificed to allow study of the muscle tissue. Holloszy found a 50 to 60% increase in mitochondrial protein, a twofold rise in the oxygen consumption of trained muscle, and enhanced ability to oxidize carbohydrate and fat (1967). These findings have been replicated in other labs and confirmed in humans, using a muscle biopsy technique.

Training Supply and Support Systems

The respiratory, circulatory, nervous, endocrine, and other systems supply and support the activities of muscles. How are they affected by aerobic training? Aerobic training

- increases the efficiency of respiration,
- improves blood volume, distribution, and delivery to muscles,
- improves cardiovascular efficiency (increases stroke volume and cardiac output while decreasing the resting and exercise heart rates), and
- fine-tunes nervous and hormonal control mechanisms.

Respiration and Oxygen Transport

Aerobic training doesn't alter the size of the lungs, but it does improve the condition and efficiency of breathing muscles, allowing greater use of the inherited capacity. Training reduces the residual volume, the portion of lung capacity that goes unused. Residual volume increases with age and inactivity, and this decline eventually reduces exercise capacity. However, the human respiratory system is overbuilt for its task, so the gradual decline isn't noticed at first. Aerobic training slows the decline, ensuring adequate respiration throughout life.

Training also enhances the efficiency of respiration, so fewer breaths are needed to move the same volume of air. Ventilation is the amount of air moving into or out of the lungs. It is the product of respiratory rate (or frequency) times the volume of air in each breath (tidal volume).

Ventilation (expired air in liters per minute) = Frequency × Tidal Volume

Consider values for trained and untrained subjects:

| Untrained | 60 L/min = 30 breaths × 2 L/breath |
| Trained | 60 L/min = 20 breaths × 3 L/breath |

The trained individual moves more air with fewer breaths and is also able to move more air at maximal ventilation (150 liters per minute or more, versus 120 or less for the untrained). Slower, deeper breaths are more efficient because they allow more of each breath to reach the portion of the lungs where oxygen and carbon dioxide are exchanged (alveolar sacs). And training improves diffusion of oxygen from the lungs into the blood. Diffusion depends on good ventilation and adequate blood flow in the capillaries.

Blood Volume

Oxygen is transported via red cells and hemoglobin. We have long known that aerobic fitness is closely associated with total hemoglobin, and that blood volume and hemoglobin improve with training. More recently we have learned that the loss of blood volume that occurs with detraining is closely correlated with the reversal of important cardiovascular adjustments (lower heart rate and increased stroke volume) (Coyle, Hemmert, & Coggan, 1986). Thus, it is likely that training-induced changes in blood volume are responsible, at least in part, for so-called cardiovascular changes, and that these changes may be secondary to changes in blood volume.

Training-induced changes in blood volume are responsible, at least in part, for so-called cardiovascular changes.

Heart and Circulation

For years we knew that endurance training led to a reduction in the heart rate at rest and at submaximal workloads, and to an increase in the stroke volume, the amount of blood pumped with each beat of the heart. That is why we used the term cardiovascular to describe training effects. Training leads to an increase in the size of the left ventricle, but only during the filling stage, or diastole (increased left ventricular end diastolic volume, LVEDV). This change takes place with little thickening of the heart muscle or alteration in its oxidative enzyme capacity. The efficient trained heart pumps more blood each time it beats, at rest or during exercise, and therefore can beat at a slower rate. The heart is a pump that ejects the blood that enters its chambers; put more blood into the chamber, and more comes out.

It appears that training has little effect on the thickness of heart muscle, and only a minor effect on aerobic enzymes and mitochondria. The trained heart is better able to use fat as a source of energy, perhaps because training enlarges the diameter of coronary arteries and improves the oxygen supply to heart muscle.

Another important contributor to stroke volume and cardiac output is a redistribution of blood from digestive and other organs to working muscles. Blood

STROKE VOLUME

Stroke volume depends on blood volume and the size of the left ventricle. But the heart is enclosed in a fibrous sac (pericardium) that may limit its size. When the sac was removed from dog hearts, the animals were able to train and increase their stroke volume and cardiac output (Cardiac Output = Heart Rate × Stroke Volume) a whopping 20% (Stray-Gunderson, 1986). You can't remove your pericardium because the operation risks a life-threatening infection of the heart, but you can increase blood volume with training, and that seems to lead to increases in stroke volume and cardiac output and decreases in resting and exercise heart rates.

vessels in active muscles dilate, while those in other organs constrict, directing blood where it is needed during exercise and helping to maintain a high stroke volume. Training actually improves this ability to redistribute blood.

Training also seems to enhance delivery of blood to muscle fibers via the capillaries. Trained muscles have a higher capillary-fiber ratio (Blomqvist & Saltin, 1983). Because trained muscle fibers increase in diameter, the rise in capillaries may be necessary to maintain a short diffusion distance from the capillary to the interior of the fiber.

Nervous System

Training has several subtle but important effects on the nervous system, including improved economy and efficiency of movement, and improved efficiency of the cardiovascular system.

The economical athlete uses less energy to perform at a given speed. Hours of practice lead to a relaxed and efficient use of force to achieve results. This economy is especially evident in complex tasks such as swimming and cross-country skiing, but it can also be found in running or cycling.

The nervous system, which controls the heart rate and constriction and relaxation of blood vessels, participates in another adjustment that may help solve the question of why heart rate and stroke volume change with training. In 1977 Saltin published a simple experiment in which subjects trained one leg on a bicycle ergometer, with the other leg serving as a control. Pre- and posttest measures of oxygen intake and oxidative enzyme activity demonstrated that changes occurred only in the trained leg—i.e., that the training was specific. Furthermore, the heart rate response to exercise was significantly lower for the trained leg, but not for the control.

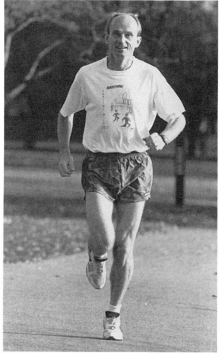

The efficient athlete uses less energy to perform at a given speed.

Training's influence on the skeletal muscle may alter cardiovascular responses.

Saltin reasoned that the improvements in the trained muscle were responsible for the lower heart rate response. Mitchell and associates (Mitchell, Reardon, McCloskey, & Wildnethal, 1977) demonstrated that small nerve endings located in muscle fibers are able to modify the heart rate response to exercise via connections to the cardiac control center in the brain. Thus, it appears that training's influence on the muscle may alter cardiovascular response—that the reduced heart rate can be traced to the improved metabolic condition in trained muscle. When the heart beats more slowly, it has more time to fill, allowing an improved stroke volume.

This interpretation suggests that some of the well-documented effects of training are actually by-products of changes in the skeletal muscles. When we consider these changes with the increase in blood volume and redistribution of blood, which combine to put more blood into the heart, we understand why training leads to a decrease in the exercise heart rate and an increase in the stroke volume. It therefore appears that some so-called cardiovascular effects of training are actually due to changes in the muscles being trained, that these changes are specific, and that training doesn't easily transfer from one leg (or one activity) to another.

Endocrine System

The endocrine system includes the many glands whose secretions—hormones—are distributed via the circulation. Effects of training include increased sensitivity to certain hormones, adjustments in hormonal response, and important metabolic adjustments.

Many hormones are involved in the regulation of energy; epinephrine, cortisol, thyroxine, glucagon, and growth hormone raise blood sugar, whereas insulin is the only hormone capable of lowering blood sugar. Insulin is secreted from the pancreas when blood sugar levels are elevated, such as after a meal, helping tissues take up the sugar. The others are secreted when levels are low, as in vigorous exercise. Epinephrine and growth hormone also are involved in the mobilization of fat from adipose tissue, while insulin helps deposit fat. Endurance training lowers the need for insulin because the muscle can take up sugar during exercise, even in the absence of insulin as in diabetes. Training seems to increase receptor sensitivity to insulin, leading to a more efficient use of hormones and energy.

Fat Metabolism

Years ago, animal and then human studies demonstrated improved fat utilization following training. The trained muscle is better suited to use fat as a source of energy, thereby conserving limited supplies of carbohydrate (glycogen) in muscle and liver. A key finding was the enhancement of beta oxidation, an enzymatic process that systematically chops two carbon fragments from fat (free fatty acids). Along with this improvement in fat metabolism is a near doubling of stored fat (triglyceride) in trained muscle fibers. On top of all this, training leads to improvements in fat mobilization.

Fat Mobilization

Epinephrine is available from two sites, the adrenal gland and the nerve endings of the sympathetic nervous system. Like most other hormones, epinephrine acts on receptors located in the surface membrane of its target organ, in this case adipose tissue. The hormone initiates a series of steps leading to the breakdown of triglyceride fat and the release of free fatty acids (FFA) into the circulation (see figure 5.2). The FFA then travel to working muscles or the heart, where they are used to fuel contractions. During very vigorous exercise, lactic acid produced in the muscles seems to block or inhibit the action of epinephrine, which reduces the FFA available for energy. Under these conditions the muscle is forced to use limited supplies of muscle glycogen for energy.

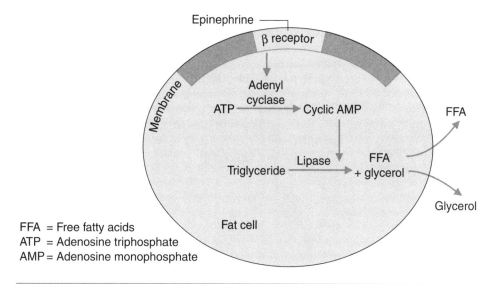

Figure 5.2 Mobilization of free fatty acids from adipose tissue. Lactic acid inhibits the influence of epinephrine on the fat cell and blocks the mobilization of fat.
Adapted from Sharkey 1975.

Training improves the oxidative ability of muscles, leading to less lactic acid production and greater fat mobilization and fat metabolism (Holloszy et al., 1986). And it appears that trained individuals are able to mobilize fat even when lactic acid is elevated (Vega deJesus & Siconolfi, 1988). The result is improved access to a major source of energy, some 50 times more abundant than carbohydrate! Further, the enhanced utilization of fat has major health benefits as well as those related to fitness and performance. I'll say it again: The utilization of fat may be one of the most important outcomes of the active life and fitness.

Other Effects of Training

Training has effects on other tissues, including adipose tissue (fat), bone, ligaments, and tendons. While some are mere adjustments that counteract the stresses of training and make more activity possible, others have health and cosmetic effects.

Body Composition

Body composition refers to the relative amounts of fat and lean weight. Although the lean body weight (body weight minus fat weight) is relatively unchanged with training, substantial loss of fat tissue is to be expected. One of the best documented effects of training is the loss of unwanted fat and a change in body composition, revealing a trim, pleasing figure. Researchers use underwater weighing or skinfold calipers to measure percent body fat.

If you have 25% fat and weigh 120 pounds, you have 30 pounds of fat and 90 pounds of lean body weight (LBW). If you jog 3 miles a day, 5 days a week, you will burn about 1,650 calories per week (3 miles × 110 calories per mile × 5 days = 1,650 calories). In just 2 weeks you'll burn 3,300 extra calories, almost a pound of fat (3,500 calories = 1 pound of fat), or almost 2 pounds a month. In the process you will lower your percent body fat and your body weight, with only a slight increase in LBW.

Bones, Ligaments, and Tendons

Bones, ligaments, and tendons respond to the stresses placed upon them. Every change in function is followed by adaptations. For bones, an increase in activity leads to a denser, stronger structure designed to counteract the new level of stress. Inactivity leads to reabsorption of calcium and loss of supportive structures. Increasing age and inactivity create a dangerous combination for females. Bone demineralization, or osteoporosis, begins early in adult life (30 to 40 years) and becomes more serious after menopause. Lack of activity hastens the weakening of bones. And while moderate activity causes bone tissue to become stronger and more dense, excessive training associated with weight loss or menstrual irregularities (e.g., amenorrhea, or absence of menstruation) can cause early and possibly irreversible osteoporosis. Calcium intake may be helpful, but it won't do much good without the stress of moderate weight-bearing exercise.

Moderate activity also strengthens ligaments, tendons, and other connective tissue, such as the covering of muscle. By gradually increasing the workload, you can make tissues tough enough to withstand the normal demands of activity and to resist damage during slips, trips, and falls.

Specificity of Training

An activity such as jogging recruits muscle fibers uniquely suited to the task. Slow fibers are recruited for slow jogging. The metabolic pathways and energy sources are also suited to the task. Daily jogging recruits the same fibers and pathways over and over, leading to the adaptive response known as the training effect.

The outcomes of training are directly related to the activity employed as a training stimulus. We've shown that training has effects on muscle fibers as well as on the supply and support systems, such as the cardiovascular system. In general, the effects of training on muscle fibers are very specific, meaning that they are unlikely to transfer to activities unlike the training. So, the benefits of run training will not transfer to swimming or cycling. On the other hand, because the effects on the respiratory or cardiovascular systems are more general, they may transfer to other activities (Sharkey & Greatzer, 1993).

Training leads to changes in aerobic enzyme systems in muscle fibers, so it is easy to see why those changes are specific. In the early stages of training, the muscles' inability to use oxygen limits performance. Later on, as the fibers adapt and can utilize more oxygen, the burden shifts to the cardiovascular system, including the heart, blood, and blood vessels. Then the cardiovascular system becomes the factor that limits performance (Boileau, McKeown, & Riner, 1984).

Training gains don't automatically transfer from one activity to another. Training effects can be classified as *peripheral* (in the muscle) and *central* (heart, blood, lungs, hormones). Central effects may transfer to other activities, but peripheral changes are unlikely to transfer. Endurance running, for example, leads to improvements in the oxidative enzymes in active muscle fibers, changes unlikely to help a swimmer or a cyclist who uses different muscle fibers. However, central changes in blood volume and redistribution may aid performance in another endurance activity. But remember, some part of the heart rate (and stroke volume) change is due to conditions within the muscle fibers, conditions that are relayed to the cardiac control center. These changes are specific and will not transfer from one activity to another.

The responses to exercise and the adaptations to training are specific. Although some effects of training may be generalized to similar types of activity, all peripheral and some central effects are specific. It makes sense to concentrate training on the movements, muscle fibers, metabolic pathways, and supply and support systems that will be used in the particular activity and sport. This does not imply that athletes should ignore other exercises and muscle groups, of course. Additional training is necessary to avoid injury, to achieve muscle balance, and to provide backup for prime movers when they become fatigued. In spite of the widespread affection for the term cardiovascular fitness, the evidence suggests that the concept is overrated. Muscle is the target of training.

Finally, if exercise and training are specific, it stands to reason that testing must be specific if it is to reflect the adaptations to training. This means you should not use a bicycle to test a runner, or vice versa. Training is so specific that hill runners are best tested on an uphill treadmill test. How do we test the effects of training on dancers? We don't. When studies compare runners and dancers on a treadmill test, the runners exhibit higher $\dot{V}O_2$max scores. If that is true, why do runners poop out in aerobic dance? Because the effects of training are specific. At present there is no widely accepted way to accurately assess the effects of aerobic, ballet, modern, or other dance forms.

> Many of the effects of training are specific and will not transfer from one activity to another.

Summary

In this section we've looked at the effects of aerobic training. I've shown that muscles undergo specific adaptations when they are recruited in exercise that lasts long enough to overload their oxidative pathways. As aerobic pathways are improved, muscles use oxygen more efficiently, raising the lactate threshold and enhancing the metabolism of fat. The metabolic efficiency is relayed to the cardiac control center in the brain, which results in a slower heart rate, more filling time, and a greater stroke volume. Increased blood volume and improved distribution provide ample blood for the heart to pump. Since so many adaptations take place in the muscle, training should be specific to its intended use.

Because training is so specific, it is important that you select an appropriate activity for aerobic training. Fat metabolism and cardiovascular benefits are enhanced in regular moderate activity that employs major muscle groups for extended periods, but not when different muscles are engaged in a series of short lifting bouts (i.e., circuit weight training). Bone mineral content is maintained when bones are subjected to regular moderate stress, as in weight-bearing and resistance exercises.

Choose an activity you enjoy, or one you want to improve. Long-slow training improves the ability of slow oxidative fibers to use fat as an energy source. Faster and necessarily shorter training recruits fast twitch (fast oxidative glycolytic) fibers. High-intensity training may also have more effect on the cardiovascular system. Your approach to training depends on your goals. Train more slowly for distance, faster for speed. You can combine both by going easy and then increasing pace near the end of the workout. German distance coach Ernst Van Aaken advocated a 20:1 slow:fast ratio for his elite athletes (1976). For example, on a 5-mile run, pick up the pace for the last quarter mile. This short distance provides some speed training at a time when you are well warmed. I like this approach because it limits the discomfort associated with elevated lactic acid. Training doesn't have to hurt to be good.

CHAPTER 6

Improving Your Aerobic Fitness

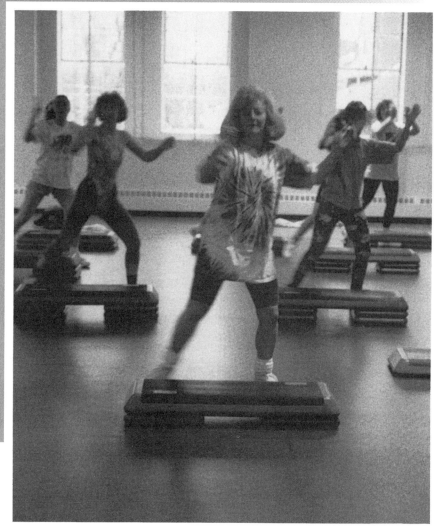

"Fitness can neither be bought nor bestowed. Like honor it must be earned."

© Terry Wild Studio

Years ago, before exercise physiologists knew how to prescribe exercise, we were faced with a number of unproven training systems that were based on the ideas and experience of well-known physicians, coaches, and educators. Then researchers began to identify the factors associated with improvements in fitness. Today's exercise prescriptions are based on the results of hundreds of studies. The dose of exercise that safely promotes the training effect is usually represented in terms of the intensity, duration, and frequency. Research and clinical experience are adding to a carefully developed methodology for the safe and effective prescription of exercise.

Aerobic fitness is earned minute by minute, day by day, as you engage in appropriate training exercises. As with any treatment or drug, the exercises must be prescribed and taken with care if the benefits are to be realized and if potentially harmful side-effects are to be avoided.

THIS CHAPTER WILL HELP YOU

- utilize your heart rate or perceived exertion to determine exercise intensity;
- determine exercise duration using calories, minutes, or miles;
- develop a personalized aerobic fitness prescription based on your age, level of fitness, and training goals; and
- understand how to achieve, maintain, and regain aerobic fitness.

The Fitness Prescription

Throughout recorded history people have sought the health benefits believed to be associated with exercise, with prescriptions dating back to centuries-old Chinese and Roman documents. In the late 1800s Dr. Dudley Sargent, physician and director of the Harvard College Gymnasium, tested students and prescribed exercises to rectify weaknesses. Subsequently, prescriptions improved only slightly until the 1950s when researchers established the link between lack of activity and heart disease. Since then, we have agreed on a definition of aerobic fitness, identified the factors that contribute to its improvement, and become more aware of the benefits and limitations of exercise as a modality for the prevention and rehabilitation of disease. We now know how hard (intensity), how long (duration), and how often (frequency) one must exercise to achieve the aerobic training effect. We'll discuss the prescription, then learn how to proceed.

Intensity

Intensity is the most important factor in the development of the maximal oxygen intake ($\dot{V}O_2max$); it reflects the energy requirements of the exercise, the amount of oxygen consumed, and the calories of energy expended. While intensity is usually defined with the training heart rate, other measures also can be used (see table 6.1).

TABLE 6.1   Measures of Exercise Intensity[a]

Intensity	Heart rate (bpm)	$\dot{V}O_2$ (L/min)	Cal/min[b]	METs[c]
Light	100	1.0	5	4.0
Moderate	135	2.0	10	8.1
Heavy	170	3.0	15	12.2

The number of calories burned per minute depends on body weight; therefore, a heavier individual burns more during a given exercise. Each MET equals 3.5 ml/kg · min, so the MET is adjusted for weight. The aerobics point system popularized by Dr. Kenneth Cooper is a close relative of the MET. Each aerobic point is worth 7 ml/kg · min), or 2 METs.

[a]For 70-kg individual, fitness score = 45.

[b]1 L of oxygen is equivalent to 5 cal/min.

[c]The MET, or metabolic equivalent, is a multiple of the resting metabolic rate. The resting rate is 1.2 cal/min (1 MET), so 12 cal/min = 10 METs.

Aerobic Threshold

Early training studies agreed that training had to exceed a certain minimum level or threshold if significant changes in fitness were to occur (see figure 6.1). In one study we trained young men at heart rates of 120, 150, and 180 beats per minute (bpm). The higher-intensity groups improved similarly, but the low-intensity subjects did not (Sharkey & Holleman, 1967). Then we learned that training intensity depended on one's level of fitness,

TRAINING HEART RATE

Early training studies focused on the metabolic demands of training. The heart rate was then used as a simple, inexpensive way to translate training information to the lay public. The heart rate was merely a by-product of the metabolic activity. Unfortunately, over the years the public and some fitness professionals have lost sight of the point. Today many consider the training heart rate, and not the sustained metabolism of a large muscle mass (e.g., legs), to be the goal of training. They believe that raising the heart rate, no matter how it is done, will result in improvements in fitness. For example, the elevation of the heart rate during weight training has led some to believe that circuit weight training could be used to improve aerobic fitness. They ignore the fact that each muscle group is engaged for only 20 to 30 seconds, far too short a time to prompt changes in the oxidative pathways of muscles. The training heart rate is a convenient external indicator of oxygen consumption, a simple way to gauge exercise intensity, but it isn't an end in itself.

with low-fit subjects making progress at lower intensities, while high-fit subjects had a higher training threshold (Sharkey, 1970). This training threshold is called the aerobic threshold.

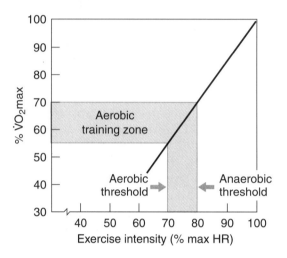

Figure 6.1   Aerobic exercise: The training zone. Aerobic fitness improves when you exercise within the aerobic training zone.

Anaerobic Threshold

Studies also defined an upper limit to training intensity. They showed that training above that level didn't yield additional benefits. In recent years we recognized that the upper limit of the training zone coincides with the anaerobic or lactate threshold. When the activity exceeds the muscle's ability to produce energy aerobically and blood lactate accumulates, the exercise's contribution to aerobic fitness diminishes. Stated another way, anaerobic exercise does not contribute to the development of aerobic fitness.

Thus, there is an aerobic training zone that ranges from the aerobic threshold to the anaerobic (lactate) threshold, the point of diminishing returns. Training at the low end of the zone leads to improvements in fat metabolism and changes in slow oxidative muscle fibers. Training at the high end of the zone recruits and benefits fast oxidative glycolytic muscle fibers, and leads to central circulatory (cardiovascular) benefits. Also, the high-intensity interval training used by athletes has been shown to raise the anaerobic (lactate) threshold. This improvement sometimes takes place without an increase in the already high $\dot{V}O_2max$, especially in athletes who have undergone long-term training.

The Training Zone

Both thresholds are related to your level of activity and fitness. Inactive individuals have a low aerobic threshold. If normal daily activity seldom exceeds a slow walk, a brisk walk will exceed the threshold and elicit a training effect. Regular participation in high-intensity activity raises the anaerobic threshold, so highly active individuals have an elevated threshold and a higher training zone.

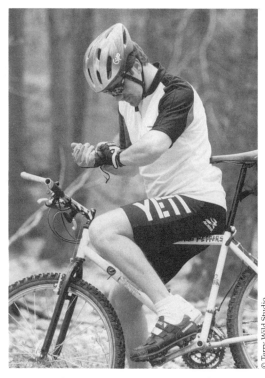

© Terry Wild Studio

Use your heart rate as a measure of exercise intensity.

The training zone is based on a percentage of your estimated maximal heart rate (max HR). Because the max HR declines with age, we use both fitness level (see chapter 4) and age to determine the training zone (see figure 6.1).

Fitness (ml/kg · min)	Training Zone (% max HR)
Low (under 35)	60-75%
Medium (35 to 45)	70-85
High (over 45)	75-90

If your max HR hasn't been measured, estimate it with the formula: max HR = 220 – age. Since there is such variability in the estimation of the max HR (see chapter 3) you should view the estimated HR with caution. If your training zone feels too high, back off to a more comfortable level. Your max HR may be lower than expected. If it feels far too easy, inch it up a bit. Because of this variability I like to use the rating of perceived exertion (RPE) along with the training zone. The RPE is a simple 20-point rating scale designed to provide an estimate of exercise intensity (see table 6.2). It has been shown to be a physiologically valid tool for the prescription of exercise (Steed, Gaesser, & Weltman, 1994). Training should feel "somewhat hard" in the early stages. The "talk test" is another way to determine if you are within your zone: You should be able to carry on a conversation while you train. Exercise doesn't have to hurt to be good.

In time you won't need to check your heart rate because you'll know how it feels to be in the zone.

In time you won't need to check your heart rate because you'll know how it feels to be in the zone. We begin with a prescription, but as you learn more about exercise and your body, improve your fitness, and decide on your goals, you will outgrow heart rates and training zones.

TABLE 6.2 Borg's RPE Scale

6	No exertion at all
7	Extremely light
8	
9	Very light
10	
11	Light
12	
13	Somewhat hard
14	
15	Hard
16	
17	Very hard
18	
19	Extremely hard
20	Maximal exertion

Reprinted from Borg 1985.

HEART RATE RANGE

A given percentage of your max HR (e.g., 70%) is not equivalent to the same percentage of your maximal oxygen intake ($\dot{V}O_2$max). To resolve this, the heart rate range formula calculates a heart rate that is equal to the same percent of the $\dot{V}O_2$max. So, for 70% of the $\dot{V}O_2$max:

$$HR = [70\% \times (max\ HR - resting\ HR)] + resting\ HR$$
$$= [70\% \times (170 - 70)] + 70$$
$$= 140\ bpm$$

In this example, 70% of the max HR (170) equals 119 bpm, which is approximately equal to 55% of the $\dot{V}O_2$max. The heart rate range is sometimes used to adjust for measured differences in the resting and maximal heart rates, and to avoid errors in the estimation of the training heart rate.

Duration

Exercise duration and intensity go hand in hand: An increase in one requires a decrease in the other. Duration can be prescribed in terms of time, distance, or calories. I'll mention all three to show how they relate, but I prefer to use the calorie because it is so educational. Food labels tell you how many calories you gain when you eat and drink (e.g., double burger = 550 calories, one beer = 150 calories). You should also know how much exercise it takes to balance your energy intake (e.g., at about 100 calories per mile, you'd have to jog almost 7 miles to burn the calories consumed with the beer and burger).

THE CALORIE

The calorie (technically a kilocalorie) is a unit of energy defined as the amount of heat required to raise the temperature of 1 kilogram of water 1 degree Celsius. We store calories when we eat, and burn them when we exercise. Caloric expenditure during exercise is influenced by body weight. For instance, a 180-pound person burns more calories running at a certain pace than one who weighs 150 pounds (136 calories per mile versus 113). In this book caloric expenditures are based on a weight of 150 pounds: Add or subtract 10% for each 15 pounds over or under 150. For example, add 20% to 113 calories to determine the cost for the 180-pound example ($113 \times .20 = 22.6 + 113 = 135.6$ calories).

An early training study showed that low-fit individuals can improve their fitness with as little as 100 calories of exercise per session (10 minutes at 10 calories per minute) (Bouchard, Holimann, Venrath, Herkenrath, & Schlussel, 1966). Low-fit subjects do not respond to long-duration or high-intensity training, but in time, as fitness improves, they should extend duration to 200 calories or more. Fitness pioneer Dr. Tom Cureton found that higher expenditures were needed to bring about significant changes in cholesterol levels (Cureton, 1969). And more recent studies have shown that longer workouts (more than 35 minutes) produce greater fitness benefits (Wenger & Bell, 1986), perhaps because the proportion of fat metabolized continues to rise for the first 30 minutes of exercise.

A study of 17,000 Harvard graduates noted earlier in this book provides another way to assess the importance of exercise duration. Paffenbarger, Hyde, and Wing (1986) found a significant reduction in the risk of heart disease for graduates who averaged more than 2,000 calories of exercise per week. That translates into about 300 calories daily (400 calories per day in 5 days, etc.). Longer-duration training leads to improved fat metabolism, which may be the major health benefit of exercise. Increase duration to gain significant fitness, weight control, and fat metabolism benefits, and to lower blood lipids. However, there is no conclusive health evidence to recommend workouts that exceed 60 minutes (or 600 calories). Endurance athletes participate in longer workouts to improve stamina and performance, not for enhanced health benefits. In fact, a recent study suggests that falling mortality rates start to go back up at very high levels of energy expenditure (more than 3,500 calories per week—or 700 per day) (Lee, Hsieh, & Paffenbarger, 1995).

Fitness (ml/kg · min)	Duration (calories per session)
Low (under 35)	100-200
Medium (35 to 45)	200-400
High (over 45)	Over 400

Overload is the key to improvements in training. As fitness improves we need to increase intensity and duration if we hope to continue improvements in $\dot{V}O_2$max and the lactate threshold. Now let's see how training frequency must be adjusted as training progresses.

Frequency

For low-fit individuals, three sessions per week on alternating days are sufficient to improve fitness (Jackson, Sharkey, & Johnston, 1968). But as training progresses in intensity and duration, it must also increase in frequency if improvements are to continue (Pollock, 1973). An extensive review of training studies found that changes in fitness are directly related to frequency of training, when it is considered independent of the effects of intensity, duration, program length, and initial level of fitness (Wenger & Bell, 1986). Six days per week is more than twice as effective as three. So, for fitness or weight control, consider more frequent exercise.' Athletes engage in long sessions or train two or more times, two to three times per week. But they also observe the hard-easy principle, following hard or long sessions with easy or short ones. Failure to allow adequate time for recovery from training nullifies its effects; it can lead to overuse injuries or illness via suppression of the immune system.

The body needs time to respond to the training stimulus, and some people find that they need more than 24 hours. As I approach my 60th year I find that I take more time to recover from extremely long or strenuous activity. Experiment with schedules to find one that suits you. Work out daily if you prefer, or try an alternate-day plan and increase duration. Whatever you do, be sure to schedule at least 1 day of relative rest or diversion each week. A colleague and training partner once wrote, "We should approach running not as if we are trying to smash our way through some enormous wall, but as a gentle pastime by which we can coax a slow continuous stream of adaptations out of the body" (Frederick, 1973, p. 20).

Fitness (ml/kg · min)	Frequency (days per week)
Low (under 35)	3-4
Medium (35 to 45)	5-6
High (over 45)	6+

Now let's put all the factors together in your personalized prescription for fitness.

Your Prescription

A comprehensive review of training studies showed that maximal gains in aerobic fitness ($\dot{V}O_2max$) were achieved with high intensity (90% of $\dot{V}O_2max$ or 95% of max HR), a duration of 35 to 45 minutes, and a frequency of four times per week (Wenger & Bell, 1986). Lesser intensities produced very respectable results with much less risk of injury. But keep in mind that all these conclusions were based on changes in the $\dot{V}O_2max$, acknowledged as a measure of intensity (Sharkey, 1991). While $\dot{V}O_2max$ is important, there are even better measures of endurance, such as the lactate or ventilatory thresholds. And improved fitness and performance aren't the only goals; health benefits, weight control, and improved appearance may be achieved with lower levels of intensity, duration, and frequency. Use the prescription in table 6.3 as a starting point, but don't be a slave to training. Adapt the program to meet your personal style and goals.

TABLE 6.3   The Aerobic Fitness Prescription

Fitness (ml/kg · min)	Intensity (% max HR)	Duration (calories)	Frequency (days/wk)
Low (under 35)	60-75	100-200	3-4
Medium (35-45)	70-85	200-400	5-6
High (over 45)	75-90	400+	6+

Figure 6.2 illustrates how the prescription is carried out on a given day. Begin every session with a warm-up to reduce any soreness and the risk of injury. Start with a gradual increase in exercise activity, and then stretch. Pay attention to stretching for the lower back, hamstrings, calf muscles, and any sore muscles. Muscle soreness shows up at the start of a program but diminishes soon thereafter. It won't return unless you lay off for weeks or do a new activity. Follow the prescription during the aerobic portion of the session, then be sure to cool down before you hit the shower. Easy jogging, walking, and stretching help lower the body temperature, reduce metabolic by-products such as lactic acid, and dissipate the hormone norepinephrine, which could cause irregular rhythms.

To vary the program, take different routes, work at the upper edge of the zone for shorter periods (i.e., hard-short) and at the lower edge for longer periods (easy-long), or use another activity for variety (cross-training). As training progresses, the same pace will feel easier and more enjoyable. As fitness improves, the prescription changes, calling for more intensity, duration, and frequency. By then you will have an idea of what you want to achieve from fitness, and you can decide what works best and feels best to you.

As training progresses, the same pace will feel easier and more enjoyable.

Use the nomogram developed by my friend Dr. Jeffrey Broida (figure 6.3) to determine the details of your prescription and to become familiar with how intensity, duration, and frequency interact. It will help you see how you can vary your program and meet your daily and weekly caloric expenditure goals.

To use it you choose a heart rate within your training zone and draw a horizontal line connecting with your fitness level. Then drop to the lower graph and intersect the line that describes your daily caloric expenditure goal. Finally, draw a horizontal line to the left until it indicates exercise duration in

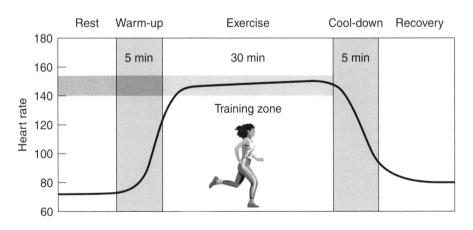

Figure 6.2   The aerobic training session.
Adapted from Sharkey 1977.

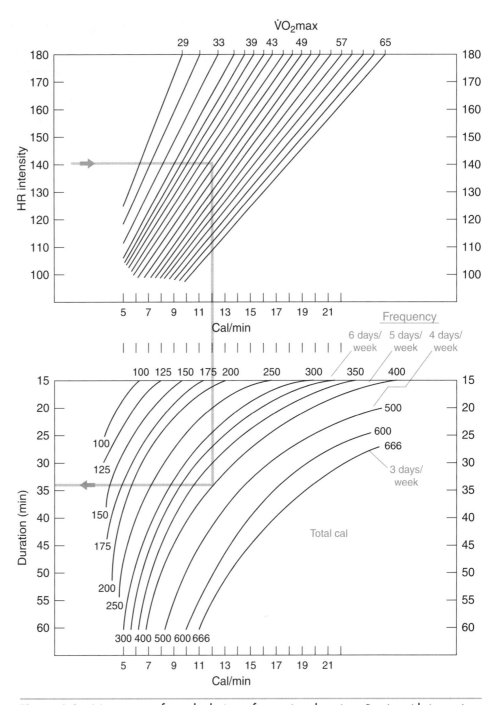

Figure 6.3 Nomogram for calculation of exercise duration. Begin with intensity, move across to fitness level ($\dot{V}O_2$max), then move down to total calories and across to duration (min).

minutes. In our example in the figure, a 40-year-old with a fitness score of 45 and a training HR of 140 needs 400 calories, which can be achieved with less than 35 minutes of exercise at that intensity. The nomogram also shows several ways to get at least 2,000 calories per week, using more days and shorter sessions or fewer days and longer sessions. The subject in the example chose the 2,000-calorie-per-week level, since it has been associated with a lower risk of heart disease.

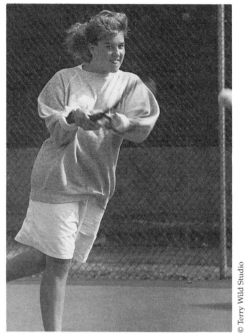

© Terry Wild Studio

The best exercise is the one you enjoy and continue to do regularly.

Mode of Exercise

Health benefits occur regardless of the exercise you select. Dr. Michael Pollock and associates (Pollock, Dimmick, Miller, Kendrick, & Linnerud, 1975) compared the fitness and weight control benefits of walking, running, and cycling. Sedentary middle-aged men trained for 20 weeks, all using the same prescription. Tests administered at the conclusion of the study indicated that all three groups improved similarly in fitness, body weight, and fat. No one mode of exercise is superior to others when the prescription is the same. The best exercise is the one you enjoy and will continue to do regularly (see table 6.4 for sample activities). However, as discussed earlier, improvements in fitness are specific to the manner of training. So, if you want to improve your running, that is the way to train. Swimming and cycling do surprisingly little to improve running, and vice versa, because many of the really important changes take place only in the muscles used in training.

TABLE 6.4   Sample Aerobic Activities

Fitness category (ml/[kg · min])*	Running		Jogging		Cycling		Walking	
	Distance (mi)	Time (min)	Distance (mi)	Time (min)	Distance (mi)	Time (min)	Distance (mi)	Time (min)
Low (under 35)	0.8-1.7	7-14	0.8-1.7	10-20	1.9-3.9	12-24	1.0-2.1	18-36
Medium (35-45)	1.7-3.4	14-27	1.7-3.4	20-40	3.9-7.8	24-47	2.1-4.2	36-72
High (over 45)	3.4+	27+	3.4+	40+	7.8+	47+	4.2+	72+

*Distance and time remain the same regardless of age.

Adapted from Sharkey 1977.

Achievement

The key to the achievement of fitness goals is to make haste slowly. Rush the process, and the result may be painful, injurious, or worse. It takes time to coax that slow, continuous stream of adaptations from the body. You'll experience improved energy and vigor within weeks, improved self-concept and body image will follow, and performance will show change within a month. But don't view these exciting changes as a license for imprudent behavior. Athletes train for years to achieve dramatic results. Why, then, do older, less adaptable adults attempt to undo years of inactivity or expect to remove a decade's accumulation of fat in a few short weeks?

What progress can you expect when you follow your prescription? Although the ultimate achievement will depend on your genetic endowment, with time and effort you can reach your potential. The rate of improvement is influenced by age and initial level of fitness. Training during or just after puberty, a period of intense growth and development, leads to the greatest adaptations in your ability to take in, transport, and utilize oxygen. Trainability declines slowly thereafter, but even a 70-year-old can expect a 10% improvement in fitness ($\dot{V}O_2$max). Adolescent training may prompt a 30 to 35% improvement in aerobic fitness. Young adults are able to improve 20 to 25%. Improvements are possible at any age when significant weight loss is involved.

Because active individuals are closer to their genetic potential, they will not improve as much as their less active and less fit contemporaries. Complete inactivity, such as prolonged bed rest, provides a clean canvas for the demonstration of dramatic changes, perhaps as much as 100% improvement above bed rest levels. Sedentary folks may improve more than 30%, whereas already trained athletes may have to accept 5% improvement or less, depending on age, proximity to the genetic potential, and level of training.

The rate of improvement is dramatic at first, 3% per week for the first month, 2% per week for the second, and slowing to 1% or less thereafter. But even though the improvements in aerobic fitness begin to plateau after several months, the capacity to perform submaximal work continues to grow (see figure 6.4). Both the submaximal capacity (aerobic threshold) and the upper limit of aerobic endurance (the anaerobic or lactate threshold) continue to increase after the $\dot{V}O_2$max has plateaued. And it is these submaximal capacities and not the $\dot{V}O_2$max that define our capacity for work or sport, respectively.

> Because active individuals are closer to their genetic potential, they will not improve as much as their less active and less fit contemporaries.

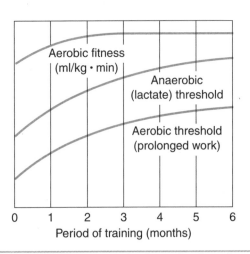

Figure 6.4 Training, aerobic fitness, and submaximal work capacity. With prolonged training, aerobic fitness begins to plateau, but the capacity to perform submaximal work continues to improve.

A normally active middle-aged adult male with a fitness score of 40 ml/kg · min may improve to 50. If he had started as an adolescent, with a fitness score of 55, and achieved a 30% improvement, he may have scored more than 70 and been an outstanding athlete. If you started late, don't despair; you can still achieve dramatic improvements in endurance and energy. Most important are the improvements in the submaximal capacities, changes that allow a once sedentary individual to climb a mountain, or to run a marathon. In addition to improvements in fitness, you are able to sustain a higher percentage of your max and continue once-fatiguing activities indefinitely, without fatigue or discomfort. And the benefits will extend beyond your regular mode of exercise to all your daily tasks. Fitness expands your horizons.

Maintenance

If you ever attain a level of fitness and performance that meets your needs, you may want to switch to a maintenance program. You'll be able to maintain your fitness with three sessions per week, allowing time to apply your new-found fitness in new pursuits. Maintenance has been studied several ways. One is to train to a level of fitness, then use various frequencies of training to see how much is required. Another is to cease training to see how quickly it is lost. With some activity, fitness doesn't decline too rapidly, but with complete bed rest it may drop as much as 10% per week (Greenleaf, Greenleaf, VanDerveer, & Dorchak, 1976). You can maintain fitness with two or three sessions weekly, but the effort must be of the same intensity and duration used to achieve the improvements (Brynteson & Sinning, 1973). Exercise of lower intensity but longer duration also seems to work, but it won't keep you tuned for a race. One workout of very long duration each week may help maintain

CROSS-TRAINING

The popular triathlon gave rise to the "theory" of cross-training, and the suggestion that running or cycling could enhance swim performance, and so forth. Unfortunately, cross-training doesn't work that way; training must be specific to improve performance (Sharkey & Greatzer, 1993). But there are several good reasons to use variety in training. One obvious reason is to train for a multisport event such as the triathlon. Another is to add variety and interest to your training. But the most important reason is to reduce impact and overuse in activities such as running.

I run year-round, even in the dead of the Montana winter. I've found that cross-training relieves the tendency to get nagging overuse injuries. And the variety eliminates the boredom of unrelenting training. I run, swim, and mountain bike in the summer, with tennis, hiking, and paddling for diversion. The winter includes cross-country skiing, running, and swimming. Winter diversions include back-country ski trips and downhill skiing. I do one or two muscular fitness sessions most weeks to maintain muscular fitness and to try to improve performance. Fall and spring serve as transition periods, enhanced by new activities, new weather, and new locales. Try more than one mode of exercise to train some muscles while resting others. You'll like it!

fitness for a while, but a combination of activities plus two or three training sessions is certain to do the job.

More recently researchers have used a more complex approach to study maintenance. By observing the effect of a single dose of training on specific aerobic enzymes, the researcher can plot the influence of training and determine its half-life, the time it takes to lose one-half of the benefit. These studies suggest that the half-life of training ranges from 4.5 to 9.4 days (Watson, Srivastava, & Booth, 1983). The half-life is used because it is difficult to tell when a biological effect, such as an increase in enzyme activity, returns to pretraining levels. So, one measures the increase and the time it takes to return to half of that value. If half of the training effect is lost in 4.5 days, you'll want to train more frequently to maintain or improve fitness.

Regaining Fitness

Instead of worrying about how little it takes to achieve, maintain, or regain fitness, find activities you enjoy and make them part of your life.

Does a previously fit individual regain fitness more quickly than one who has not been fit? Although the limited work in this area says probably not, my experience argues for a tentative maybe. The answer may depend on such factors as genetic potential, the initial level of fitness, and the extent of previous training. An extensive period of previous training may lead to structural changes that are retained longer than alterations in aerobic enzymes and blood volume. And the repetitions of training will certainly lead to skill and economy of motion that makes subsequent activity seem easier.

But instead of worrying about how little it takes to achieve, maintain, or regain fitness, find activities you enjoy and make them part of your life. Then you'll view activity as an essential and enjoyable component of every day. You'll be hooked on activity, and the rest will take care of itself.

Summary

This chapter summarizes the findings of hundreds of studies that have contributed to our knowledge of the factors associated with the development of aerobic fitness. Intensity, duration, and frequency of exercise are manipulated to bring about improvements in fitness. Virtually all of the studies relied on the same measure of improvement, the $\dot{V}O_2max$, which has been acknowledged as a measure of exercise intensity. So, it is not surprising that most studies favor intensity as the most important factor in the training prescription. If your goal is to raise the $\dot{V}O_2max$, by all means emphasize intensity (e.g., the training heart rate), at least some of the time.

However, if your goal is health, or the capacity to endure for extended periods, you should give equal attention to exercise duration. Longer-duration exercise ensures the utilization of fat as a source of energy, and that has distinct health benefits. And if your goal is endurance you should include sufficient duration in your training. Remember that training must be specific to its intended purpose if you are to achieve optimal results.

Intensity is important, but excessive emphasis on intensity can take the joy out of regular activity. Athletes don't train hard every day, and you shouldn't either. That is why I encourage you to move beyond the objective approach of heart rates and training zones to the subjective, where you utilize perceived exertion and learn to listen to your body. Adopt the active life gradually, enjoying the experience and savoring the adaptations.

CHAPTER 7

Aerobic Fitness Programs

"You will never find time for anything. If you want time you must make it."
Charles Buxton

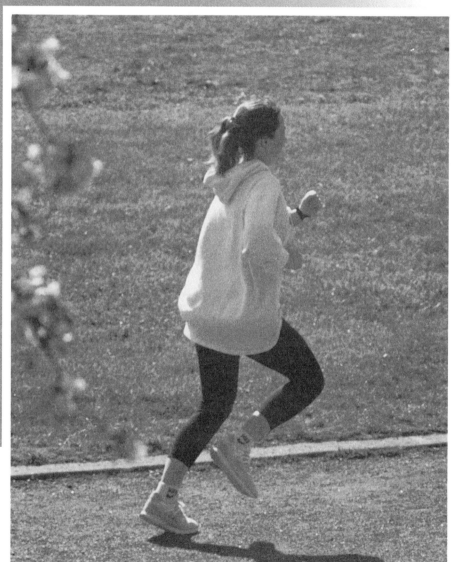

People often tell me they would like to become more fit but they just haven't got the time. I tell them how others make time for regular exercise, including our last five presidents and many other busy people. The time has come for you to make time for regular fitness training. This chapter provides training tips, training programs, and other information you'll need to make training safe, enjoyable, and effective. The programs in this chapter have been proven to be cost-effective, providing maximum benefit for the time invested.

THIS CHAPTER WILL HELP YOU

- understand how to make training safe and enjoyable;
- apply your aerobic fitness prescription via walk-jog-run programs, cycling or swimming programs, or advanced aerobic training;
- select alternative ways to remain active and fit; and
- deal with common exercise problems.

Training Tips

The time has come for you to make time for regular fitness training.

We'll begin with walking and running as modes of exercise because, for the time and cost, they provide a great training stimulus. Intensity and duration are easy to control, and the activities can be done at any time, in almost any weather, with little investment in equipment. The equipment is light and easily transported on vacation or a business trip. You can participate alone or in a group, and continue throughout life. For these reasons and more, walking and running are fine ways to achieve and maintain aerobic fitness.

What to Wear

Nothing is more important to your enjoyment than comfortable shoes, so don't economize when you purchase footwear. Go to a reputable sporting goods dealer and seek advice from a knowledgeable salesperson. Avoid sale shoes at discount outlets unless you know something about the product. Buy a training shoe, not one built for competition. A firm, thick sole, good arch support, and a well padded heel are essential. The sole should be firm but not terribly difficult to flex. A firm heel counter is also important. If blisters are a problem try tube socks, a thin sock under a heavier one, or petroleum jelly on potential hot spots.

Walking and jogging don't require fancy clothing. Nylon or cotton gym shorts and a T-shirt are adequate in summer. For winter, a sweatshirt or jogging suit serves until temperatures fall below 20 degrees Fahrenheit. Some runners prefer tights or long underwear. Several layers of lighter apparel are preferable to a single heavy garment. Add gloves and a knit cap in colder temperatures. When the wind blows, a thin nylon windbreaker helps to reduce heat loss. A cap is particularly important in cold weather, because you lose a great deal of body heat from your head. When temperatures fall below 20, you may choose to wear both the long underwear and a sweat suit. Many runners continue to run in subzero temperatures, which is safe provided you are properly clothed, warmed up, and sensitive to signs of wind chill and frostbite. (Many runners and skiers appreciate polypropylene underwear that wicks perspiration away from skin, thereby avoiding rapid cooling.)

Never wear a rubberized sweat suit in *any weather*. The water lost through perspiration doesn't contribute to long-term weight loss, and your body's most effective mode of heat loss is blocked.

Technique

An upright posture conserves energy. Run or walk with your back comfortably straight, your head up, and your shoulders relaxed. Bend your arms and hold your hands in a comfortable position. Keep arm swing to a minimum during jogging and slow running; pumping action should increase with speed. Your legs should swing freely from the hip with no attempt to overstride. Many successful runners employ a relatively short stride. Lab studies show that the stride that feels best is usually the most efficient as well.

No aspect of running technique is violated more often by neophytes than the foot strike. Many beginners say they don't like to jog. Observation of their foot strike often reveals the reason: They run on the balls of their feet. Although appropriate for sprints and short distances, this foot strike is inappropriate for distance runs and will probably result in soreness. I recommend the *heel-to-toe* foot strike for most new runners. Upon landing lightly on the heel, the foot rocks forward to push off on the ball of the foot. For faster running, employ a slight forward lean, more knee lift, a quick forceful push off the ball of the foot (toe-off), and more vigorous arm action. The heel-to-toe technique is the least tiring of all, and a large percentage of successful distance runners use it. The flat foot strike is a compromise: The runner lands on the entire foot and rocks onto the ball for push-off. Check your shoes after several weeks of running; if you're using the correct foot strike, the outer border of the heel will show some wear.

Time of Day

Exercise whenever it suits your fancy. Some people like to do several miles before breakfast. Others elect to train during lunch hour, then eat a sandwich at the desk. Many prefer to exercise after work to help cleanse the mind of the day's problems. A few night owls brave the dark in their quest for fitness; they are quick to point out that the run and shower help them sleep. I caution you to avoid vigorous activity 1 or 2 hours after a meal, when the digestive organs require an adequate blood supply and when fat in the circulation hastens the risk of clotting.

Unless you enjoy spending time by yourself, consider training with a companion. When you find one with similar abilities, interest, and goals, you aren't likely to miss your workout.

Exercise whenever it suits your fancy.

Where to Walk or Run

Where should you go? Almost anywhere you please. Avoid hard surfaces for the first few weeks of training. Walk or run in the park, on playing fields, on golf courses, or on running tracks. After a few weeks, you'll be ready to try the back roads and trails in your area. Varying your routes will help you maintain interest. When the weather prohibits outdoor exercise, try a mall, YMCA, or school gym, or choose an exercise supplement you can do at home, such as running in place or skipping rope.

Now let's consider programs for beginning, intermediate, and advanced fitness training.

Sample Aerobic Fitness Programs

Your fitness prescription gives you the freedom to tailor a fitness program to meet your specific needs. You have a wide choice of exercises and also many options in the length of time you want to exercise and the intensity of that activity. Some people prefer a more detailed, step-by-step approach. For this reason, I've included some walk-jog-run programs.

I'll describe programs for three levels of ability: A starter program for those in low-fitness categories (aerobic fitness score under 35 ml/kg · min), an intermediate program (35 to 45), and one for those in the high-fitness categories (46 or better). The starter program was prepared by the President's Council on Physical Fitness and Sports and appears in the booklet "An Introduction to Physical Fitness."

Starter Programs (Walk-Jog-Run)

Take the walk test to determine your exercise level.

Walk Test

The object of this test is to determine how many minutes (up to 10) you can walk at a brisk pace, on a level surface, without undue difficulty or discomfort.

If you can't walk for 5 minutes, begin with the *red* walking program.

If you can walk more than 5 minutes, but less than 10, begin with the third week of the *red* walking program.

If you can walk for the full 10 minutes but are somewhat tired and sore as a result, start with the *white* walk-jog program. If you can breeze through the full 10 minutes, you're ready for bigger things. Wait until the next day and take the 10-minute walk-jog test.

Walk-Jog Test

In this test you alternately walk 50 steps (left foot strikes ground 25 times) and jog 50 steps for a total of 10 minutes. Walk at the rate of 120 steps per minute (left foot strikes the ground at 1-second intervals). Jog at the rate of 144 steps per minute (left foot strikes ground 18 times every 15 seconds).

If you can't complete the 10-minute test, begin at the third week of the *white* program. If you can complete the 10-minute test but are tired and winded as a result, start with the last week of the *white* program before moving to the *blue* program. If you can perform the 10-minute walk-jog test without difficulty, start with the *blue* program.

Red Walking Program

Start with this program, doing each activity every other day at first (see figure 7.1). The first week you'll walk at a brisk pace for 5 minutes, or for a shorter time if you become uncomfortably tired. Walk slowly or rest for 3 minutes. Then walk briskly again for 5 minutes or until you become uncomfortably tired. The second week of the program is the same, but increase your pace as soon as you can walk 5 minutes without soreness or fatigue. During the

WEEK	Sunday	Monday	Tuesday	Wednesday	Thursday	Friday	Saturday
1	Brisk walk 5 min Slow walk / rest 3 min Brisk walk 5 min		Brisk walk 5 min Slow walk / rest 3 min Brisk walk 5 min		Brisk walk 5 min Slow walk / rest 3 min Brisk walk 5 min		Brisk walk 5 min Slow walk / rest 3 min Brisk walk 5 min
2		Brisk walk 5 min Slow walk / rest 3 min Brisk walk 5 min		Brisk walk 5 min Slow walk / rest 3 min · Brisk walk 5 min		Brisk walk 5 min Slow walk / rest 3 min Brisk walk 5 min	
3	Brisk walk 8 min Slow walk / rest 3 min Brisk walk 8 min		Brisk walk 8 min Slow walk / rest 3 min Brisk walk 8 min		Brisk walk 8 min Slow walk / rest 3 min Brisk walk 8 min		Brisk walk 8 min Slow walk / rest 3 min Brisk walk 8 min
4		Brisk walk 8 min Slow walk / rest 3 min Brisk walk 8 min		Brisk walk 8 min Slow walk / rest 3 min Brisk walk 8 min		Brisk walk 8 min Slow walk / rest 3 min Brisk walk 8 min	

Figure 7.1   Red walking program.

third week of the program you'll increase your brisk walking to 8 minutes. Increase your pace in the fourth week. When you've completed week 4 of the red program, begin at week 1 of the white program.

White Walk-Jog Program

In this program you'll begin by walking at a brisk pace for 10 minutes, or for a shorter time if you become uncomfortably tired (see figure 7.2). After a slow walk or rest you'll resume the brisk pace. The second week will increase the amount of time spent walking at a brisk pace; the third and fourth weeks will incorporate jogging short distances. Do each activity four times a week. When you've completed week 4 of the white program, begin week 1 of the blue program.

Blue Jogging Program

In this program you'll increase the amount of time spent jogging each week (see figure 7.3). Do each activity five times a week, as indicated.

WEEK	Sunday	Monday	Tuesday	Wednesday	Thursday	Friday	Saturday
1	Brisk walk 10 min Slow walk / rest 3 min Brisk walk 10 min	Brisk walk 10 min Slow walk / rest 3 min Brisk walk 10 min		Brisk walk 10 min Slow walk / rest 3 min Brisk walk 10 min		Brisk walk 10 min Slow walk / rest 3 min Brisk walk 10 min	
2	Brisk walk 15 min Slow walk / rest 3 min Brisk walk 10 min		Brisk walk 15 min Slow walk / rest 3 min Brisk walk 10 min		Brisk walk 15 min Slow walk / rest 3 min Brisk walk 15 min		Brisk walk 15 min Slow walk / rest 3 min Brisk walk 15 min
3	Jog 10s (25 yd) Walk 1 min (100 yd) 12x		Jog 10s (25 yd) Walk 1 min (100 yd) 12x		Jog 10s (25 yd) Walk 1 min (100 yd) 12x		Jog 10s (25 yd) Walk 1 min (100 yd) 12x
4		Jog 20s (50 yd) Walk 1 min (100 yd) 12x		Jog 20s (50 yd) Walk 1 min (100 yd) 12x		Jog 20s (50 yd) Walk 1 min (100 yd) 12x	Jog 20s (50 yd) Walk 1 min (100 yd) 12x

Figure 7.2 White walk-jog program.

Intermediate Jog-Run Program

If you've followed the starter program or are already reasonably active, you're ready for the intermediate program (see figure 7.4). You're able to jog 1 mile slowly without undue fatigue, rest 2 minutes, and do it again. Your sessions consume about 250 calories.

You're ready to increase both the intensity and the duration of your runs. You'll be using the heart rate training zone for those of medium fitness (35 to 45 ml/[kg · min]). You'll begin jogging 1 mile in 12 minutes, and when you finish this program you may be able to complete 3 miles or more at a pace approaching 8 minutes per mile. Each week's program includes three phases—the basic workout, longer runs (overdistance), and shorter runs (underdistance). If a week's program seems too easy, move ahead; if it seems too hard, move back a week or two. On most of the days, you'll jog in intervals and walk to recover. For example, on Tuesday of the first week, begin by jogging 1/4 to 1/2 mile slowly. Then try to jog 1/2 mile in 5 minutes 30 seconds, walk to recover, and repeat. Next, jog 1/4 mile in 2 minutes 45 seconds, walk to recover, and repeat three times. Finally, jog 1/4 to 1/2 mile as

WEEK	Sunday	Monday	Tuesday	Wednesday	Thursday	Friday	Saturday
1	Jog 40s (100 yd) Walk 1 min (100 yd) 9x	Jog 40s (100 yd) Walk 1 min (100 yd) 9x		Jog 40s (100 yd) Walk 1 min (100 yd) 9x	Jog 40s (100 yd) Walk 1 min (100 yd) 9x		Jog 40s (100 yd) Walk 1 min (100 yd) 9x
2	Jog 1 min (150 yd) Walk 1 min (100 yd) 8x	Jog 1 min (150 yd) Walk 1 min (100 yd) 8x	Jog 1 min (150 yd) Walk 1 min (100 yd) 8x		Jog 1 min (150 yd) Walk 1 min (100 yd) 8x	Jog 1 min (150 yd) Walk 1 min (100 yd) 8x	
3	Jog 2 min (300 yd) Walk 1 min (100 yd) 6x	Jog 2 min (300 yd) Walk 1 min (100 yd) 6x		Jog 2 min (300 yd) Walk 1 min (100 yd) 6x	Jog 2 min (300 yd) Walk 1 min (100 yd) 6x		Jog 2 min (300 yd) Walk 1 min (100 yd) 6x
4	Jog 4 min (600 yd) Walk 1 min (100 yd) 4x		Jog 4 min (600 yd) Walk 1 min (100 yd) 4x	Jog 4 min (600 yd) Walk 1 min (100 yd) 4x		Jog 4 min (600 yd) Walk 1 min (100 yd) 4x	Jog 4 min (600 yd) Walk 1 min (100 yd) 4x
5	Jog 6 min (900 yd) Walk 1 min (100 yd) 3x	Jog 6 min (900 yd) Walk 1 min (100 yd) 3x		Jog 6 min (900 yd) Walk 1 min (100 yd) 3x	Jog 6 min (900 yd) Walk 1 min (100 yd) 3x		Jog 6 min (900 yd) Walk 1 min (100 yd) 3x
6	Jog 8 min (1,200 yd) Walk 2 min (200 yd) 2x		Jog 8 min (1,200 yd) Walk 2 min (200 yd) 2x	Jog 8 min (1,200 yd) Walk 2 min (200 yd) 2x		Jog 8 min (1,200 yd) Walk 2 min (200 yd) 2x	Jog 8 min (1,200 yd) Walk 2 min (200 yd) 2x
7	Jog 10 min (1,500 yd) Walk 2 min (200 yd) 2x	Jog 10 min (1,500 yd) Walk 2 min (200 yd) 2x		Jog 10 min (1,500 yd) Walk 2 min (200 yd) 2x	Jog 10 min (1,500 yd) Walk 2 min (200 yd) 2x		Jog 10 min (1,500 yd) Walk 2 min (200 yd) 2x
8	Jog 12 min (1,760 yd) Walk 2 min (200 yd) 2x		Jog 12 min (1,760 yd) Walk 2 min (200 yd) 2x	Jog 12 min (1,760 yd) Walk 2 min (200 yd) 2x		Jog 12 min (1,760 yd) Walk 2 min (200 yd) 2x	Jog 12 min (1,760 yd) Walk 2 min (200 yd) 2x

Figure 7.3 Blue jogging program.

WEEK	Monday	Tuesday	Wednesday	Thursday	Friday	Saturday/Sunday
1	1 mi (12 min) Walk 2x	1/4 - 1/2 mi slow 2 x 1/2 mi (5.30 min) 4 x 1/4 mi (2.45 min) 1/4 - 1/2 mi jog	2 mi slow jog	1 mi (12 min) Walk 2x	1/4 - 1/2 mi slow 2 x 1/2 mi (5.30 min) 4 x 1/4 mi (2.45 min) 1/4 - 1/2 mi jog	2 mi slow jog
2	1 mi (11 min) Walk 2x	1/4 - 1/2 mi slow 1/2 mi (5 min) 2 x 1/4 mi (2.30 min) 2 x 1/4 mi (2.45 min) 4 x 220 yd (1.20 min) 1/4 - 1/2 mi slow	2 1/4 mi slow jog	1 mi (11 min) Walk 2x	1/4 - 1/2 mi slow 1/2 mi (5 min) 2 x 1/4 mi (2.30 min) 2 x 1/4 mi (2.45 min) 4 x 220 yd (1.20 min) 1/4 - 1/2 mi slow	2 1/4 mi slow jog
3	1 mi (10.30 min) Walk 2x	1/4 - 1/2 mi slow 1/2 mi (4.45 min) 4 x 1/4 mi (2.30 min) 4 x 220 yd (1.10 min) 4 x 100 yd (.30 min) 1/4 - 1/2 mi slow	2 1/2 mi slow jog	1 mi (10.30 min) Walk 2x	1/4 - 1/2 mi slow 1/2 mi (4.45 min) 4 x 1/4 mi (2.30 min) 4 x 220 yd (1.10 min) 4 x 100 yd (.30 min) 1/4 - 1/2 mi slow	2 1/2 mi slow jog
4	1 mi (10 min) Walk 2x	1/4 - 1/2 mi slow 2 x 1/2 mi (4.45 min) 4 x 1/4 mi (2.20 min) 4 x 220 yd (1 min) 1/4 - 1/2 mi slow	2 3/4 mi slow jog	1 mi (10 min) Walk 2x	1/4 - 1/2 mi slow 2 x 1/2 mi (4.45 min) 4 x 1/4 mi (2.20 min) 4 x 220 yd (1 min) 1/4 - 1/2 mi slow	2 3/4 mi slow jog

Figure 7.4   Intermediate jog-run program. Times are given in minutes and seconds (e.g., 2.45 min is 2 minutes and 45 seconds).

WEEK	Monday	Tuesday	Wednesday	Thursday	Friday	Saturday/ Sunday
5	1 mi (9.30 min) Walk 2x	1/4 - 1/2 mi slow 1/2 mi (4.30 min) 4 x 1/4 mi (2.20 min) 4 x 220 yd (1 min) 4 x 100 yd (0.27 min) 1/4 - 1/2 mi slow	3 mi slow jog	1 mi (9.30 min) Walk 2x	1/4 - 1/2 mi slow 1/2 mi (4.30 min) 4 x 1/4 mi (2.20 min) 4 x 220 yd (1 min) 4 x 100 yd (0.27 min) 1/4 - 1/2 mi slow	3 mi slow jog
6	1 1/2 mi (13.30 min) Walk 2x	1/4 - 1/2 mi slow 2 x 1/2 mi (4.30 min) 4 x 1/2 mi (2.10 min) 4 x 220 yd (1 min) 4 x 100 yd (0.25 min) 1/4 - 1/2 mi slow	3 mi slow jog—increase pace last 1/4 mi	1 1/2 mi (13.30 min) Walk 2x	1/4 - 1/2 mi slow 2 x 1/2 mi (4.30 min) 4 x 1/2 mi (2.10 min) 4 x 220 yd (1 min) 4 x 100 yd (0.25 min) 1/4 - 1/2 mi slow	3 mi slow jog—increase pace last 1/4 mi
7	1 1/2 mi (13 min) Walk 2x	1/4 - 1/2 mi slow 2 x 1/2 mi (4.15 min) 4 x 1/4 mi (2 min) 4 x 220 yd (0.55 min) 1/4 - 1/2 mi slow	3 1/2 mi slow jog	1 1/2 mi (13 min) Walk 2x	1/4 - 1/2 mi slow 2 x 1/2 mi (4.15 min) 4 x 1/4 mi (2 min) 4 x 220 yd (0.55 min) 1/4 - 1/2 mi slow	3 1/2 mi slow jog
8	1 mi (8 min) Walk 1 mi (8.30 min) Walk 2x	1/4 - 1/2 mi slow 2 x 1/2 mi (4 min) 4 x 1/4 mi (1.50 min) 4 x 220 yd (0.55 min) 4 x 100 yd (0.23 min) 1/4 - 1/2 mi slow	3 1/2 mi slow jog	1 mi (8 min) Walk 1 mi (8.30 min) Walk 2x	1/4 - 1/2 mi slow 2 x 1/2 mi (4 min) 4 x 1/4 mi (1.50 min) 4 x 220 yd (0.55 min) 4 x 100 yd (0.23 min) 1/4 - 1/2 mi slow	3 1/2 mi slow jog

(continued)

Figure 7.4 *(continued)*

WEEK	Monday	Tuesday	Wednesday	Thursday	Friday	Saturday/ Sunday
9	1 mi (8 min) 3x	1/4 - 1/2 mi slow 1/2 mi (4 min) 4 x 1/4 mi (1.50 min) 4 x 220 yd (0.50 min) 4 x 100 yd (0.20 min) 4 x 50 yd (0.10 min) 1/4 - 1/2 mi slow	4 mi slow jog	1 mi (8 min) 3x	1/4 - 1/2 mi slow 1/2 mi (4 min) 4 x 1/4 mi (1.50 min) 4 x 220 yd (0.50 min) 4 x 100 yd (0.20 min) 4 x 50 yd (0.10 min) 1/4 - 1/2 mi slow	4 mi slow jog
10	1 1/2 mi (12 min) 2x	1/4 - 1/2 mi slow 2 x 1/2 mi (3.45 min) 6 x 1/4 mi (1.50 min) 2 x 220 yd (0.45 min) 1/4 - 1/2 mi slow	4 mi slow jog—increase pace last 1/2 mi	1 1/2 mi (12 min) 2x	1/4 - 1/2 mi slow 2 x 1/2 mi (3.45 min) 6 x 1/4 mi (1.50 min) 2 x 220 yd (0.45 min) 1/4 - 1/2 mi slow	4 mi slow jog—increase pace last 1/2 mi
11	1 mi (7.30 min) 3x	1/4 - 1/2 mi slow 4 x 1/2 mi (3.30 min) 4 x 1/4 mi (1.45 min) 2 x 220 yd (0.45 min) 1/4 - 1/2 mi slow	4 mi slow jog	1 mi (7.30 min) 3x	1/4 - 1/2 mi slow 4 x 1/2 mi (3.30 min) 4 x 1/4 mi (1.45 min) 2 x 220 yd (0.45 min) 1/4 - 1/2 mi slow	4 mi slow jog
12	1 1/2 mi (11.40 min)			1 1/2 mi (11.40 min)		

Figure 7.4 *(continued)*

in the beginning of the workout. On Thursday, jog 1 mile in 11 minutes, walk to recover, and repeat. Table 7.1 is a pace guide for gauging your speed over various distances. Remember to warm up and cool down as part of every exercise session.

TABLE 7.1   Pace Guide for Gauging Speed Over Various Distances

	Pace	1 mi	1/2 mi	1/4 mi	220 yd	100 yd	50 yd
					(minutes:seconds)		
Slow jog	10 cal/min (120 cal/mi)[a]	12:00	6:00	3:00	1:30	0:40	0:20
Jog	12 cal/min (120 cal/mi)	10:00	5:00	2:30	1:15	0:34	0:17
Run	15 cal/min (120 cal/mi)	8:00	4:00	2:00	1:00	0:27	0:13
Fast run	20 cal/min (120 cal/mi)	6:00	3:00	1:30	0:45	0:20	0:10

[a]Depends on efficiency and body size; add 10% for each 15 lb over 150; subtract 10% for each 15 lb under 150.

Advanced Aerobic Training

This section is for the well-trained individual. I'll provide some suggestions for advanced training, but keep in mind that there is no single way to train. If you enjoy underdistance training, by all means use it. If you find that you prefer overdistance, use that approach.

Simply pick up the pace as you approach the end of a long run, and you'll receive an optimal training stimulus. Moreover, because the speed work is limited to a short span near the end of the run, discomfort is brief.

Consider the following suggestions:

There is no single way to train.

• Always warm up before your run.
• Use the high-fitness heart rate training zone.
• Vary the location and distance of the run (long-short, fast-slow, or hilly-flat).
• Set distance goals:

Phase 1	20 miles per week
Phase 2	25 miles per week (ready for 3- to 5-mile road races)
Phase 3	30 miles per week
Phase 4	35 miles per week (ready for 5- to 7-mile road races)
Phase 5	40 miles per week
Phase 6	45 miles per week (ready for 7- to 10-mile road races)
Phase 7	More than 50 miles per week (consider longer races such as the marathon—26.2 miles)

• Don't be a slave to your goals, and don't increase weekly mileage unless you enjoy it.
• Run 6 days per week if you like; otherwise, try an alternate-day schedule with longer runs.
• Try one long run (not more than one-third of weekly distance) on Saturday or Sunday.

- Try two shorter runs if the long ones seem difficult: 5 + 5 instead of 10.
- Keep records if you like. You'll be surprised! Record date, distance, and comments. Note morning pulse and body weight. At least once per year, check your performance over a measured distance to observe progress (use a local road race or the 1.5-mile run test [see chapter 4, page 81]). Check your fitness several times per year.
- Don't train with a stopwatch. Wear a wristwatch so you'll know how long you've run.
- Increase speed as you approach the finish of a run.
- Always cool down after a run.

Walking, Cycling, and Swimming

This section provides training programs for walkers, cyclists, and swimmers. The programs combine the training concepts outlined earlier and the principles of training described in chapter 16 to provide safe, effective, and interesting approaches to fitness. Use the programs to improve fitness, but when you are satisfied with your level of fitness, switch to a maintenance program. It isn't necessary to improve fitness to a high level; the health benefits are available to those who remain active.

Walking Program

Begin with the walk test included earlier in this chapter. If you can walk for the full 10 minutes, you are ready for this program. If not, complete the 4-week red walking program.

The weekly training menu includes the following:

Monday	Easy distance—walk at a comfortable pace (PE = 12).*
Tuesday	Pace—stride briskly (PE = 15).
Wednesday	Hills (or stairs)—walk briskly uphill to build stamina (PE = 13).
Thursday	Intervals—walk intervals at PE = 16. Increase to PE = 17 after 4 weeks.
Friday	Overdistance—walk slowly for a long distance (PE = 11).
Saturday	Variety—try a different activity or hike a trail at a leisurely pace.
Sunday	Rest—or try light activity (e.g., gardening).

* PE = perceived exertion, from table 6.2, p. 102

After you have completed the 8-week program (see figure 7.5), design your own using this or another format or switch to a walk-jog program. If you prefer one type of training, such as easy distance, use that and forget the other items I've mentioned. Remember, you should enjoy your regular activity.

Plan a hiking trip with friends, and train together to prepare for the outing. You may even want to take up race walking, that curious gait that requires the heel of one foot to touch the ground before the toe of the other foot leaves the ground.

Your Weekly Walking Program

| | WEEK | | | | | | | |
	1	2	3	4	5	6	7	8
Monday	15 min	20	25	20	25	30	35	30
Tuesday	2 × 8 min*	2 × 9	2 × 10	3 × 7	3 × 8	3 × 9	3 × 10	4 × 10
Wednesday	10 min	11	12	13	2 × 10	2 × 12	2 × 14	3 × 10
Thursday	3 × 2 min	3 × 3	3 × 4	4 × 2	4 × 3	4 × 4	5 × 2	5 × 3
Friday	30 min	35	40	35	40	45	50	60

*2 sets at 8 min each

Always warm up and stretch before each workout.

Pace: Do one set, walk slowly to recover, and do the next.
Hills: Optional; try not to exceed PE = 13.
Intervals: Do one set, walk slowly to recover, and do another.

Figure 7.5   Your weekly walking program.

Cycling Program

This program utilizes a training menu to guide your progress (see figure 7.6). The weekly training menu includes the following:

Monday	Easy distance—ride at a comfortable pace (PE = 13).
Tuesday	Pace—cycle at a brisk pace (PE = 15).
Wednesday	Hills—include hills to build stamina (PE = 14).
Thursday	Intervals—push harder for brief intervals (PE = 16). Increase to PE = 17 after 4 weeks.
Friday	Overdistance—go easy to develop endurance (PE = 11).
Saturday	Variety—try a different activity (e.g., tennis or hiking) or ride a trail.
Sunday	Rest—or try a light activity (e.g., gardening or walking).

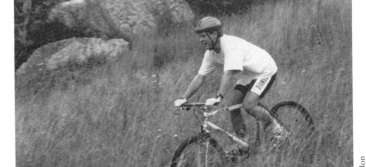

© W. Lynn Seldon

Train to prepare for enjoyable trail rides.

Your Weekly Cycling Program

	WEEK							
	1	2	3	4	5	6	7	8
Monday	30 min	40	50	40	50	60	70	60
Tuesday	2×10 min	2×15	2×20	3×10	3×15	3×20	4×10	4×15
Wednesday	15 min	20	25	20	2×15	2×20	2×25	3×20
Thursday	3×3 min	3×4	3×5	3×6	4×3	4×4	4×5	5×5
Friday	60 min	70	80	75	90	100	110	120

Always wear a helmet; ride easy to warm up.

Pace: Ride 10 min, relax and recover, ride another set.
Hills: Include some standing but try to keep PE = 14.
Intervals: Ride one, cycle easy to recover, and ride the next.
Overdistance: Ride easy; stop for rest and fluids every 30 min.

Figure 7.6   Your weekly cycling program.

After 8 weeks design your own program using elements from this plan or others you enjoy. Plan a long trip with friends, and do training rides together.

Swimming Program

This program assumes a certain amount of skill in swimming (see figure 7.7). If the program seems too difficult for your level of ability, scale down the program and take lessons to improve your skill and efficiency.

The weekly training menu includes the following:

Monday	Easy distance—go easy at a comfortable pace (PE = 12).
Tuesday	Pace—swim at a firm pace (PE = 15).
Wednesday	Arms/legs—swim with arms or legs only (PE = 13).
Thursday	Intervals—swim harder for brief intervals (PE = 16). Increase to PE = 17 after 4 weeks.
Friday	Overdistance—relax on a longer swim (PE = 11).
Saturday	Variety—try a different activity or water games (e.g., water polo).
Sunday	Rest—or try a light activity (e.g., gardening or walking).

When you have completed 8 weeks, design your own program using the types of training you most enjoy. You could even decide to take up triathlon training.

Your Weekly Swimming Program								
	WEEK							
	1	2	3	4	5	6	7	8
Monday	15 min	20	25	20	25	30	35	30
Tuesday	2 × 5 min	2 × 6	2 × 7	2 × 8	3 × 6	3 × 7	3 × 8	4 × 5
Wednesday	5 min/each	6/e	7/e	8/e	9/e	10/e	11/e	12/e
Thursday	3 × 3 min	3 × 4	3 × 5	3 × 4	4 × 3	4 × 4	4 × 5	5 × 4
Friday	25 min	30	35	40	35	40	45	50

Use good goggles; warm up well on Tuesday, Wednesday, and Thursday, and swim easy laps after those workouts.

Pace: Swim slowly or walk in the water to recover between sets.

Arms/Legs: Use a kickboard or flotation device for support.

Intervals: Swim slowly or walk to recover between sets.

Figure 7.7   Your weekly swimming program.

Triathlon Training Tips

This combination of swimming, cycling, and running has become very popular in recent years. The variety in training makes it a safer sport than the marathon. For those who crave a challenge, the triathlon is just the ticket.

The triathlon requires a high level of performance in each event. Although some enthusiasts are able to train for each event four or more times per week, most participants are happy to train for each event three times each week (nine training sessions per week is about all the time most can afford). Because it takes more than three sessions per week to improve in each event, I recommend that you raise your best event to a high level with five training sessions per week (leaving only two sessions each for the other events). Then switch to maintenance (two to three times per week) and raise the next best event. When this event is satisfactory, place it on a maintenance schedule and focus on your weakest event.

When you feel ready to experience the entire triathlon, enter a small, local event, preferably one in which the swimming is conducted in a pool. Then hone your sports and transitional skills and conditioning in more competitive events. Along the way you'll probably also want to upgrade your equipment in order for you to be more competitive in your age group. Someday you may be ready for the grueling Ironman Triathlon in Hawaii (more than 2 miles of swimming, 116 miles of cycling, and a full marathon—26.2 miles—of running). Even if you never compete in the Ironman, training for the triathlon will certainly make you a more fit, versatile, and adaptable athlete.

Aerobic Alternatives

Be certain that you are ready to utilize the device you intend to purchase. Then purchase a good basic machine with only those features you know you'll use.

When you are unable to engage in your regular aerobic activity because of weather or injury, consider an alternative. These examples can also serve as supplements for a weight-loss program, or as part of a cross-training program. There are many types of aerobic exercise devices on the market. You should know that most devices end up gathering dust in the basement within a year of purchase. Be certain that you are ready to utilize the device you intend to purchase. Then purchase a good basic machine with only those features you know you'll use. Avoid paying hundreds more for expensive electronics or heart rate monitors you may not need. Use a fan to make the experience of stationary exercise more enjoyable.

• **Bicycle:** Riding a bike is a great way to get aerobic exercise. I've done more biking and less running as my knee, injured in high school football, tells me to cut back. Now I'm hooked on long mountain rides. Less desirable but sometimes necessary is indoor cycling. The best and least expensive alternative is a stand for your bicycle. The stand provides stability and resistance for less than $200. A good stationary bicycle should be comfortable and offer good controls and sufficient resistance to provide a training stimulus, now and in the future. Be sure the bike is comfortable for your significant other if he or she plans to use it. Several companies make fine machines that combine cycling with arm exercise. The best of these allow leg, arm, or combined exercise along with a flywheel fan for resistance and cooling. These devices are particularly useful for individuals with disabilities such as multiple sclerosis.

• **Treadmill:** Treadmills range from less expensive nonmotorized devices, to sturdy motor-driven machines, and devices that combine leg and arm exercise. Be certain that you like the feel of the machine, that it is well built and guaranteed, and that it is capable of sufficient elevation and speed to provide a training stimulus, now and in the future.

• **Cross-country ski devices:** Ski simulators are widely advertised in magazines and on TV. Be sure you try the device several times before you make a purchase. As with all long-term purchases, you are wise to buy a reputable brand, known for durability, rather than a low-cost look-alike.

• **Rowing machines:** Less expensive models of rowing machines use adjustable shock absorbers to control resistance, while better devices use a fan flywheel or electronic brake. Rowing machines combine upper and lower body exercise, as do ski devices and some bicycles and treadmills. The combined exercises allow you to burn more calories than you do in leg exercise at a given level of perceived exertion.

• **Stair climbers:** These devices gained popularity at health clubs. Moderate-priced units are now available for home purchase. Look for a sturdy, brand-name device with a good warranty.

• **Skipping rope:** Skipping rope is a full-time aerobic activity for some. The equipment is inexpensive and easy to transport, and you can skip rope anywhere, even in a hotel room. The exercise allows a wide range of intensities. Rope length is important; the ends of the rope should reach your armpits when you hold the rope beneath your feet. Commercial ropes with ball bearings in the handles are easier and smoother to use, but a length of number 10 sash cord from your local hardware store serves quite well. Rope skipping requires a degree of coordination and if done inappropriately can quickly raise the heart rate above your training zone. If this happens, walk or jog in place slowly, then resume skipping. Besides the aerobic benefits, rope skipping could improve your tennis or racquetball game, where rapid footwork is important.

• **Race walking:**   Race walking has not yet taken the country by storm, but if you are a jogger with an injury or a fitness walker in search of a greater challenge, race walking may be for you. The difference between regular walking and race walking is form. The rules require that the toe of one foot remain on the ground until the heel of the other foot touches, producing the distinctive rolling style of competitive walking. This excellent form of aerobic exercise provides all the benefits of jogging, but because there is less pounding on the feet and knees, it is easier to tolerate. If you like to jog but can't, or if you are in an area where race walking is becoming popular, give it a try.

• **Other alternatives:**   Other aerobic alternatives include slide boards, rebound exercise, aerobic dance, step aerobics, dancing, and the best of low-impact activities, swimming. Runners can run in the deep end of the swimming pool while they wait for injuries to heal. In short, there is no excuse for stopping exercise because of weather or injury.

Exercise Problems

Previously inactive adults often encounter problems when they begin exercise. You'll avoid such problems if you vow to make haste slowly. It may have taken you 10 years to get in the shape you're in, and you won't be able to change it overnight. Plan now to make gradual progress. At the start, too little may be better than too much. After several weeks, when your body has begun to adjust to the demands of vigorous effort, you'll be able to increase your exercise intensity. Another way to avoid exercise problems is to warm up before each exercise session. Careful attention to pre-exercise stretching and warming eliminates many of the nagging complications that plague less patient individuals. Never forget to cool down after each workout. Use good equipment (e.g., shoes

Plan now to make gradual progress.

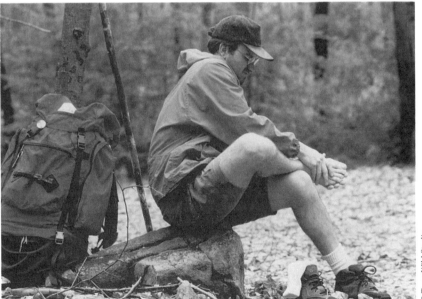

© Terry Wild Studio

Prevention is the most effective way to deal with exercise problems.

and socks), don't start out on hard surfaces, and get plenty of rest. In short, prevention is the most effective way to deal with exercise problems. When problems do arise, the next rule is to treat the cause, not just the symptom. If your knee hurts, put ice on it, but don't stop there. Find out why it hurts, and correct the problem once and for all.

Minor Problems

You can deal easily with many of the minor problems that threaten to diminish your enjoyment of training.

Blisters

Foot blisters are really minor burns caused by friction. Blisters may be prevented by using good-quality, properly fitted footwear. Runners, as well as tennis and handball players, should consider the tube sock with no heel, which seems to reduce the incidence of blisters. Hikers or skiers can wear thin inner liners with their heavy wool socks. Use petroleum jelly on potential hot spots.

At the first hint of a blister, cover the skin with some moleskin or a large bandage. Advanced cases can be treated with a sterilized hollow needle. Release the accumulated fluid, treat the area with an antiseptic, cover it with gauze, circle it with foam rubber, and go back to work. It is wise to keep the items needed for blister prevention in your locker or gym bag, and always carry a blister prevention kit on hiking trips.

Muscle Soreness

Soreness usually develops within 24 hours after exercise. It occurs in the muscles involved and may be due to microscopic tears in the muscle or connective tissue or to localized contractions of muscle fibers. Any professional baseball player will say that it is almost impossible to avoid soreness at the beginning of the season. You can minimize the pain and stiffness of muscle soreness by phasing into a program or sport gradually and by engaging in mild stretching exercises when soreness does occur. Stretch the affected muscles gradually. These stretching movements can be used to relieve the discomfort of soreness or as a warm-up for exercise on the following day. Massage seems to reduce the discomfort of soreness, and it helps to keep sore muscles warm during subsequent activity.

Muscle Cramps

A cramp is a powerful involuntary contraction. Normally, the nervous system tells the muscle when to contract and when to relax. Cramps result when, for some reason, the muscle refuses to relax. Normal control mechanisms fail, and the contraction often becomes painful. Immediate relief comes when the cramped muscle is stretched and massaged. However, that does not remove the underlying cause of the involuntary contraction. Salt and calcium are involved in the chemistry of contraction and relaxation. Cold muscles seem to cramp more readily. It is always wise to warm up sufficiently before vigorous effort and to attend to fluid and electrolyte replacement during hot weather.

Bone Bruises

Hikers and joggers sometimes get painful bruises on the bottoms of their feet. Such bruises can be avoided by careful foot placement and by quality footwear.

Cushioned inner soles also help; air sole shoes or shock-absorbing inner soles aid in reducing the shocks that cause soreness, bruises, and other side effects of running on hard surfaces. A bad bruise can linger, delaying your exercise program many weeks. There's no instant cure once a bruise has developed, so prevention seems the best advice. Ice may help to lessen discomfort and hasten healing. Padding may allow exercise in spite of the bruise.

Ankle Problems

A sprained ankle should be iced immediately. Immersion in a bucket of ice water in the first few minutes may allow a return to activity the next day. A serious sprain should be examined by a physician. High-topped gym shoes reduce the risk of ankle sprains in games such as basketball and handball, whereas low-cut shoes with thick soles invite sprains in such games. Ankle wraps, lace-on supports, or tape often will allow exercise after a sprain, but again, prevention is a more prudent course. First aid for sprains includes RICES:

R est

I ce

C ompression

E levation

S tabilization

Achilles Tendon Injuries

Achilles tendon injuries have become quite common. Some high-backed shoes have been implicated in the rash of bursa injuries. The bursa is located beneath the tendon and serves to lubricate its movements. When rubbed long enough, the bursa becomes inflamed. Once inflamed, it may take weeks to return to normal. Ice helps, but continued activity is often impossible for several weeks. Rupture of the Achilles tendon seems to have become more frequent in recent years. Partial rupture occurs when some of the fibers of the tendon are torn. Complete rupture results when the tendon, which connects the calf muscles to the heel, is completely detached. Prevention is the only approach to these problems, because surgery is the only cure. An inflammation of the tendon could lead to partial or complete rupture if abused or left untreated. Also, individuals with high serum uric acid level, as determined in a laboratory blood test, seem more prone to Achilles tendon injuries; they should have ample warm-up before exercising and should avoid sports with sudden starts, stops, and changes of direction.

Shinsplints

Pains on the front portion of the shinbone are known as shinsplints. They can be caused by a lowered arch, irritated membranes, inflammation of the tibial periosteum (the outer layer of the shin bone), tearing of the tibialis anterior muscle from the bone, a muscle spasm due to swelling of that muscle, hairline fracture of the tibia or fibula, muscle imbalance, or other factors. Rest is the best cure for shinsplints, although taping or a sponge heel pad seems to help some cases. Preventive measures include gradual adjustment to the rigors of strenuous training, light resistance exercises, stretching, avoidance of hard running surfaces, occasional reversal of direction when running on a curved track, and use of the heel-to-toe foot strike, which is the least tiring and least wearing on the rest of the body. Treatment might involve deep massage, anti-inflammatory drugs, or ultrasound. Surgery may be required when the tibialis muscle outgrows its connective tissue compartment.

Knee Problems

As knee injuries and subsequent knee operations become more common in sport, more adults will be plagued with knee problems during exercise. The trauma of an injury often leads to early signs of arthritis. Thus, a high school football injury may lead to signs of arthritis in the 20s or early 30s. These degenerative changes often restrict the ability to run, ski, or engage in other vigorous activities. The problems of prevention are being studied by specialists in sports medicine. Possibilities include rule changes, better cleats and playing surfaces, and considerable attention to preseason conditioning. I will identify some potentially dangerous knee exercises in a subsequent section. Anyone with established problems should consult a physician for ways to relieve the limitations imposed by knee problems. Some people have found that aspirin effectively suppresses the inflammation and pain often associated with exercise. If you forget to take the aspirin, ice helps to reduce the inflammation and speed the return to activity. Maintenance of thigh and hamstring strength helps stabilize the knee (try cycling as well as weight training).

Distance runners often develop knee problems for no apparent reason. So-called runner's knee, characterized by pain around the kneecap, and some other problems may result from a condition known as pronation, in which the foot rolls to the inside. Problems arise when you engage in a considerable amount of exercise, such as distance running; foot, knee, and even back problems may result from the structural and postural adjustments required.

If you have experienced runner's knee or some other problem, correct the cause, not the symptom. Various do-it-yourself treatments are available. Plastic heel cups, arch supports, or foam rubber pads or doughnuts help solve a number of problems. A new pair of shoes may also help. (Two good pairs are better yet—get one pair with thick soles to wear when your feet are sore, another with flexible soles to wear when your legs are sore.) If these treatments don't help, consult an experienced athletic trainer or a podiatrist. Specialists may recommend special supports to help the problem, but try the low-cost solutions before you resort to orthotics (plastic inserts designed to correct problems such as pronation), cortisone injections, or surgery.

Overuse Syndromes

Don't be alarmed by overuse syndromes, which we all suffer at one time or another. If you go too far or too fast too soon, if you forget to do your stretching, if you have serious muscle imbalances, if one leg is shorter than the other, or if you have weak feet, you are bound to have problems now and then. You will soon become adept at first aid. Muscle pulls and bruises get ice for several days. Ice helps relieve shinsplints and heel spurs (inflammation of the tissue of the plantar ligament, which fans outward from the heel to the toes). In fact, when in doubt use ice to relieve pain and swelling. You can also use it after exercise to minimize subsequent swelling. I keep an ice "popsicle" frozen in a small soup can: Just tape a tongue depressor upright in the can of water and put it in the freezer. When you need ice, take out your popsicle and go to work. Ice works best when you use it several times a day, rubbing the problem area until it becomes numb. You'll be amazed by the quick results.

ASPIRIN

I have found that judicious use of aspirin and other nonsteroidal anti-inflammatory drugs (NSAIDs) can minimize many nagging problems. With my doctor's advice I have taken one pill a day for 15 years to quiet a painful knee, the result of a high school football injury and a later operation. In recent years we have learned that one pill a day reduces the clotting and little strokes (transient ischemic attacks) that become more prevalent with age. Aspirin also seems to reduce the risk of subsequent heart attacks. Now we are learning that aspirin may have additional benefits for those engaged in vigorous exercise.

Aspirin reduces pain and inflammation by inhibiting the production of cell hormones called prostaglandins. Exercise causes prostaglandin production, which may lead to soreness and fatigue. Because prostaglandins cause the breakdown of muscle protein during an infection, they may be involved in the soreness and breakdown associated with prolonged vigorous effort, such as a long-distance run.

I have found that a single aspirin or ibuprofen tablet before exercise (with lots of water) is worth many more after soreness develops. Aspirin is especially helpful on long downhill runs that are a sure bet to cause soreness. Of course, you should know that some people are allergic to aspirin, and that it causes some stomach irritation. In large doses it could even alter enzyme activity. But small doses in advance of exercise reduce the need for larger doses afterward. And aspirin and ibuprofen keep many of us aging athletes active long after others give up. Do these drugs carry some risk? Perhaps, but aspirin has been shown to reduce the risk of heart disease and stroke, and recent studies indicate that regular use of ibuprofen may reduce the risk of Alzheimer's disease.

Exercise Hazards

Regular, moderate physical activity is an established aid to health, fitness, weight control, and perhaps longevity. The term *regular* is easily understood by all, but the concept of *moderate* requires further definition. Moderate exercise for the athlete may be hazardous for the sedentary adult. Moderate activity for the unfit individual could be less than a warm-up for the distance runner. Moderate can be defined as a level of exercise likely to bring about improved fitness without exposing the individual to the hazards of more strenuous effort. The heart rate training zone is an excellent guide to moderate exercise, as is the talk test. If you can carry on a conversation during exercise, the level is not too intense.

If you can carry on a conversation during exercise, the level is not too intense.

Sudden Vigorous Exercise

Failure to warm up before vigorous exercise results in electrocardiogram abnormalities, regardless of the fitness or age of the subjects. Dr. R.J. Barnard of the UCLA School of Medicine found such abnormalities in 31 of 44 healthy firemen tested on a vigorous treadmill test. The findings indicated inadequate blood flow in the coronary arteries and a lack of oxygen to the heart muscle. This momentary lack of oxygen could account for the occurrence of heart attacks in those with normal coronary arteries. A warm-up consisting of an easy 4- to 5-minute jog prevented the occurrence of the oxygen deficit and the electrocardiogram abnormalities (Barnard, Gardner, Diaco, & Kattus, 1972).

Athletes and coaches have long appreciated the contribution of the warm-up to the quality of performance in sport. We are now beginning to realize the value of warm-up for a variety of workers such as firefighters, police, and even factory and construction workers. A law enforcement officer may not be able to warm up before jumping from the cruiser to chase a suspect, but there is no reason why assembly line employees cannot do calisthenics before beginning work. Calisthenics are common among factory workers in some European countries and in Japan.

Stressful Exercise

Physiologically speaking, stress is something that is perceived as a threat by the individual. We react to the threat by secreting a group of hormones that assist the mobilization of energy sources and prepare the body for combat or retreat (fight or flight). Many things can be perceived as physical or psychological threats to the body. The body does not differentiate between physical and mental threats; it reacts similarly to each. A difficult exam or an important job interview may be stressful to a student. Swimming or a canoe trip may be stressful to a nonswimmer, and unfamiliar exercise can be stressful to unfit or uncoordinated individuals.

One interesting reaction to stress is an acceleration of the clotting time of the blood. A faster clotting time likely is useful to a soldier on the battlefield or a fighter in the ring, but to an adult with advanced atherosclerotic pathology, with already developed blockage of the blood vessels of the heart, a blood clot could be fatal. Thus, it is important to recognize the types of exercise that accelerate clotting time.

Unfamiliar Exercise

The first experience on a treadmill or in some other unfamiliar situation may be threatening. Studies show that the first exposure to a treadmill test is stressful, and that continued exposure to the situation results in a removal of the threat. One of these studies (Whiddon, Sharkey, & Steadman, 1969) indicated that blood clotting accelerated during the early phase of the study but returned to normal when the test was no longer perceived as a threat.

Although little data has been collected to prove the point, it is likely that other unfamiliar or threatening exercise situations also prove stressful. The first experience on skis, the first parachute jump, white water in a canoe, rappelling, and similar examples come to mind. For the previously inactive adult, the first trip to the health club, gym, or pool could also be stressful.

For the previously inactive adult, the first trip to the health club, gym, or pool could be stressful.

Exhaustive Exercise

Japanese researchers conducted a noteworthy experiment with dogs indicating that exhaustive exercise can be stressful (Suzuki, 1967). The animals were taken for runs of various intensities and durations along the paths of a park with a bike-riding attendant. Post-exercise hormone analyses indicated that only the exhaustive runs were stressful. The researchers concluded that nonexhaustive exercise need not be stressful.

Competitive Exercise

Some years ago, researchers at the Harvard University School of Medicine studied the stress responses to various types of competition in rowing (eight-oar crew). Crew members did not perceive the strenuous effort of a practice session as a threat, but did have increased hormone levels after a time trial and an actual competitive race. The nonexercising coxswain (who steers) also exhibited a stress response after the competitive event. The researchers concluded that exercise, by itself, was not stressful, but that the excitement of competition did elicit the stress response—with or without exercise (Hill, Goetz, & Fox, 1956).

The hormones of the stress response are required for the full mobilization of resources and the optimal performance of the athlete. No one would suggest the need for healthy young men or women to avoid the excitement of competitive sport; however, for the sedentary adult, stress poses additional problems.

Does this mean that adults must avoid the excitement of the unfamiliar, the challenge of the exhaustive, or the thrill of competition? It does not. Your perception of exercise or any other event or consequence can be modified. Over a period of gradual exposure, the exercise neophyte becomes familiar with the demands of an activity. After several months the sedentary adult becomes more fit and finds a particular exercise less exhaustive. With months and years of practice and play, the athletic adult learns to live with the physical and psychological requirements of competition.

Adults can and do engage in potentially stressful activities. For many, the excitement of sport keeps them regularly active. Those who seem to thrive on challenge, excitement, or exhaustion do so after a long period of preparation. The first men to scale Mount Everest engaged in years of physical and mental preparation. Aging but successful professional athletes must continue to practice and train if they are to remain competitive. If you desire to return to competitive tennis, softball, golf, or handball, give yourself time to adjust to the demands of competition. Improve your fitness and skill as you prepare for your first casual competition. Set reasonable competitive goals, and never, never, never take the results too seriously.

> Set reasonable competitive goals, and never, never, never take the results too seriously.

Problem Exercises

I have discussed the potential dangers of highly competitive, exhaustive, or unfamiliar exercise. Now let's consider some common calisthenic-type exercises that may do more harm than good.

Toe Raises

Do toe raises (standing on toes and raising up with contraction of calf muscles) cause development of excessive power in the calf, a situation that could lead to Achilles tendon rupture? Possibly, but not likely. The calf is one muscle group in which muscle imbalance is impossible to avoid. However, problems can be minimized by stretching the tendon and by turning the toes inward during the exercise. Also, standing with the balls of the feet on a 2-inch platform ensures the stretch of the tendon.

Knee Bends

Deep knee bends tend to stretch the ligaments of the joint and lead to instability. Unless you are an Olympic-style weight lifter you don't need to do full knee bends. The half knee bend (until the thighs are parallel to the floor) is a safe and acceptable way to exercise for quadriceps strength or endurance.

The muscular strength of the quadriceps (and the hamstring muscles) aids joint stability as well as performance.

Abdominal Exercises

The leg lift is often recommended for abdominal development. This exercise should be avoided unless the lower back can be kept on the floor to prevent forward rotation of the pelvis, which tends to aggravate lower back pain. The ever-popular sit-up also tends to lead to lower back problems unless it is performed with the knees bent as in an inverted "V" or hook position. The outmoded straight-leg sit-up develops the psoas muscle. This powerful hip flexor tilts the pelvis forward unless it is counteracted by abdominal or other muscle groups. The curl-up is a good abdominal exercise, and the basket hang is useful for advanced abdominal training.

Toe Touches

Toe touches have been used with the erroneous belief that they exercise the abdominal muscles. As a hamstring or back muscle stretcher, toe touches are all right as long as you curl down slowly, avoid bouncing, and bend your knees. The slow, sitting toe touch is probably a better way to stretch the muscles on the back of the thigh, and the chair-sit toe touch may be a safer way to stretch tight back muscles.

Summary

This chapter has presented training tips; walking, running, and other training programs; aerobic alternatives; and advice on how to handle some common problems. You are welcome to adopt one of the programs, or to use your aerobic prescription and fashion your own approach. I'm often amazed by the ingenious and personal approaches that some folks devise—such as the retired zoology professor who regularly climbs the mountain behind our campus, both for exercise and to observe the flora and fauna. Years ago, before it was in vogue, he decided to utilize ski poles to exercise the arms while lowering the load on the legs. The poles become even more important on the return trip, relieving stress on the knees during the steep descent. His creative adaptation has extended his range and saved his knees for many more years of enjoyable outdoor exercise. Recently I've added a telescoping ski pole to my hiking and backpacking gear, and I wonder why I didn't do it years ago.

An addition to my personal program has been regular attention to muscular fitness. It too has helped me up and over many a steep trail. Let's see how it can help you.

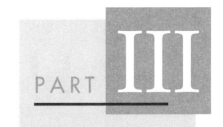

Muscular Fitness

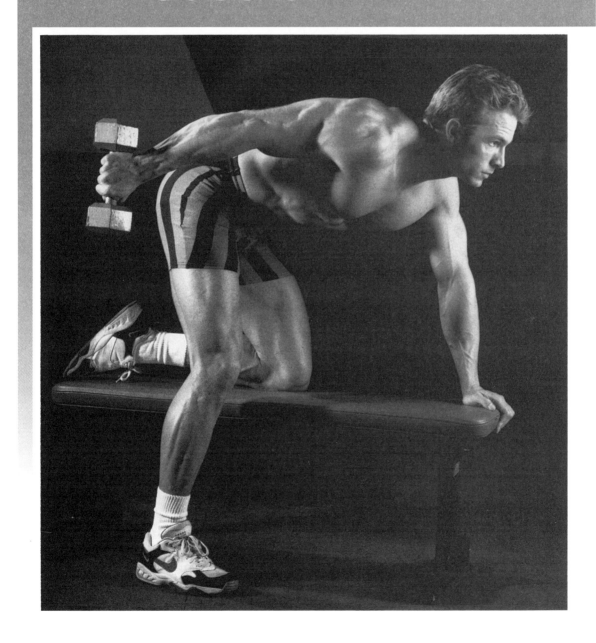

Until recently muscular fitness occupied an awkward position on the fringe of the fitness movement. We recognized its value in athletics and for some physically demanding jobs, but we lacked conclusive evidence linking muscular fitness with health and the quality of life. That has now changed, and we can say with confidence that both aerobic and muscular fitness contribute substantially to health. Muscular fitness increases muscle mass, the furnace that burns fat. Exercises that improve muscular fitness help you avoid the crippling bone demineralization known as osteoporosis. Attention to muscular fitness is essential if you are to avoid the low back problems that plague millions of Americans. And continued participation ensures the capacity for independence and mobility in postretirement years.

The essential components of muscular fitness are strength, muscular endurance, and flexibility. Other important components include power, speed, agility, and balance. As with most physiologic capabilities, you either use them or lose them, and that is certainly true for muscular fitness. Strength, endurance, flexibility, agility, and balance all decline with age. However, the rate of decline is much slower for people who remain active. And recent studies show that we have the capability to build strength even into our 90s!

But don't wait until you are 90 to experience the pleasures and rewards of muscular fitness. Begin now and you will soon notice that tasks are easier, your muscles are firmer, your tummy is flatter, and you just feel better about yourself and life.

CHAPTER 8

Understanding Muscular Fitness

"Enough work to do, and strength enough to do the work."

Rudyard Kipling

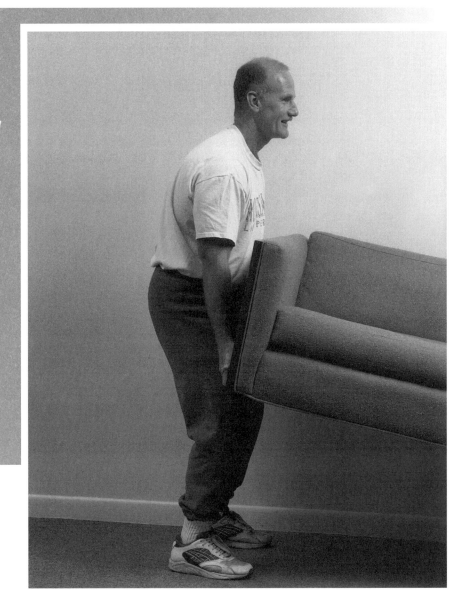

For many years muscular fitness occupied a tenuous position on the fringe of the fitness movement, due in part to images of overdeveloped, muscle-bound physiques. Now we can honestly say that aerobic and muscular fitness both contribute to health, but they do so in different ways and at different times. Young folks utilize muscular fitness to improve performance in a favorite sport or activity, or to look good in a bathing suit. Middle-aged individuals rely on abdominal tone and flexibility exercises to prevent or minimize low back problems. And older folks employ strength and endurance activities to retain bone density and to remain active and independent, capable of performing the essential activities of daily living. Again, muscular fitness is the key deterrent to low back problems that plague millions of people. In recent years we have learned that muscular fitness training (e.g., resistance or weight training) is a good way to avoid osteoporosis. And we've learned that muscular fitness helps maintain muscle to burn fat and to sustain mobility well into retirement years. So, if you intend to remain active after retirement, you'd better add muscular fitness training to your fitness program.

We begin with a consideration of the primary components of muscular fitness: strength, muscular endurance, and flexibility. They're called primary components because they are the ones most related to health. Other components, such as speed, power, agility, balance, and coordination, are covered later in the chapter.

THIS CHAPTER WILL HELP YOU

- identify the components of muscular fitness,
- understand the factors that influence strength,
- differentiate between strength and muscular endurance,
- understand the importance of flexibility, and
- determine how muscular fitness contributes to health, total fitness, and performance.

Strength

Strength is obviously important when your occupation demands it, in certain sports, and—it may be surprising—for those over 60 years of age. During the early part of our lives, as we age, strength declines at a slow pace, especially if it is used. But somewhere after 55 to 60 years, the decline becomes more rapid. Throughout life we need some strength to avoid acute or chronic injury, to meet emergencies, and to engage fully and independently in daily activities. It takes strength to change a flat tire; to shovel the walk; and to lift and carry infants, the laundry, or the groceries. Lack of muscular fitness leads to lack of activity, which hastens the loss of strength, and so on in a vicious cycle that ends in a nursing home. But you can reverse this vicious circle and remain strong and independent well into your eighth decade.

Strength is defined as the maximal force that can be exerted in a single *voluntary* contraction. Most of us possess more strength than we are able to demonstrate. In a fascinating experiment, Ikai and Steinhaus (1961) showed that significant increases in strength could be elicited with a gunshot, shouting, drugs,

Strength is defined as the maximal force that can be exerted in a single *voluntary* contraction.

or hypnosis during a contraction. Untrained individuals inhibit the full expression of strength. Inhibitions reside in the brain and in inhibitory muscle receptors. One effect of training is to reduce inhibitions and allow a fuller expression of available strength.

Strength, then, is not an absolute value. It is subject to change, and this is what makes strength training so interesting. When strength improves, how much is due to reduced inhibitions and how much to changes in the muscle tissue? Can we find a way to increase strength without spending a lot of time with weights?

Factors Influencing Strength

The force you exert in a maximal voluntary contraction depends on a number of factors, such as inhibitions, girth or cross-sectional area, the number of contracting fibers and their contractile state (length, fatigue), and the mechanical advantage of the bony lever system. Most of these are easy to explain. More fibers equal more girth and more force; the stretched muscle exerts more force (probably because of elastic recoil and a favorable alignment of contractile proteins); the unfatigued muscle exerts more force; and mechanical factors conspire to magnify force or speed. Several other influences, however, including gender, age, and fiber type deserve more attention.

Gender

Until 12 to 14 years of age, boys are not much stronger than girls. Thereafter, the average male gains an advantage that persists throughout life. Is the difference due to the increase in the male hormone testosterone at puberty? Perhaps; the average male has 10 times the testosterone found in the average female. Testosterone is an anabolic (growth-inducing) steroid that helps muscles get larger. College women have half the arm and shoulder strength of male counterparts and 30% less leg strength. But a relationship doesn't imply cause and effect. The relationship of strength and testosterone might also be related to a third factor. For example, the hormone may make the individual more aggressive and willing to train harder.

Consider another confounding possibility: body fat. Young women average twice the percentage of fat as men (25% versus 12.5%). When you look at strength per unit of lean body weight (body weight minus fat weight), women have slightly stronger legs, while arm strength remains 30% below the men's values. Wilmore (1983) suggests that since women use their legs as men do (to walk, climb stairs, bicycle), their leg muscles are similar in strength. However, since fewer women use their arms in heavy work or sport, their strength lags behind in this area. Thus, it is too early to judge women the weaker sex. As more women engage in upper body strength training for sport or occupational purposes (police work, fire fighting, construction), their strength may well come closer to that of men.

However, muscle size and strength do go together, for males and females, and the average male is larger than the average female. Most studies indicate a force of 4 to 6 kilograms per square centimeter of muscle girth, regardless of gender. To estimate muscle girth in the upper arm, you should measure subcutaneous fat and bone size as well, since they will be part of the total circumference. All other things being equal, the larger muscle is the stronger one, but not necessarily the most successful in work or sport.

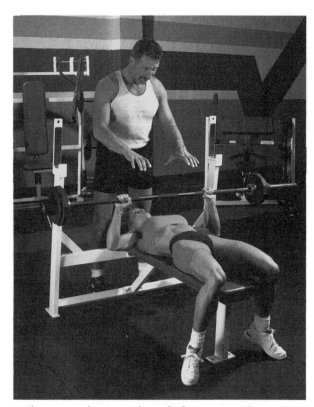

Both men and women benefit from strength training.

Age

Strength reaches a peak in the early 20s and declines slowly until age 60 or above. Thereafter the rate of decline usually accelerates, but it doesn't have to. When strength is used, it hardly declines at all, even into the 60s. Champion weight lifters have achieved personal records in their 40s. Mechanics retain grip strength into their 60s. Training before puberty leads to improvements that are mostly due to changes in the nervous system (neurogenic factors include reduced inhibitions and learning how to exert force). Training after puberty combines nervous system changes with changes in the muscle tissue (myogenic changes). Since testosterone levels decline in old age, many physiologists thought that senior citizens would be limited to neurogenic changes. However, a study of very elderly people (72-98 years) has shown that resistance training leads to increased strength, muscle mass, and mobility (Fiatarone et al., 1994). Training at any age maintains or improves strength, especially when the diet is adequate. We'll say more about both later on.

Muscle Fiber Types

I have discussed the presence of two fiber types: slow twitch and fast twitch. The larger, faster-contracting fast twitch fibers are capable of exerting more force. Individuals with a higher percentage of fast twitch fibers have a greater potential for force development. Studies of human muscle tissue reveal that weight lifters have twice the area of fast twitch fibers as nonlifters. The size can be attributed to heredity and to training. The effect of strength training on muscle fiber types has yet to be completely resolved; current evidence indicates that both types grow larger with training, but growth of the fast fibers is more pronounced. Strength training improves the capabilities of both types but doesn't seem to change one type into another.

Types of Strength

Strength can be measured and developed in several ways, each of which is highly specific. How the strength will be used should dictate the mode of training and testing.

Dynamic Strength

Also called isotonic, dynamic strength is defined as the maximal weight that can be lifted one time. This is actually a measure of strength at the hardest part of the lift, usually the beginning. Since the mechanical advantage of your muscle-lever system changes, the lift becomes easier after you overcome the initial resistance and angle of pull. Dynamic strength measurements are related to performance in sport and work. Weight lifting with weight machines or free weights is the common form of isotonic training. (*Iso* means "same," and *tonic* means "tone"; so *isotonic* means "same tone.")

Static Strength

The measure of static strength is achieved when one exerts maximal force against an immovable object. Also called isometric strength, it is specific to the angle at which it was trained; it doesn't tell much about dynamic strength or strength throughout the range of motion. Static contractions are used in rehabilitation, and to gain strength at the "sticking point" of a lift. (*Metric* means "length"; *isometric* means "same length.")

Isokinetic Strength

Isokinetic strength is measured with an expensive electronic or hydraulic apparatus. It allows display of force output throughout the range of motion. While such devices have become popular testing and training aids, it is not yet clear to what extent strength throughout the range of motion is related to performance. (*Kinetic* means "movement"; *isokinetic* implies movement at a fixed speed.)

A number of sophisticated devices are available for the measurement of muscle force and power. Sports medicine specialists evaluate knee extension and flexion strength, power, and endurance and then use isokinetic devices to rehabilitate athletes following knee surgery. Variable and accommodating resistance devices are used to strengthen muscles and to prevent injuries. Examples of these devices include variable resistance (resistance varies with speed of contraction) and accommodating resistance (resistance accommodates to available force). While each type of apparatus has some interesting features, no method or system has proven superior in the development of strength in subjects with little previous muscular fitness training. More experienced lifters will use the method suited to and specific for the task or activity. Athletes may use free weights, isokinetic machines, and even isometric contractions in an effort to improve performance. Strength is specific to the method of training, to the speed of contractions, and to the angle employed in training. Therefore, the method of testing should be specific to the mode of training if you want to accurately assess the effects of training. In other words, don't use a static strength test to reflect changes due to dynamic strength training, or vice versa.

Muscular Endurance

Muscular endurance means the ability to persist. It is defined and measured as the repetition of submaximal contractions or submaximal holding time (isometric endurance). Muscular endurance is essential for success in many work and athletic activities. Once you have the strength to perform a repetitive task, additional improvement in performance will depend on muscular endurance, the ability to persist. As you know, stronger fast twitch fibers fatigue more readily. Thus, endurance and strength are not highly related, except when a very heavy load is used in an endurance test.

> Muscular endurance is essential for success in many work and athletic activities.

Endurance and Strength

Let's spend a moment contrasting endurance and strength, which are really quite different in physiological terms. Endurance is achieved by repetitive contractions of muscle fibers. Repetitive contractions require a continuous supply of energy, and muscle fibers with aerobic capabilities (slow oxidative, fast-oxidative-glycolytic) are suited to the job. The repetitive contractions enhance anaerobic and aerobic enzymes, mitochondria, and fuels needed for endurance.

Strength comes from lifting heavy loads a few times. As explained, the effects of strength training are most noticeable in fast twitch fibers. Training effects include increases in contractile (contracting) proteins (actin and myosin) and tougher connective tissue. The increased strength comes from the increased cross-sectional area, which means more contractile protein to exert force. So the effects of endurance and strength training are quite different. Keep that in mind as you develop your program. Endurance is important for sustained practice, training, and performance. Repetition leads to skill, and repetition requires endurance, so endurance is often the key to success in sport or work.

Diet and Endurance

While training is certainly the best way to enhance endurance, there is something else you can do, something as simple as selecting the right foods. The fuel for muscular contractions depends on the intensity of exercise; muscle glycogen is the fuel used for high-intensity effort. But the supply of glycogen, the storage form of glucose, is limited in muscle, and when the supply is gone the muscle's performance drops to a level compatible with fat metabolism. That means long-duration, high-intensity endurance efforts such as a long, hard run

ENDURANCE?

I use the term *muscular endurance* to differentiate it from other uses of the term. It is possible to develop considerable endurance in small muscles, such as the finger flexors used by a pianist or barber, without having any noticeable effect on the heart or respiratory systems. My barber has great endurance in the muscles of his fingers, but his aerobic fitness is poor. Muscular endurance resides in metabolic adaptations and neuromuscular efficiency within the fibers used in the activity.

or bike ride will be enhanced if you have more glycogen stored in the working muscles. The food you eat can directly influence muscle glycogen levels and endurance performance.

In 1939 Scandinavian researchers (Christensen & Hansen, 1939) reported remarkable improvements in endurance for subjects who were fed a high-carbohydrate diet. That study virtually went unnoticed for years as coaches and trainers continued to order high-protein meals for athletes. More recently, the muscle biopsy technique has been used to study the influence of exercise and diet on endurance performance, and a series of studies has led to several firm conclusions: The best endurance performances are always attained on the high-carbohydrate diet; average performance on a typical mixed diet; and the worst performances on the low-carbohydrate (high fat and protein) diet.

Smart athletes follow the high-performance (high-carbohydrate) diet that is good for fitness, performance, and health. It includes

- 25% of total calories from fat
- 15% from protein
- 60% from carbohydrate

Compare that with the average American diet of 35 to 40%, 15%, and 45% from fat, protein, and carbohydrate respectively. The carbohydrate I advocate is called complex carbohydrate, in contrast to the simple carbohydrate (e.g., refined sugar) found in junk food. Complex carbos include corn, rice, beans, potatoes, and whole-grain products (breads, pasta). They are a good source of energy and, unlike refined sugar, include other nutrients and fiber. Together with fresh fruits, they constitute the basis of the high-performance diet. Unless you're involved in an endurance event, the diet provides all you'll need.

Flexibility

Flexibility is the range of motion through which the limbs are able to move. Skin, connective tissue, and conditions within joints restrict the range of motion, as does excessive body fat. Injury occurs when a limb is forced beyond its normal range, so improved flexibility reduces this potential.

The range of motion increases when joints and muscles are warmed.

The range of motion increases when joints and muscles are warmed. Stretching exercises are most successful after some warm-up but before vigorous effort. Stretching after exercise, during the cooldown period, may help reduce subsequent muscle soreness. Flexibility exercises are important when you are training for strength or endurance. They help you to maintain the range of motion that might otherwise be reduced. Most runners turn to stretching to make the pastime more enjoyable. Calf, hamstring, groin, and back muscles can become tight and sore, especially after an increase in intensity or duration of training, and daily stretching can mean the difference between enjoyment and discomfort.

Yoga has gained popularity as a way to achieve relaxation and meditative states. Years ago, yoga positions were viewed as painful contortions, tortuous exaggerations on the lunatic fringe of exercise. But today, stripped of its mystical elements, yoga has emerged as a safe, enjoyable, and relaxing flexibility program. Note that the benefits are limited to flexibility; there is little evidence to support claims of improved aerobic fitness or significant gains in strength or endurance.

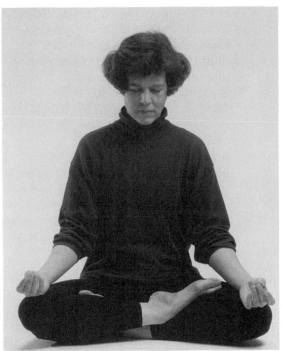

Yoga has emerged as a safe, enjoyable, and relaxing flexibility program.

Flexibility contributes to success in work and sport. Lack of flexibility is implicated in the development of acute and chronic injuries and low back problems. All of us profit from regular stretching exercises, and older folks have a special need, since connective tissue becomes less elastic with age.

Other Components of Muscular Fitness

In addition to strength, endurance, and flexibility, muscular fitness includes speed, power, agility, balance, and neuromuscular coordination or skill. While these attributes are often important to success in sport or work, and may help one to avoid serious injury (especially agility and balance), they are not believed to be health-related components of muscular fitness.

Speed and Power

Both speed and power are important and related components of most sports. Both are somewhat related to muscular strength, and both can be improved.

Speed

Speed may be the most exciting ingredient in sport. Total speed of movement includes reaction time and movement time. Reaction time (the time from the stimulus—such as a starting gun—till the beginning of the movement) is a function of the nervous system. We can't change the speed of nerve impulse transmission along a neuron. Thus, any significant improvement in reaction time must be achieved by increasing awareness of appropriate stimuli and by repetition of appropriate responses, which reduces central nervous system processing time. In sports, coaches use special drills to improve reaction time.

Movement time, the interval from the beginning to the end of the movement, may often be improved (decreased) with appropriate strength training. The key to success lies in the principle of specificity: The movement must be specific to the sport. If you want to throw a baseball with greater velocity, train with light weights at a fast speed. If you are a shot putter, throw heavier weights as fast as possible. Specificity applies to the rate of movement and the resistance employed, which means that the training should simulate the action as closely as possible.

How much can you improve? Remember what I've said about fast twitch fibers: You'll need a high percentage to be fast. However, if you don't have more than 50% fast fibers, don't despair. You may never be as fast as those who do, but you can improve your movement time by following the principles presented in the next chapter. Also, don't conclude that continued improvements in strength will always lead to improvements in movement time; strength is more related to speed when the movement is resisted (as in football, shot put, etc.). And remember that speed, like strength, is extremely task-specific. The speed of arm movement, for example, is not necessarily related to the leg speed. Some people may be quick with their hands but, because of lack of training or skill or because of excess fat, may be slow of foot. Improved skill and strength training reduce the time it takes to complete a movement.

Power

Power is something football coaches often talk about. A lineman needs explosive power to move his opponent. But power is also important in other sports, such as cycling and cross-country skiing. Power is defined as work divided by time, or the rate of doing work.

$$\text{Power} = \frac{\text{Force} \times \text{Distance}}{\text{Time}} \left(\frac{F \times D}{T} \right) = \text{Force} \times \text{Velocity} \left(\text{Velocity} = \frac{D}{T} \right)$$

It combines strength (force) and velocity or speed (distance/time). A person who is able to do more work than another in the same unit of time has more power. If I move 100 kilograms 1 meter in 1 second, I've done 100 kilogram meters of work per second. If you move the same load 2 meters in 1 second or 1 meter in half a second, you've exhibited twice as much power. Thus, power is related to movement time; improve movement time and you'll increase power, or vice versa.

Power is important in a number of sports, but it is seldom required of nonathletic adults. If you want to increase your power for cycling, skiing, basketball, or some other sport, remember the principle of specificity. Even runners can increase power by running uphill, running against resistance, or using high-speed repetitions in weight training. I'll provide a power prescription in chapter 10.

Agility

Agility is the ability to change position and direction rapidly, with precision and without loss of balance. It depends on strength, speed, balance, and coordination. Agility is undeniably important in the world of sport, but it is also useful if you hope to avoid embarrassment or injury in recreational activities, and in potentially dangerous work situations. Since agility is associated with specific skills, no one test predicts agility for all situations. It can be improved with practice and experience. Excess weight hinders agility for obvious reasons. Extreme strength isn't a prerequisite, nor is aerobic fitness; however, since agility deteriorates with fatigue, aerobic and muscular fitness should help maintain agility for extended periods, such as a long tennis match.

Balance

Dynamic balance is the ability to maintain equilibrium during vigorous movements. Balance depends on the ability to integrate visual input with information from the semicircular canals in the inner ear, and from muscle receptors. It is difficult to measure and predict how dynamic balance contributes to or detracts from sport performance. Evidence indicates that balance can be improved through participation in sports and a variety of movement experiences, especially during childhood. Since it is likely that balance is also task-specific, practice of the specific activity should be the best way to improve balance and performance.

Having football or basketball players engage in aerobic dance or ballet classes is likely to result in a profound cultural experience, for both the players and the teacher, and it is sure to make the athletes better dancers. However, whether or not it will improve their performance on the field or court has yet to be demonstrated. It is safe to say that few, if any, of the top basketball professionals developed their moves around an arabesque, entrechat, or glissade. And none I've seen shoot fouls in the fifth position!

Coordination or Skill

Coordination implies a harmonious relationship, a smooth union or flow of movement in the execution of a task. In striking the tennis serve, one develops force sequentially. As momentum from body turn approaches its peak, the arm extends at the elbow, and maximum racquet speed is finally achieved with the snap of the wrist. If the forces are added in the wrong sequence, the movement appears uncoordinated.

Coordination or skill is achieved with hours of practice. Repetition of a skill leads to decreases in synaptic resistance in the nervous system, increasing the likelihood and accuracy of the practiced movement, and eventually making the movement automatic. It is important to practice properly; repetition of the wrong movement will lead to formation of a habit that is hard to break. Seek professional instruction as you endeavor to improve your skill.

Because every skill is specific, each must be learned individually. Ability in tennis doesn't assure success in badminton, squash, or racquetball; skill doesn't transfer readily from one sport to another. Another feature of coordination or skill will become apparent as you train for fitness: Skilled individuals work efficiently—they don't waste movement or energy. A skilled runner uses less energy at a given speed. A skilled worker often can outproduce a stronger or more fit co-worker. Skill, coordination, and technique can be learned. With proper skill we make best use of leverage and large muscle groups, thereby avoiding injury and fatigue of smaller muscles.

Because every skill is specific, each must be learned individually.

Muscular Fitness Tests

You may wonder how you stack up in terms of muscular fitness. If so, you can assess your muscular fitness with some simple tests (see table 8.1). The tests provide an indication of your current status and provide a benchmark for future comparisons. Select the component of muscular fitness you wish to evaluate (e.g., strength or speed) and the part of the body to be tested (upper body, trunk, legs). Compare your score with typical values for young men and women as categorized in the table. The muscle fiber type estimation may help you understand your capabilities and select activities suited to them. Note that chin-ups, push-ups and sit-ups are in repetitions; leg strength is in pounds; vertical jump is in inches; and, of course, aerobic fitness is in ml/kg · min.

Be sure to warm up and do some stretching before you attempt a vigorous test. Or you may prefer to engage in some training before you perform the tests. The chapters that follow describe the effects of training and provide proven training prescriptions to help you improve your scores.

Summary

I've introduced the components of muscular fitness and discussed their contributions to health and performance. I hope you have decided to integrate muscular fitness into your activity program. You won't be sorry you did. With improved muscular fitness I'm better able to do yard work, to hike with a pack, to peddle or run uphill, to paddle a canoe, to cross-country and downhill ski, and more. And the effects are more pronounced with every passing year. See what muscular fitness can do for you!

TABLE 8.1   Muscular Fitness Tests

			Men			Women		
			Low	Medium	High	Low	Medium	High
Upper body	Strength	Chin-up[a]	< 6	6-10	> 10	< 20	20-30	> 30
	Endurance	Push-up	< 20	20-40	> 40	< 10	10-20	> 20
Trunk	Endurance	Sit-up	< 30	30-50	> 50	< 25	25-40	> 40
Leg	Strength	Leg press	< 400	400-550	> 550	< 300	300-450	> 450
Flexibility (Sit & reach)	Reach toes		No	Yes	Beyond	No	Yes	Beyond
Power	Vertical jump		< 17	17-23	> 23	< 10	10-15	> 15
Speed (50 yd)	Seconds		> 7.5	7.5-6.0	< 6.0	> 9.0	9.0-7.5	< 7.5
Muscle fiber type estimation								
Fast twitch	Vertical jump		< 17	17-23	> 23	< 10	10-15	> 15
Slow twitch	Aerobic fitness (1 mi walk or 1.5-mi run)		< 40	40-60	> 60	< 35	35-50	> 50

[a]Women do modified chin-up.

CHAPTER 9

Benefits of Muscular Fitness

"... power waits
upon him who
earns it."
John Burroughs

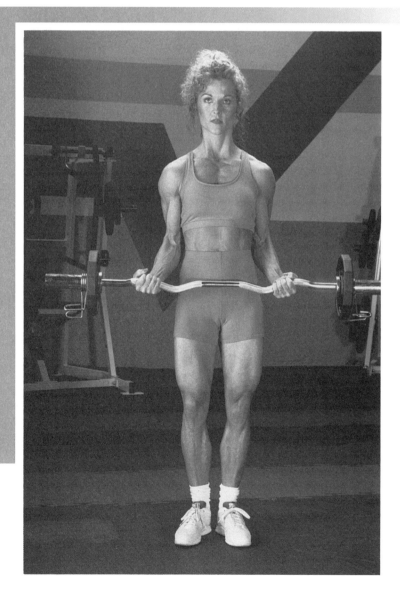

How does training lead to changes in the muscles? How does a muscle fiber know the difference between strength and endurance training? Part of the answer to these questions is related to the training stimulus, the characteristic of training that leads to specific adaptations. Strength improves when sufficient *tension* is applied to the muscle fiber and its contractile proteins. The tension required seems to be above two-thirds of the muscle's maximal force. If you do contractions that require less tension, you won't gain much strength. Contraction *time*, the total number of contractions—or metabolism—also seems to influence the development of strength (Smith & Rutherford, 1995). Do more contractions, and you obtain better results, up to a point. The number of contractions probably depends on your level of training, nutrition, and your hereditary endowment. You will receive benefits from any form of strength training, as long as you exert enough tension for a sufficient number of repetitions (or time).

THIS CHAPTER WILL HELP YOU

- understand how a bout of training leads to changes in muscles,
- identify the specific changes that result from strength or endurance training,
- recognize the importance of flexibility exercises,
- understand how to minimize muscle soreness, and
- see how speed and power training improve performance.

The Training Stimulus

In training we often speak of the overload principle, which states:

- For improvements to take place, workloads have to impose a demand (overload) on the body system (above two-thirds of maximal force for strength).
- As adaptation to loading takes place, more load must be added.
- Improvements are related to the intensity (tension for strength), duration (repetitions), and frequency of training.

Overload training leads to adaptations in the muscles according to the type of training. Here again, the principle of specificity applies, as it did with aerobic training. The adaptation to strength training includes increased size, due to increases in contractile proteins (actin and myosin) and tougher connective tissue. These and other adaptations allow the muscle to exert more force.

The specific adaptations to muscular endurance training include improved aerobic enzyme systems, larger and more numerous mitochondria (increased mitochondrial density), and more capillaries. All these changes promote oxygen delivery and utilization within the muscle fiber, thereby improving endurance (Jackson & Dickinson, 1988). Fatiguing repetitions somehow stimulate the muscle fiber to become better adapted to use oxygen and aerobic enzymes for the production of energy (ATP) to sustain contractions. Do many repetitions, and you become better able to use fat as a source of energy.

Table 9.1 reviews the effects of each type of training. It shows that high-resistance training leads to the development of strength and that low-resistance repetitions lead to muscular endurance, and suggests that there are still

TABLE 9.1   The Strength-Endurance Continuum

	Strength	Short-term (anaerobic) endurance	Intermediate endurance	Long-term endurance
For	Maximum force	Brief (2-3 min) persistence with heavy load	Persistence with intermediate load	Persistence with lighter load
Prescription	6-8 RM 3 sets	15-25 RM 3 sets	30-50 RM 2 sets	Over 100 RM 1 set
Improves	Contractile protein (actin and myosin) ATP and CP Connective tissue	Some strength and anaerobic metabolism (glycolysis)	Some endurance and anaerobic metabolism Slight improvement in strength (for untrained)	Aerobic enzymes Mitochondria Oxygen and fat utilization
Doesn't improve	Oxygen intake Endurance	Oxygen intake		Strength

RM = repetitions maximum
ATP = adenosine triphosphate
CP = creatine phosphate

questions regarding the effects of training that falls between strength (high resistance/low repetitions) and endurance (low resistance and high repetitions). Use the table to help reach your training goals.

Strength Training

Strength will certainly help you lead an active and vigorous life, well beyond retirement years.

Strength contributes to performance in work and sport, and strength training puts stresses on bones that reduce the risk of osteoporosis. Strength training can also be used to improve your appearance and, within limits, your shape. And strength will certainly help you lead an active and vigorous life, well beyond retirement years. How does this simple mode of exercise get such remarkable results?

Strength training, sometimes called resistance training, involves high resistance and low repetitions, and leads to increased contractile protein (actin and myosin), tougher connective tissue, contractile efficiency and reduced inhibitions, and possible increase in number of muscle fibers.

Contractile Protein

Some years ago, Gordon (1967) compared the effects of strength and endurance training on muscle proteins. The results have since been corroborated in labs throughout the world. Strength training adds to the portion of the muscle that generates tension, the contractile proteins, while endurance training enhances the energy supply system, the aerobic enzymes (all enzymes are constructed of proteins). But the most surprising outcome of his study was the observation that strength training brings about a decline in endurance enzyme, and that endurance training led to a decline in contractile protein. Thus, if you

THE STIMULUS

Just how the strength or endurance training stimuli bring about the appropriate changes is not entirely known. But from what is known about how cells work, it is likely that the training stimulus signals the nucleus to make messenger RNA (mRNA). This messenger is shaped by the DNA and sent into the muscle fiber to order the production of protein (contractile protein for strength training, aerobic enzyme protein for endurance training). Structures in the muscle fiber called ribosomes receive the message and begin to produce the protein needed to adapt to the training stimulus. Another RNA (transfer RNA, or tRNA) is used to gather up the amino acids needed to construct the protein, bring them to the ribosome, and place them in the growing chain of amino acids that become a specific protein. Since RNA is formed by DNA, the training stimulus must somehow influence the nucleus. Because we don't know if the nucleus is signaled by tension, electrolytes, metabolic waste products, or hormones, we are unable to trick the muscle into getting stronger or building endurance without training. So, you'll have to pursue the prescriptions in chapter 10 to improve your muscular strength or endurance.

train for only strength or endurance, you could lose a bit of the other. This aspect of specificity shouldn't be so surprising—the size and strength of thigh muscles increase during cycling or ski seasons but decline when you return to distance running.

Connective Tissue

Connective tissue and tendons grow in size and toughness when they are placed under tension. This increased toughness in tendons may help quiet the inhibitory influence of the muscle receptor known as the tendon organ. The increase in thickness of connective tissue contributes to the overall growth, or hypertrophy, of the muscle.

Nervous System

Some of the effects of strength training occur in the nervous system. With experience we seem to have fewer inhibitions, both in the central nervous system and from muscle receptors. Practice (repetition) allows us to be more efficient, more skilled in the application of force. Thus, practice alone accounts for some of the improvements in the early stages of training. This may explain why involuntary contractions brought on by an electrical stimulator do not equal the results obtained with voluntary contractions. Involuntary contractions may elicit changes in the muscle, but they don't teach the nervous system how to contract (Massey, Nelson, Sharkey, & Comden, 1965).

Muscle Fibers

The ability to look at samples of human muscle before and after training has led to some fascinating questions. Can strength training lead to the formation of additional muscle fibers?

Studies on human muscle suggest that we may be able to increase the number of muscle fibers, when overloaded fibers split to form new fibers. However, this finding is still the subject of scientific debate. And I would never suggest that you will form new fibers as the result of ordinary strength training. But for those athletes who spend hours each day lifting weights, or for those who use anabolic steroids to promote unnatural growth, increased fibers may be possible.

The available evidence does suggest some differences between the high-resistance/low-volume training of power lifters and the medium-resistance/high-volume training of body builders. The high-resistance training seems to increase the size (hypertrophy) of fast twitch fibers, while the medium-resistance/high-volume training causes selective hypertrophy of slow twitch fibers (Tesch, Thorsson, & Kaiser, 1984). Here again the response seems to be specific to the type of training.

NEW FIBERS?

For years we believed that the number of muscle fibers was set at birth and was not subject to change. Then Van Linge (1962) transplanted the tendon of a small rat muscle into a position where it would have to assume a tremendous workload. After a period of heavy training, he studied the rat muscle and found that the transplanted muscle had doubled its weight and tripled its strength. Furthermore, the heavy workload stimulated the development of new muscle fibers.

Endurance Training

Endurance training, which involves low resistance and high repetitions, leads to increased aerobic enzymes and mitochondria, increased capillaries, and more efficient contractions. I've already mentioned the effects of endurance training on aerobic enzymes, particularly those involved in fat metabolism, on mitochondria, and on capillaries. More efficient aerobic pathways are able to provide more energy from fat, thereby conserving muscle glycogen and blood glucose, which is needed by the nervous system. As a result, muscles that once fatigued in minutes become able to endure for hours. Some of the effects of endurance training take place in the nervous system. Skilled, more efficient movements conserve energy, thereby contributing to endurance. But the most documented effects of muscular endurance training seem to focus on the muscle fibers.

FIBER TYPE TRANSFORMATION

Recent evidence suggests that the aerobic enzyme improvements noted in endurance training may be a stage in the eventual transformation of fast twitch to slow twitch fibers. Pette (1984) has reported metabolic (enzyme) and then structural changes in muscle following prolonged endurance training (electrical stimulation). In studies of rat and rabbit muscle, fast-twitch fibers first take on the oxidative capabilities and eventually assume the contractile properties of slow twitch fibers. We do not yet know if these fiber type changes occur in humans.

Successful distance runners have as much as 80% slow twitch fibers. Is that due to fiber type transformation or to heredity? At present it appears that endurance training can improve the aerobic or oxidative capabilities of all fibers, and that fast twitch fibers become more able to utilize oxygen. These studies do show that muscle is extremely adaptable and is able to adjust to the demands imposed upon it.

Short Versus Long Muscles

Did you ever hear that running gives you short muscles, while swimming gives you long ones? The truth is that the length of a muscle is fixed by its bony attachments. Running on the toes can develop the size of the calf muscle, but it isn't likely to shorten the muscle itself. Similarly, the long muscle belly seen in the calf of the swimmer could be a product of specific swim training, but it is also possible that the difference existed before training, and that it had something to do with the athlete's success in the sport.

Methods of Training

If you want to gain strength to improve performance in work or sport, your training should be specific to your goal.

What is the best way to train for strength or endurance: isometric, isotonic, or isokinetic methods? The answer depends on what you are training to accomplish, the goal of your training. If you just want to get stronger, almost any method will work. If you want to gain strength to improve performance in work or sport, your training should be specific to your goal. We conducted a study in which college women trained with weights (isotonic), isokinetic devices, or calisthenics. The isotonic group did best on lifting tests, and the calisthenics group scored best on calisthenics tests. The isokinetic training group, which gained strength on the isokinetic devices, came in third on the other two tests. This study showed how important it is to train in the manner in which the strength will eventually be used (Sharkey, Wilson, Whiddon, & Miller, 1978).

Isometric Training

Also called static contractions, isometrics were the rage of the early 1960s. Professional athletes were using the technique that promised dramatic results in just 6 seconds a day (most unproven techniques resort to the use of celebrity claims to try to fool unsuspecting consumers). Based on an early study conducted in Germany (Hettinger & Müller, 1953), the technique was popular until studies finally compared isometrics with traditional weight lifting, and isometrics came in a distant second. Isometric contractions don't provide a sense of increased strength, they elevate blood pressure, and they are seldom specific to the training goal. Isometrics do have some uses: In rehabilitation, when that is all that can be done; for work at the sticking point of a lift; and in activities in which static strength or endurance is required (e.g., archery). More recently, isometrics have been used in conjunction with weight lifting to get better results. The weight is lifted and held against an immovable object for several counts in a technique known as functional isometrics.

Isotonic Training

Isotonic contractions (weight lifting) were established when DeLorme and Watkins (1951) outlined a formula for success. Simply stated, the formula called for high-resistance/low-repetition exercise. Variations of that formula are still used to develop dynamic strength. Since the resistance is high only at one point of the lift (usually the start), there has been some question about the value of the technique. Isotonic programs compare well with isokinetic training, especially when tested on isotonic tests. Free weights and weight machines are readily available in most health clubs. And weight lifting with free weights remains the method of choice for most serious athletes and body builders. While fitness buffs usually lift 3 days per week, serious athletes increase the strength training stimulus by doing five or more sets of each exercise and by training 5 or 6 days per week.

Isokinetic Training

Isokinetic exercises combine the best features of isometric (near maximal force) and isotonic (full range of motion) training. With the appropriate device it is possible to overload the muscles with a near maximal contraction throughout the range of motion, and to control the speed of contraction. Theoretically, this method should lead to strength throughout the range of motion. The problem, if there is one, seems to be the lack of specific devices for many sports skills (see figure 9.1). But as more devices are developed for specific sports, isokinetic training will become even more popular.

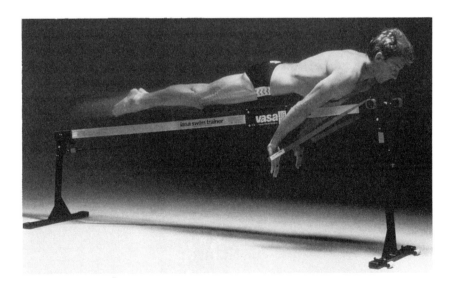

Figure 9.1   The swim bench provides a sport-specific way to train.

Which Method Is Best?

There is no best method for strength or endurance training. Free weights are inexpensive and versatile but require more supervision for safety and to prevent theft. Weight machines are convenient and require less supervision. More expensive isokinetic devices are effective but limited in application. Isokinetic variations (variable resistance, accommodating resistance) are popular in health clubs. They are useful for fitness and sport and have one special advantage: Unlike weight lifting, isokinetic training doesn't cause muscle soreness. Thus, it can be done in conjunction with other activities without adversely affecting performance.

A note of caution before we go on: Be sure the training program you adopt is appropriate to your level of fitness and ability. What is best for beginners doesn't work for athletes, and vice versa. In psychology many theories are based on research conducted on college freshmen and rats. In exercise physiology, numerous studies have been conducted on "gym rats," college students enrolled in activity classes. When various forms of strength training are compared on gym rats, they all seem to yield similar results; in other words, follow the prescription and anything works—with beginners. But that doesn't predict how the method will work on athletes or others with higher levels of strength. And it doesn't prove that the increased strength will improve performance. We know how to improve strength; now we need to find out how much is needed to improve performance, and how best to train to get results (chapter 10).

Flexibility

To consider the effect of training on range of motion, first we must consider the limits of flexibility. Muscles are covered with tough connective tissue, and this tissue is a major restriction to the range of motion, as are the joint capsule and tendons. Training, therefore, must concentrate on altering these limits. Flexibility decreases with age and inactivity. Some injuries may be more likely as flexibility decreases, and low back problems are associated with poor flexibility (back, hamstrings) and weak abdominal muscles. On the other hand, enhanced flexibility may improve performance in some sports, especially those with obvious flexibility components (gymnastics, diving, wrestling).

Increased muscle and joint temperatures increase flexibility, as do specific stretching exercises. Stretching gradually leads to minor distensions in connective tissue, and the summation of these small changes can be a dramatically improved range of motion.

In the past, flexibility exercises conjured up images of vigorous bobbing and jerking movements, but times have changed. Today we engage in static stretching or, at most, light bobbing movements. The reason for the change is the stretch reflex. Rapid stretch invokes a stretch reflex, and the reflex calls forth a vigorous contraction of the stretched muscle. Since a vigorous contraction is the opposite of what we are seeking, we must forget this rapid, forceful, or ballistic (bouncing) stretching and learn the gentle art and science of static stretching.

Static Stretching

Static stretching involves slow movements to reach a point of stretch, holding the position (5 to 10 seconds), and relaxing. The stretch may be repeated, and very light bobbing may be employed. A variation of the static stretch is the contract/relax technique. Do a static stretch, relax, then contract the muscle for a few seconds. Then repeat the static stretch. When performed on muscles such as those in the calf, the technique seems to help the muscle relax so you can better stretch the tendon. These methods are at least as effective as dynamic stretching, and they provide other advantages such as low risk of injury and reduction of tightness and lingering muscle soreness.

Warm up a bit with light exercise or calisthenics, then do your stretching. Finish the warm-up with more vigorous effort, or if you prefer, begin your run or other exercise at a slow pace. Never substitute skill rehearsal, such as tennis strokes, for stretching. Do your warm-up and stretching before you begin to compete. When flexibility training is done correctly, the results are quite persistent. Your improved range of motion should remain for at least 8 weeks. But once you have learned to enjoy stretching, you may get hooked on its subtle sensations and move on to esoteric forms such as yoga. If not, just remember to do the stretches you need to minimize soreness, to reduce the risk of injury, and to avoid low back problems.

Muscle Soreness

Delayed onset muscle soreness (DOMS) becomes evident 24 hours after you overdo.

The muscle soreness that becomes evident 24 hours after you overdo (delayed onset muscle soreness, or DOMS) may be due to slight tears in connective tissue, to uncontrolled contractions or spasms of individual muscle fibers, to muscle fiber damage, or to the lingering effects of metabolic by-products. We are reasonably certain that soreness is not due to leftover lactic acid; that by-product is eliminated within an hour of the cessation of effort. We do know that certain types of exercise (but not isokinetic) lead to soreness that often persists for days and that can make subsequent activity less enjoyable. Komi and Buskirk (1972) compared two types of strength training: concentric (as in ordinary flexion) and eccentric (the muscle is under high tension as it lowers an overload). Subjects in the eccentric group, the group that lowered the weight, complained of muscle soreness, while the other group did not. So, if you begin a weight training program and plan to lower the weights, be prepared for some soreness.

Soreness can be diminished by beginning with light weights and progressing gradually. Avoid maximal lifting, all-out running, or ballistic movements such as hard throwing or serving, at the start of the season. It's important to be patient. But experience shows that we are seldom patient enough; therefore, we need a way to reduce soreness. Stretching has been shown to reduce muscle soreness (deVries, 1986), so stretch before and after exercise, and whenever you feel discomfort. If your legs are stiff and sore during a long flight, go to the rear

ECCENTRIC TRAINING

You may be surprised to know that the eccentric group in the Komi & Buskirk study gained a bit more strength than the concentric group, a common finding in eccentric training studies, probably because you can let down more weight than you can lift (hence, the muscle is under more tension). But before you get excited about eccentric training, remember what I keep saying about specificity: Unless your sport or job calls for letting down heavy loads, the training may not help performance as much as regular weight training, and you are certain to get muscle soreness with eccentric contractions.

of the plane and stretch. If other passengers see you trying to push down the wall of the galley, don't be embarrassed. Fitness enthusiasts will understand that you are experiencing the pleasure and relief of a good static stretch.

Muscle soreness is correlated with submicroscopic muscle damage, accumulation of fluid (edema), and diminished strength that may persist for up to 2 weeks. The damage may be to older or otherwise susceptible muscle fibers. Recovery is faster and soreness is diminished after successive bouts of exercise. Leakage of the muscle enzyme creatine kinase (CK) into the circulation, as determined by a blood test, suggests membrane damage. Since the soreness peaks 1 to 2 days after the effort, and the enzyme levels peak 2 to 3 days later, the actual cause of the muscle soreness is still unclear (Armstrong, 1984). What follows is inflammation and a repair stage that leads to recovery. Fortunately, DOMS occurs only during the start-up phase, and the symptoms disappear within a few weeks and reappear only after a long layoff followed by the vigorous start of a new activity.

Flexibility Exercises

The following 11 stretching and warm-up exercises can be used in your muscular fitness program. Remember to perform each stretch in a slow, smooth movement, rather than bouncing. Continue breathing normally throughout each exercise. Stretch both at the beginning of an exercise session to prepare the muscles for the more rigorous activity to follow, and at the end to reduce soreness.

SEATED TOE TOUCH

This exercise will stretch the back and hamstrings. With toes pointed, slowly slide your hands down the legs until you feel a stretch; hold the position. Grasp your ankles, and slowly pull until your head approaches your legs. Relax. Draw toes back, and slowly attempt to touch your toes. Repeat several times. For variety, you can try the toe touch with legs apart.

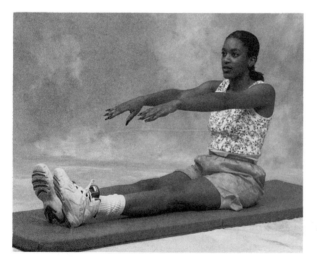 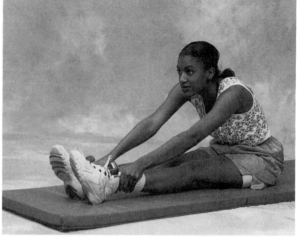

SINGLE KNEE PULL

This stretches the thigh and trunk. Pull your leg to the chest with your arms, and hold for a count of 5. Repeat with the opposite leg. Perform 8 to 10 times on each leg. As a variation, you can use a double knee pull (see page 197).

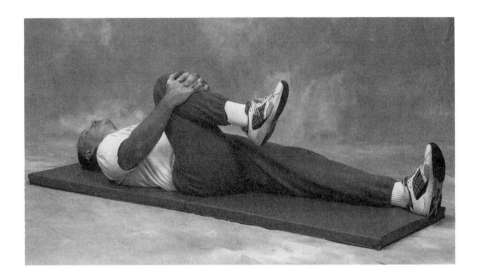

ANKLE PULL

This stretches the groin and inner thighs. Pull on your ankles while pressing the legs down with your elbows. For variety, you may lean forward and try to touch your head to your feet or the floor.

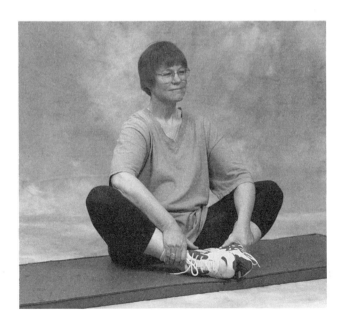

STRIDE STRETCH

This exercise works the calf and thigh muscles. Slowly slide into a stride position with the front foot flat on the floor, knee aligned over ankle, and rear foot on toes. Put your hands on a chair or the floor for balance. Hold for 10 counts. Switch legs.

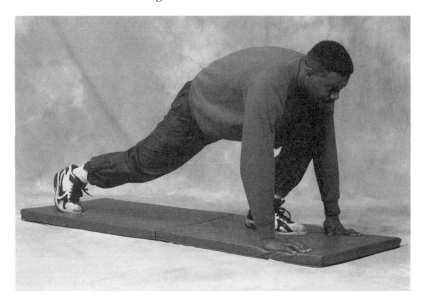

WALL STRETCH

This stretches the calf muscles. Stand 3 feet from the wall, feet slightly apart. Put both hands on the wall. With your heels on the ground, lean forward slowly and feel the stretch in your calves. Hold the position for 15 to 20 seconds. Repeat several times.

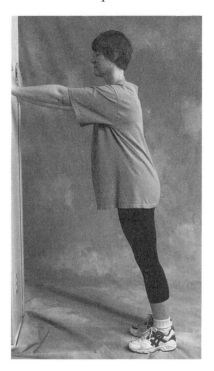
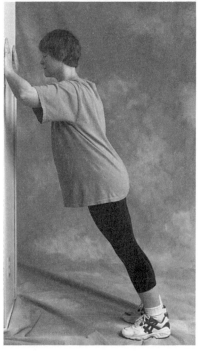

FLEXED LEG-BACK STRETCH

This exercise stretches the muscles in the legs and back. Stand erect, feet shoulder-width apart. With knees slightly flexed, slowly bend over, touching the ground between the feet. Hold for 10 seconds. Repeat several times.

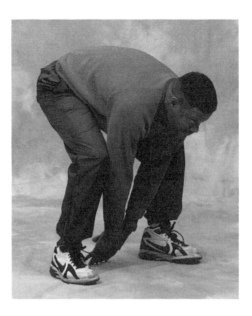

SIDE BENDER

This exercise stretches the trunk. Extend one arm overhead, the other on your hip, and keep your knees slightly bent. Slowly bend to the side; bob gently. Repeat 5 times on each side.

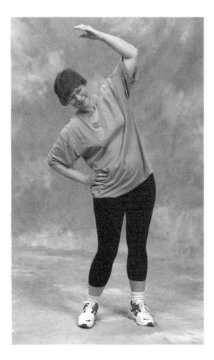 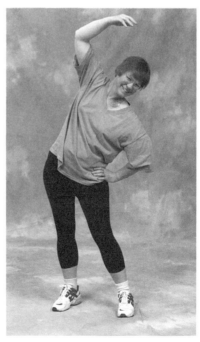

SIDE TWISTER

This stretches the trunk. With your feet comfortably apart, extend the arms palm down. Twist to one side as far as possible. Repeat to other side; do 5 repetitions on each side.

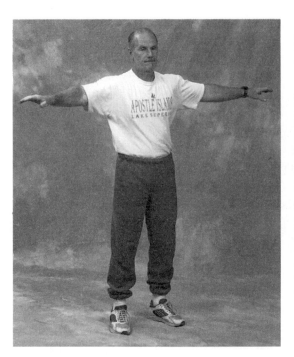 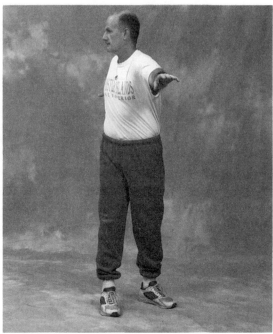

ELBOW THRUST

This stretches the shoulder and back. Keep your feet apart, arms bent, hands in front of the chest, and elbows out to the side. Without arching your back, rhythmically thrust your elbows backward, then return to the starting position. Repeat 15 times.

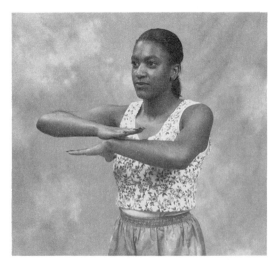 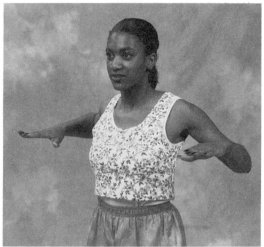

JUMPING JACKS

These stretch arms and legs and warm up the muscles. Hold your arms at the sides. On count 1, jump and spread your feet apart while simultaneously swinging your arms over your head. On count 2, return to the starting position. Use a rhythmic, moderate cadence. Repeat 15 to 25 times.

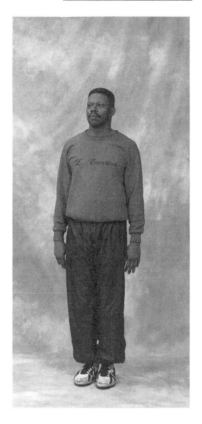
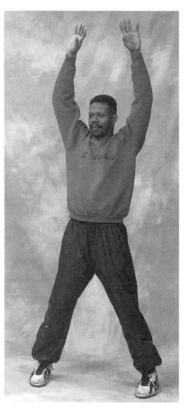

RUNNING IN PLACE

Start slowly, then increase the rate, the height of your leg lift, or both. As training progresses, run in place between subsequent conditioning exercises.

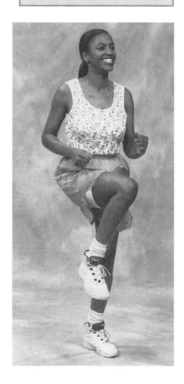

Speed and Power

Years ago, as I was attempting to make some sense of the confusing and sometimes contradictory research on strength and speed, I noticed that strength and speed seemed to be related when heavy loads were used in the test of speed. When little resistance was used, strength and speed were not related. In an effort to generalize the findings to other areas of work and sport, I turned to a well-known physiological principle, the force-velocity relationship.

Force-Velocity Relationship

It has long been known that velocity of shortening in a contraction is greatest with no load or resistance. As the resistance is increased, the velocity of shortening decreases (see figure 9.2). I thought the force-velocity relationship could help simplify basic principles about how and why muscles should be trained for force, speed, or power. From reading the available literature I concluded that strength training would improve heavily loaded movements but would have little effect on the velocity of unloaded movements, and speed training would improve the velocity of unloaded movements with little effect on heavy loads. I was delighted when I happened upon studies that confirmed my hypotheses!

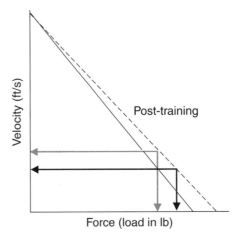

Figure 9.2 Strength training and the force-velocity relationship. The benefits of strength training are more pronounced in events involving loaded or resisted movements.

Ikai (1970) demonstrated that training for strength alone led to increased strength and velocity with heavy loads. He also found that training for speed alone improved velocity with light loads but did nothing for strength or velocity with heavy loads. Most interesting of all was the finding that training with intermediate loads (30 to 60% of maximal strength) at the highest speed possible led to improvements in force, speed, and power. Years later, this finding was corroborated when Kanehisa and Miyashita (1983) confirmed the specificity of velocity in training. They trained three groups at either slow-, medium-, or high-speed contractions. The slow-speed group improved in leg extension strength at slow speeds, and the fast group improved in the force they could exert at fast speeds. But only the intermediate-speed group was able to improve at all speeds. It appears that power training (15 to 25 repetitions at 30 to 60% of maximal strength, as fast as possible) may be the way to train when speed or power is desired. Does that throw out the concept of specificity?

If you are preparing for the shot put, in which force and speed are both important, you will need considerable strength, so train for strength. If high speed is your primary goal, as in pitching a fast ball, train for speed. Power training could help both performances. And the power prescription is ideal for sports such as cross-country skiing, a power/endurance sport that requires hundreds of little explosions to power the skier up the hills. The principle of specificity does not imply that other types of training should be avoided, only that training must eventually focus on the movements of the sport if best results are to be obtained.

A final note concerning the use of isotonic and especially isokinetic training for speed, strength, and power development is in order. Both techniques adapt to the advice I've just provided. By reducing the resistance below 30% of maximal, you can increase the velocity of contractions. Increase the resistance above 60% and you'll focus on force development. When power (force × velocity) is required, contract as fast as possible with weights in the 30-to-60%-of-maximal range. While isokinetic contractions seem ideally suited for strength or power development, it is possible that both strength and power can be developed using weight training equipment, or even with calisthenics.

Pre-Load/Elastic Recoil

Before we leave the subject of power, I want to acquaint you with one of the secrets of athletic performance. It took me years to realize that a well-known fact of muscle physiology—that a muscle exerts more force when it is stretched just before contraction—described how muscles should be used. The stretch, or pre-load, does several things: It aligns contractile elements (cross bridges) in muscle for maximal force, takes slack out of the system, and stores elastic energy in the muscle/tendon complex. From studies of the force and efficiency of contraction, it would appear that this stretch-shortening cycle is the way that muscle works most efficiently (Komi, 1992).

Here's how it works, for example, in a vertical jump. You sink at the knees to put the thigh muscles on stretch. Simultaneously you contract the muscles during the stretch and quickly convert the pre-load into elastic recoil as you jump. To see how effective pre-load/elastic recoil is, compare that jump with one in which you eliminate the pre-load. Sink to the starting position, then stop for a full second. Then jump. Without pre-load and elastic recoil, the results are inferior. The pre-load/elastic recoil works whenever you are able to pre-load just before contraction. It happens in running—at the ankle and thigh—in cross-country skiing, in tennis during the serve, and of course in weight lifting, where it has been called cheating! Often it happens automatically, but if it doesn't, see if it can be employed to provide more power, or the same power with less effort. Done properly, it contributes to the power and efficiency or economy of movement.

Summary

A muscle exerts more force when it is stretched just before contraction.

Research has shown that tension × time is the stimulus for strength development. It doesn't seem to matter how the tension is produced. Legend tells of Milo from Crete, who began daily lifts of a young calf. As time passed and the animal grew, so did Milo's strength. More recently, studies have lifted weights, pulled rubber bands, squeezed bags of water, and suffered electrical stimulation to build strength, and they all worked. We are beginning to understand how the stimulus leads to stronger, tougher, more efficient muscles. More important is our growing understanding of the distinction between strength and endurance, in terms of training and cellular outcomes. And we may soon be able to say how much strength or endurance is required to perform a sport or job.

As you pursue muscular fitness, remember the importance of flexibility in your training program. And be aware of muscle soreness and its causes, eccentric exercises such as downhill running and lowering weights, and ballistic contractions that use eccentric contractions to stop a forceful movement (such as pitching a baseball or serving a tennis ball).

By now you are ready to design and carry out a muscular fitness program that will improve your appearance, health, and everyday performance. If you want to improve performance in work or sport, you'll find help in Part V.

CHAPTER 10

Improving Your Muscular Fitness

"The two kinds of people on earth . . . are the people who lift and the people who lean."

Ella Wheeler Wilcox

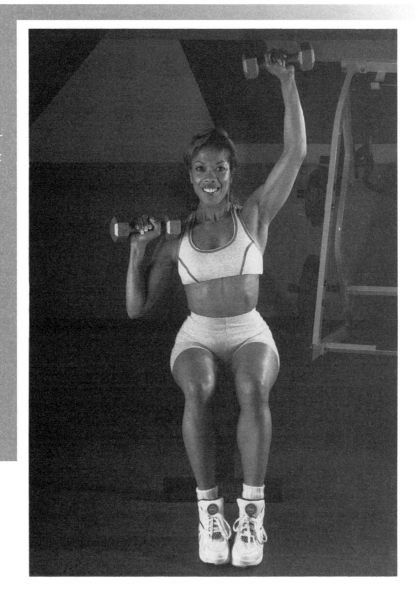

By now you have some idea of the benefits and applications of lifting (muscular fitness). First and foremost are the health benefits: All of us need to do exercises to prevent low back problems. Without regular attention to back and hamstring flexibility and abdominal tone, you risk becoming one of the millions of Americans whose days are diminished by this preventable problem. Those at risk for osteoporosis should plan a prevention program that consists of moderate weight lifting along with weight-bearing aerobic activity. And middle-aged individuals must understand how muscular fitness contributes to muscle mass, mobility, and the quality of life after retirement, and realize that they should begin before they retire and continue the rest of their days.

Of course, there are many other reasons to improve muscular fitness; many people become involved to correct posture or perceived deficiencies of figure or physique (e.g., to look good at the beach). Body shaping and body building motivate many participants. To help decide on a program, you may also want to evaluate your current level of muscular fitness. If you are dissatisfied, if there is room for improvement, or if you want to enhance performance in work or sport, use the prescriptions, select your mode of exercise, and get going. You'll be happy to learn that muscular fitness doesn't have to take a lot of time. Unless you are seeking high levels of strength or endurance, you should be able to achieve health and other goals with two to three short weekly sessions. And you can maintain muscular fitness with one or two sessions per week.

THIS CHAPTER WILL HELP YOU

- develop training prescriptions for muscular strength, endurance, speed, and power;
- take precautions and follow guidelines to make training safe and effective; and
- adopt a program to improve or maintain low back fitness.

Prescriptions for Muscular Strength

Research has identified safe, proven prescriptions for each component of muscular fitness, and they will be presented in this chapter. You may fulfill the strength prescription with calisthenics, weights, or weight machines. You'll get results with hydraulic devices, accommodating or variable resistance equipment, or with old-fashioned free weights. The key is to place the muscle under tension (at least two-thirds of maximal strength) for a sufficient period of time (or repetitions). How you intend to use the strength will dictate how you should train. Training is specific in terms of angle, range of motion, even velocity of contractions. Train the muscles and movements you are eager to improve. Consider the factors described in the following sections in designing a program.

Repetitions

We've known how to prescribe strength training since the early '50s, when DeLorme and Watkins (1951) published their analysis of progressive resistance exercise. This report and more recent studies have confirmed the need to use a resistance that can be lifted as many as 10 times (repetitions maximum or RM);

when more repetitions are possible the load must be increased (hence the term progressive resistance). A recent review of the literature leads to the conclusion that there is no one optimal number of repetitions. Anything between 2 and 10 RM yields success, so long as each set is in fact the maximal number of repetitions possible (Fleck & Kraemer, 1987).

Sets

In spite of what the manufacturers of some strength training equipment have said, the research shows that three sets of 2 to 10 repetitions (RM) is about right for newcomers to weight lifting. Later in this chapter I'll point out how more sets are used in advanced weight training. Most programs begin with one set of each exercise, then progress to two and then three as strength develops.

Frequency

One of the early studies to compare different training frequencies (Barham, 1960) found that 3- or 5-day-per-week formats were superior to 2 per week; but the 3- and 5-day programs were not significantly different from each other. In their 1987 review, Fleck and Kraemer conclude: "The majority of research indicates that three training sessions per muscle group per week is the minimum frequency which causes maximum gains in strength." Apparently, it takes untrained individuals 48 hours to recover from a training bout and to adapt to the training stimulus. The basic prescription for strength is

In practice many lifters prefer to vary the program by changing the number of repetitions per set.

- 3 sets of 6 to 10 repetitions maximum
- 3 times per week (every other day)

In practice many lifters prefer to vary the program by changing the number of repetitions (or reps) per set. Some begin at 10 RM, then go to 8 and end at 6; others prefer to begin low and go up (e.g., 6, 8, and 10 RM). For safety's sake I prefer to begin with more reps and less weight, and avoid high weights (low RM).

WARM-UP

A warm-up is as important for you as it is for your car. During winter months you can't just jump into the old pickup and expect instant performance; you start slowly and avoid overloading the engine until it heats up. In the case of the body, muscle is the engine, and increased muscle temperature improves enzyme activity and combustion. By slowly increasing heart rate, respiration, and muscle temperature, you avoid wasteful and uncomfortable anaerobic metabolism early in the workout. And by slowly stretching and warming the muscles, you greatly reduce the risk of injury (use the exercises in chapter 9). A 5-minute warm-up before and a cool-down after exercise will enhance your enjoyment of the experience and increase the likelihood that you will be able to participate tomorrow, without soreness. And remember, muscular fitness is only part of total fitness; no program is complete without a well-planned aerobic fitness regimen.

Just remember to increase the resistance when you are able to do more than 10 reps in all three sets. Keep in mind that most of the studies that led to these conclusions were done on "gym rats," previously untrained (novice) students enrolled in physical education classes. The prescription for advanced lifting is more demanding. The basic prescription can be used with a variety of methods.

Guidelines

If you engage in calisthenics, weight training, or isokinetics, keep the following points in mind:

- Ease into the program with lighter weights and fewer sets.
- Avoid holding your breath during a lift. This can cause a marked increase in blood pressure and the work of the heart. It also restricts the return of blood to the heart and the flow of blood in the coronary arteries that serve the heart muscle (just when your heart needs more oxygen, it gets less—a dangerous situation, especially for older, untrained individuals). Breath-holding can also increase intra-abdominal pressure and cause a hernia.
- Exhale during the lift and inhale as you lower the weight.
- Always work with a companion or spotter when using free weights.
- Alternate muscle groups during a session; for example, don't do several arm exercises in a row. Allow recovery time between sets of the same exercise.

Also, you should keep records of your progress. Test for maximum strength every few weeks (see figure 10.1 for a log to keep track of progress). Also record body weight and fat, and some dimensions (chest, waist, biceps, etc.).

Vary the program. Experienced athletes use a process called cycling that usually includes four cycles of up to 12 weeks each. For example, Fleck and Kraemer (1987) suggest this program for athletes in high-strength sports. Simply follow each of the 4-week cycles:

1. 10 to 20 reps, low resistance—for hypertrophy
2. 2 to 6 reps, medium resistance—for strength
3. 2 to 3 reps, high resistance—for added strength
4. 1 to 3 reps, very high resistance—peaking phase

Each cycle can be as short as 4 weeks or as long as 12. Since progress begins to plateau after 2 months, I prefer to change my program every 8 weeks. Another approach is to change exercises every 4 to 8 weeks, or when you plateau or get bored.

While strength doesn't increase rapidly, you can expect that your rate of increase will range from 1 to 3% per week, with previously untrained individuals increasing at a faster rate. With hard training, some may temporarily achieve a rate of 4 to 5% per week. The rate of improvement will decrease or plateau as you approach your potential maximal strength.

Rate of improvement may be slowed if you combine strength with strenuous aerobic training. Improvements will take place only in the muscle groups you train. Gains will be minimized unless you maintain adequate protein and energy in your diet. Increase protein intake if you are on a weight-loss diet.

A sedentary individual can expect to increase strength 50% or more in 6 months. Hard training could lead to similar gains in less time.

Strength can be maintained with a lower volume and frequency of training, so long as intensity (resistance) remains high. One session per week will maintain strength for 6 weeks or more; and two sessions will ensure maintenance for a prolonged period, depending on the level of strength achieved before the maintenance program began.

Muscular Fitness Log

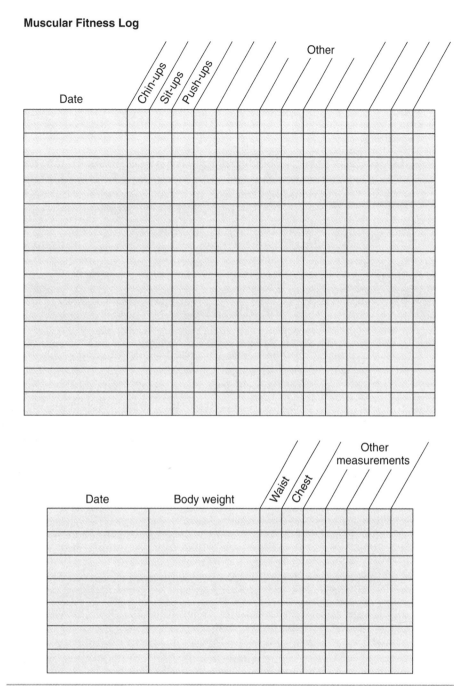

Figure 10.1 Muscular fitness log.

Detraining

Studies on older
individuals show
that strength
declines very
slowly in muscle
groups that are
used regularly.

With normal activity, newly gained strength is largely retained for up to 6 weeks after the cessation of training, and half of the strength you gain will be retained for up to a year. When you resume training, you'll return to previous levels with less effort, perhaps because of the learning that took place in earlier training. Studies on older individuals show that strength declines very slowly in muscle groups that are used regularly. Thus, an investment in strength could pay dividends later in life. I would recommend that you set aside at least 8 to 12 weeks each year to maintain or improve strength. Find a season when it suits your schedule, and follow a program. As the years pass you'll be glad you did.

Advanced Strength Training

Experienced lifters train 6 days per week. When they engage in body building, they do many sets and repetitions. Training for superior strength calls for numerous sets (more than 10) with few repetitions and very heavy loads. Some of these athletes have been known to take protein supplements or even drugs to enhance their progress. New research supports the increase of *dietary* protein when the athlete is on a weight-loss diet (Butterfield, 1987).

ANABOLIC STEROIDS

The use of steroid drugs to improve performance has become commonplace in the world of sports, especially body building, football, and professional wrestling. Though the effects of steroids have been supported by some research, their use is dangerous and unhealthy. Anabolic steroids affect glandular function, damage the liver, and lead to early heart disease via an alarming drop in HDL-cholesterol. Furthermore, they have been associated with testicular atrophy, psychological rage, and other problems. Don't depend on steroids, growth hormone, or any drug for strength or performance.

Advanced strength training guidelines include:

- Work up to 5-6 sets.
- Utilize a split program: upper body on Monday, Wednesday, and Friday, trunk and legs on Tuesday, Thursday, and Saturday.
- Eat adequate food for energy and protein, avoid rapid weight loss, and get ample rest.
- Cut back on endurance training unless you are very fit (best results may occur when serious strength training is conducted separately) (Hickson, 1980).
- Use training cycles; change your program every 4 to 8 weeks or when progress begins to plateau.

Strength may be related to performance in your work or sport. If so, by all means train to improve your strength. However, don't assume (as many have) that if some is good, more is better. In most activities, performance improves with strength, but only to a point. Thereafter, you may be wasting your time or diminishing performance with excessive attention to strength. The trick is to know how much is enough. When strength is optimal for the sport, move on to other important phases of training. Just be sure to maintain the necessary strength with one or two sessions each week.

HOW MUCH IS ENOUGH?

For endurance sports (e.g. swimming, cross-country skiing) strength in a muscle group is adequate when it exceeds 2.5 times the force used in a typical stroke. Stated another way, the load should not exceed 40% of your strength. For example, if you need 20 pounds of force in the freestyle arm pull, you should have at least 50 pounds (20 pounds × 2.5 = 50 pounds) of strength in the muscle group. Additional strength isn't likely to improve performance. So, if strength is adequate, move on to endurance training. For daylong work, strength is adequate when the force needed is at or below 20% of your maximal. Thus, if a loaded shovel weighs 10 pounds, you'll need 5 × 10, or 50, pounds of force to lift it repeatedly without undue fatigue.

Prescriptions for Muscular Endurance

I've pointed out how strength and endurance are different, and why endurance may be more important than a high level of strength, presuming that you have adequate strength. The main difference between training for strength and training for endurance is the level of tension in the muscle and, consequently, the resistance and number of repetitions. Lighter weights (less than 66% of maximum strength) don't provide much stimulus for strength development, but if you do enough repetitions, you will develop endurance.

Years ago it was believed that training with up to 10 repetitions (maximum) developed strength, while training with more than 10 repetitions developed endurance. Recent studies have added to our knowledge of strength and endurance and the territory that lies between. Studies in our lab (Washburn, Sharkey, Narum, & Smith, 1982) and others (Anderson & Kearney, 1982) show that 15 to 25 repetitions maximum will still develop some strength (1% per week versus 2 to 3% with 6 to 10 RM for strength training), along with short-term or anaerobic endurance. Table 10.1 describes the strength-endurance continuum and includes a summary of the effects of various numbers of repetitions and what they are likely to develop. As the number of repetitions increases, less strength and more endurance is developed.

The number of repetitions you need depends on several factors. What are you training for? Is it for short-term (anaerobic) or for long-term endurance? Training should be specific to the way in which it will be used. Emphasize speed when necessary. Do many repetitions when long-term endurance with less resistance is needed. When the activity involves moderate resistance, lift heavier weights and do fewer repetitions. For short (under 2 minutes) and intense activities, train with 15 to 25 repetitions maximum to get short-term or anaerobic endurance. If your goals are vague and time is short, use fewer repetitions. A friend once worked up to 400 sit-ups daily, then quit because he became bored. (Incidentally, he didn't get rid of his tummy fat until diet and aerobic exercise led to general weight loss).

TABLE 10.1　The Strength-Endurance Continuum

	Strength	Short-term (anaerobic) endurance	Intermediate endurance	Long-term endurance
Train with	High resistance Low repetitions	Medium resistance Medium repetitions		Low resistance High repetitions
Training effect	More contractile proteins (actin and myosin) Increased short-term energy (ATP and CP) Stronger connective tissue Reduced inhibitions	?		Aerobic enzymes and mitochondria Improved oxygen intake and fat utilization Increased capillaries

ATP = adenosine triphosphate

CP = creatine phosphate

Follow the appropriate endurance prescription and observe the precautions mentioned for strength training. However, since the loads are lighter, muscle endurance training is safer than strength training, and it is probably more related to the everyday activities of the average adult. Be careful, however, to breathe properly as you strain to complete the last few repetitions in a set.

Progress

Muscle endurance is very trainable. While it is difficult to go from two to four chin-ups (that takes strength), it is easy to improve from 20 to 40 push-ups (that takes endurance). When you have sufficient strength for the task, gains in endurance come with relative ease. Subjects in the Washburn study improved 10% per week in short-term endurance when they trained with 15 to 25 RM. On a laboratory endurance test, the short-term (anaerobic) endurance training was more effective than strength training, improving short-term endurance 70% versus 50% for strength training. Most adult activities are enhanced when endurance is improved. Tennis and skiing, for example, require hours of practice, and good practice requires endurance. The fatigued student usually practices a sloppy version of the skill.

Of course, your ultimate progress will be dictated by your genetic endowment and your devotion to training.

Of course, your ultimate progress will be dictated by your genetic endowment and your devotion to training. If you have a high percentage of slow twitch muscle fibers, your potential for long-term endurance is excellent. If you do not, don't despair; training will improve the endurance capabilities of all fiber types. While you may not be a world-class endurance athlete, you will come closer to your potential.

Diet and Endurance

Best endurance performances occur when muscle fibers are well supplied with muscle glycogen. And glycogen levels are highest when you follow a high-carbohydrate diet. Scandinavian studies have shown that muscle glycogen stores can be depleted in a full day of alpine skiing. If you dine on steak and salad after skiing, your muscles will not be ready to perform the following day. Do all you can to replace muscle glycogen and you will be able to ski all day and still have plenty of energy. More important, you will be less likely to fatigue, fall, and get injured. Begin carbohydrate replacement immediately after activity, and continue with a high-carbohydrate diet.

Speed and Power

As with other types of training, the key to speed and power training is specificity. Try to pattern the training after the intended use. To throw a baseball faster, train with a weighted ball, or simulate the motion with pulley weights or an isokinetic device. To improve jumping ability, do half squats with weights, jump while wearing a weighted vest, or use an isokinetic jumping device. When in doubt, be specific. Here are some ideas on speed and power training.

- **Speed (velocity):** Do high-speed contractions with low resistance. Sprinters have gained speed by running downhill, running against resistance, and assisted running (being towed). For more on speed training, consult a book on the subject (e.g., Dintiman & Ward, 1988).
- **Power (force × velocity):** Do three sets of 15 to 25 high-speed contractions with 30 to 60% of maximal resistance. You can use accommodating resistance devices to do power training, but free weights are not well suited to this high-speed training.

Another technique, borrowed from European coaches, is *plyometrics*—explosive movements designed to improve power. Sprinters do one- and two-leg hops to gain power. High jumpers, broad jumpers, volleyball and basketball athletes, and even cross-country skiers use plyometrics in an attempt to improve performance. Proponents have said that plyometrics train the capacity for pre-load/elastic recoil and build strength and explosive power (Radcliffe & Farentinos, 1985). Unfortunately, there is limited research concerning the value of plyometrics for various sports and for athletes at different levels of development. And excessive use or poor technique can lead to painful knee problems. I do recommend that you try plyometrics, if only because of the effect of practice on skill and economy. But start with a modest number, on a soft surface, and quit at the first sign of discomfort in the knee. Even if you don't gain additional power, you may become more effective in the use of the power you possess. (In chapter 9, I described the phenomenon called pre-load/elastic recoil and told how it contributes to power and performance.) The following are a few plyometrics exercises.

SQUAT JUMPS

Stand with hands on hips, one foot a step ahead of the other. Squat (drop quickly) until your front thigh is at a 90-degree angle to the lower leg, then immediately jump as high as possible, extending the knees. Switch position of feet on the way down, land, squat, and jump again. Perform 10 to 20 repetitions.

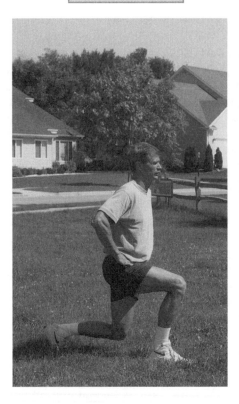 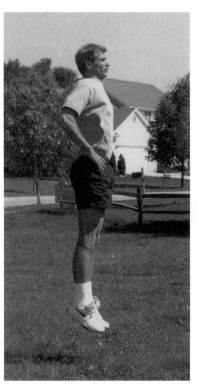

TWO-LEG JUMPS

Jump as high as possible from both legs. Do 10 to 20 explosive two-leg jumps.

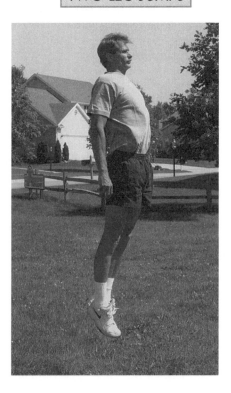

HOPS

Do one-leg hops, alternating legs with a balance step between hops. Do 10 with each leg; work up to two sets of 20.

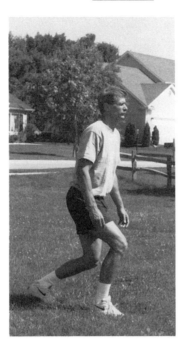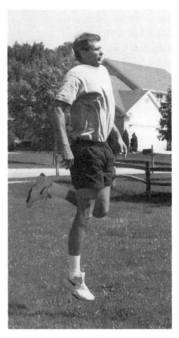

Calisthenics

Calisthenics include a wide range of exercises, such as push-ups, chin-ups, and sit-ups. The strength training prescription calls for high resistance and low repetitions, so you may have to add additional resistance when you are able to do more than 10 repetitions (more than 10 repetitions will build short-term endurance but not much strength). You can overload the push-up in several ways: For example, have someone place a hand on your back to increase the resistance, or put your feet on a chair to place more weight on the arms. You could also do variations, such as fingertip push-ups or power push-ups (push up and clap hands). Just remember, as the repetitions exceed 10, you are shifting toward endurance training. Calisthenics can be used to train for both. Try the following calisthenic exercises.

SPECIFICITY

The concept of specificity applies to muscular fitness training and testing. Training is specific in regard to angle and speed, and static tests do not reflect the effects of dynamic training (Baker, Wilson, & Carlyon, 1994). High-resistance training yields greater strength gains, while low-resistance training produces greater gains in muscular endurance (Morrissey, Harman, & Johnson, 1995). For best results, train specifically.

KNEE PUSH-UP

This is a good chest and triceps exercise for beginners. With hands outside your shoulders and knees bent, push up keeping your back straight. Do as many as possible.

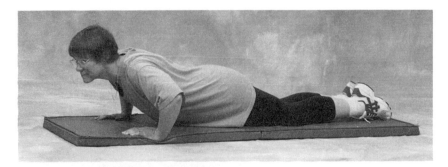

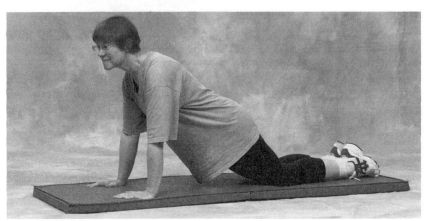

PUSH-UP

This is an intermediate exercise. With hands outside your shoulders, push up keeping your back straight; return until your chest almost touches the floor. Do as many as possible.

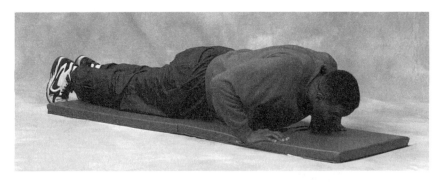

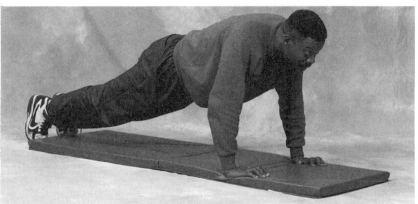

CHAIR DIPS

This is an advanced exercise. Make sure the chair used is stationary. Grasp the sides of the chair, and slide your feet forward while supporting your weight on your arms. Lower your body, and return. Do as many as possible. You can also use parallel bars if available.

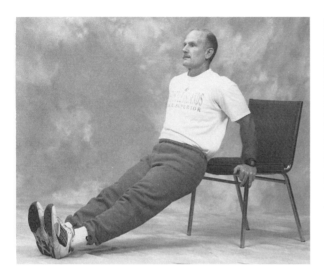 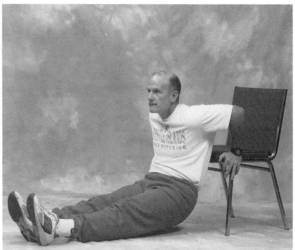

MODIFIED CHIN-UP

This is a biceps and back exercise for beginners. Stand with the bar about chest height. With an underhand grasp, hang from the bar with the body straight and feet on ground. Pull up, and return. Do as many as possible.

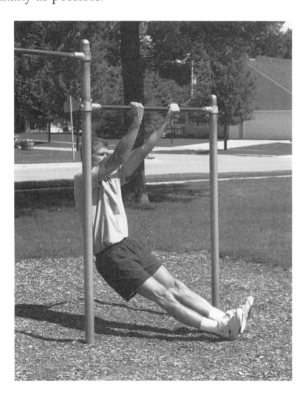 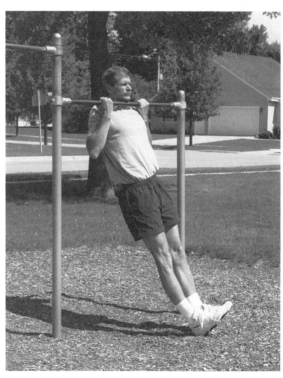

CHIN-UP

This is the intermediate version of the exercise. With the underhand grasp, pull up until your chin is over the bar; return. Do as many as possible. Variations include using an overhand grip or climbing a rope.

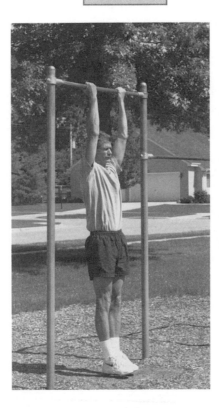
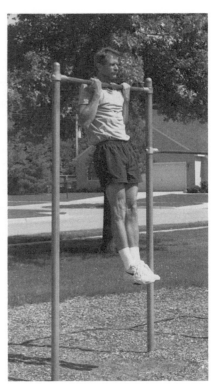

PIKE CHIN-UP

This is an advanced exercise. Perform the chin-up from the bar with legs in a pike position.

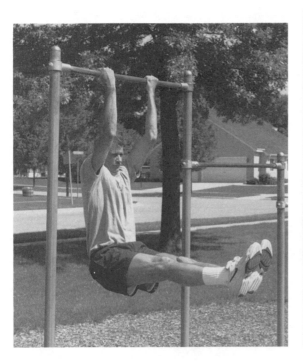
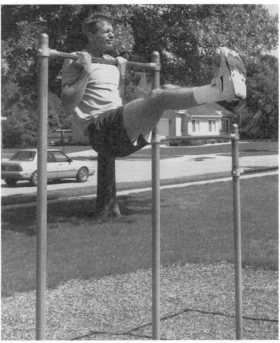

BASKET HANG

This is a more advanced exercise. Hang from the bar with an underhand grasp. Raise your legs into a "basket," and return. Do as many as possible.

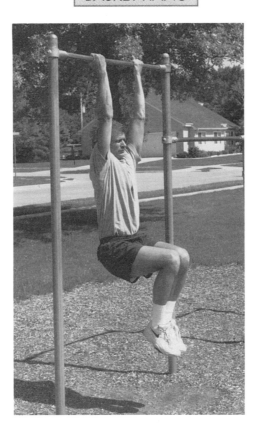

SIT-UP WITH ARMS CROSSED

This is a good exercise for abdominal strength and endurance. On your back with arms crossed on the chest and knees bent, curl up to a semi-sitting position, and return. Do 10 to 15 times. Variations: Do repetitions very fast; do the exercise on an inclined board; hold a weight on your chest.

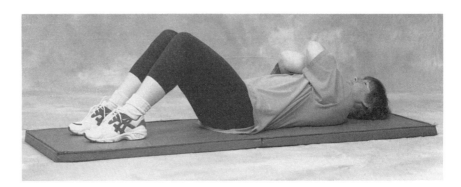

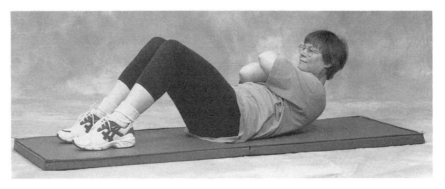

LEG LIFTS

This is a good exercise for back strength and endurance. Lying face down on the floor, with a partner holding your trunk down, raise your legs 5 to 10 times. Avoid hyperextension.

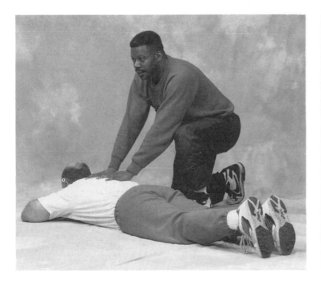
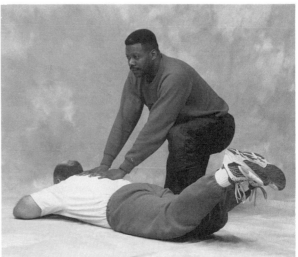

TRUNK LIFTS

Lying face down on the floor with fingers laced behind your head and ankles anchored to the ground, raise your trunk 5 to 10 times. Don't overextend.

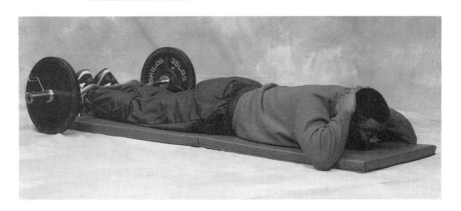

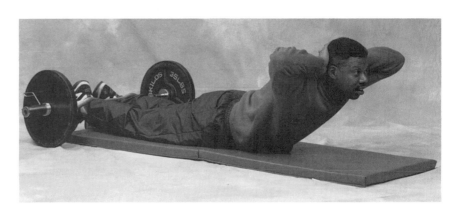

HALF KNEE BENDS

This exercise is good for leg strength and endurance. With feet apart and hands on hips, squat until your thighs are parallel to the ground; return. Do as many as possible. Try a 2-inch block under the heels to aid balance. For variety, do this exercise with a weight on your back (e.g., a backpack).

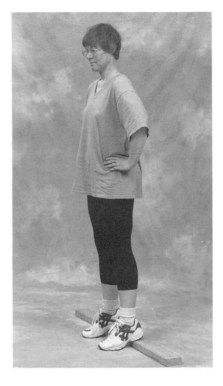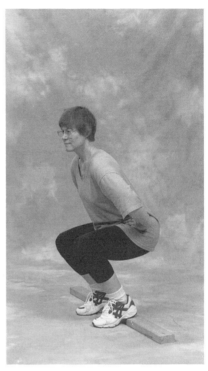

BENCH STEPPING

Step up and down on a bench as fast as possible for 30 seconds. Switch lead leg and repeat. Bench stepping can also be done with a loaded pack.

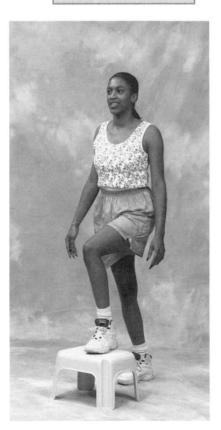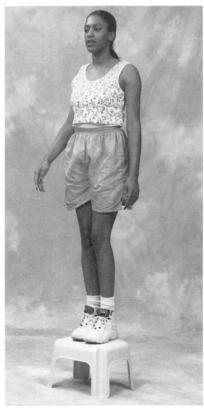

HEEL RAISES

Stand erect, hands at sides or on hips, feet close together. Raise up on your toes 20 to 40 times. Heel raises can be done with toes on a 2-inch platform; or do them with a loaded pack.

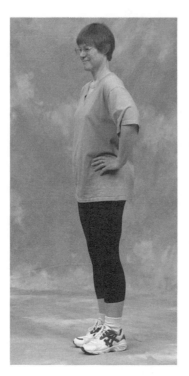 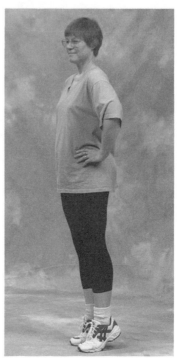

HILLS

Power walk up a steep hill, stadium steps, or office stairs. Variations: Use ski poles for balance, to aid downhill trip, or to exercise arms. Wear a weighted pack for added resistance.

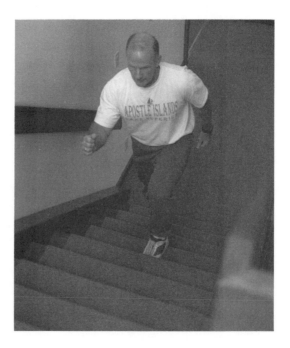

Weight Training

Weight training, sometimes called resistance training, has emerged as an essential part of the program to improve performance, fitness, and even health. Use a weight training apparatus (stack weights) or free weights (bar and weights). Though machines are expensive, they have several advantages over free weights: They are safer and more versatile, they save time, and they eliminate equipment theft. Using a machine also makes it much easier to change resistance as you move from one exercise to another. On the negative side, it restricts you to a set series of lifts and movements, and you don't learn to balance the load as well. But for general training, and especially for groups, the machines are probably the best bet. Try the weight training exercises that follow the descriptions of the apparatus in this section. Remember, for strength, do three sets of 6 to 10 repetitions, three times per week (every other day).

Weight Training Machines

Several companies manufacture weight training machines. Universal Gym, popular isotonic equipment, typically provides stations for the bench press and leg press, as well as the following:

- Abdomen and trunk exercises
- Military press and curls
- Lat pull-down
- Leg flexion and extension

Nautilus equipment utilizes a cam to adjust resistance throughout the lift. Most clubs have stations for triceps and chest exercises and the leg press, as well as the following:

- Biceps curl
- Bench press
- Lat pull-over and pull-down
- Leg flexion and extension
- Abdominals and trunk

Mini Gym makes a variety of variable-resistance devices specifically designed for certain sports such as basketball, volleyball, and swimming. Excellent equipment is also manufactured by Paramount, Hydra Gym, Kiefer, Polaris, and others. Sturdy home devices are now available for $1,000 to $2,500.

Free Weights

Advanced programs often utilize free weights to isolate and overload specific muscles. Use the appropriate prescription to achieve your goal (e.g., 6-10 repetitions maximum for strength).

TRICEPS EXTENSION

Sit astride a bench with your back straight. Grasp the bar with your hands about 2 inches apart, using an overhand grip. Bring the bar to full arm extension above your head. Lower the bar behind your head, keeping elbows stationary.

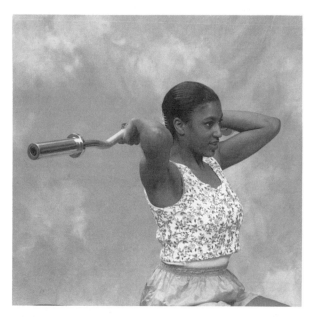 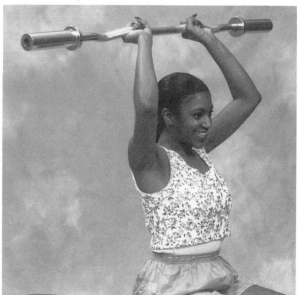

MILITARY PRESS

The military press works the arm and shoulder muscles. Stand erect with feet comfortably apart. Grasp a barbell with an overhand grip and raise it to your upper chest. Then press the bar overhead, until elbows are fully extended. Lower the bar to chest position; repeat.

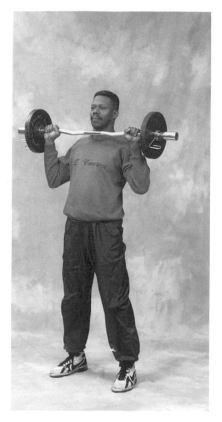 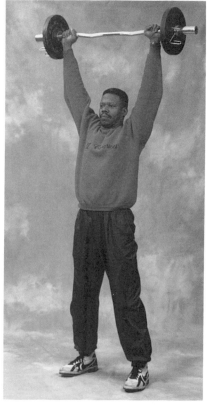

BICEPS CURLS

For the biceps curl, stand erect, feet comfortably apart, and knees slightly flexed. Hold the bar in front of your thighs with an underhand grip shoulder-width apart, arms straight. Flex your elbows fully, lifting the bar toward your chest. Keep your elbows close to your sides, and avoid raising your shoulders. Don't lean backward or bounce the bar with your leg motion. Return to the starting position.

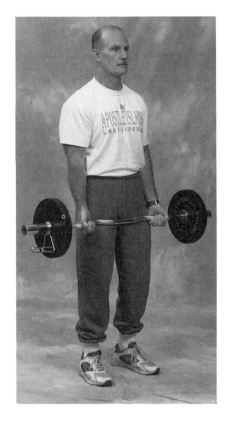
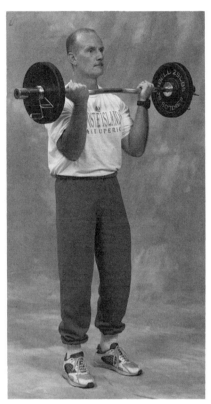

BENT ROWING

Work the back muscles with bent rowing. Stand in a bent-over position; your back is flat and slightly above parallel with the floor. Spread your feet shoulder width apart, with knees comfortably bent. Grasp a barbell with an overhand grip; hands should be slightly wider than shoulder width. Keep your buttocks lower than your shoulders. Pull the bar to your chest, then lower it to the starting position. Keep your upper body stationary.

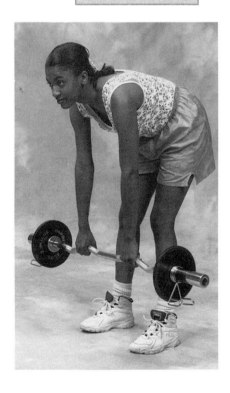
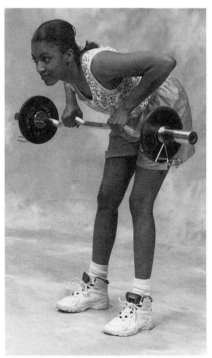

BENCH PRESS

Bench presses exercise the chest and arm extensor muscles. Lie flat on your back with feet on the floor astride the bench. Grasp the bar wider than shoulder width, with arms extended. Lower the bar to your chest, then press it back up to the starting position. Inhale while lowering the weight, and exhale while pressing it. A partner should assist with weights before and after the exercise.

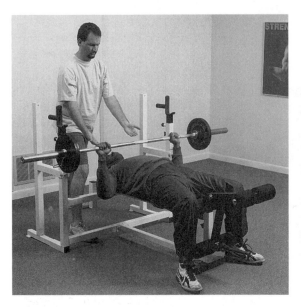 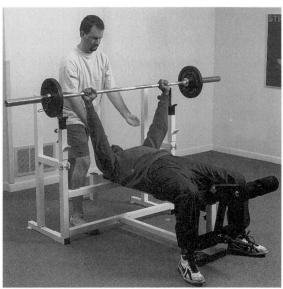

PULL-DOWN

This exercise works the lats. Kneel on one or both knees, or sit on a bench if one is available, and grasp the handles. Pull the bar down, and return to the starting position.

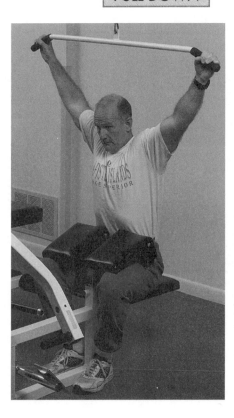 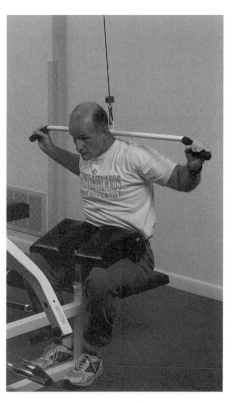

LEG PRESS

Leg presses work the quadriceps. Place your feet on the pedals, and grasp the handles of the seat. Press your feet forward to elevate the weight, and return. Inhale while lowering weight, and exhale while lifting it.

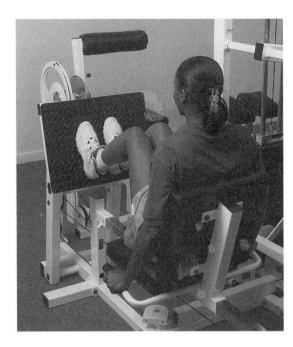
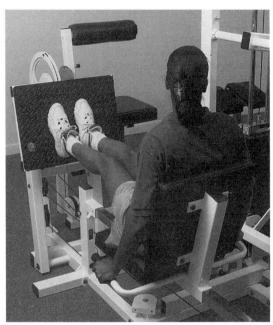

LEG FLEXION

This exercise works the hamstrings. Lie face down on the table with heels positioned behind the padded bar. Flex your legs to elevate the weight. Return to the starting position. Watch for leg cramps.

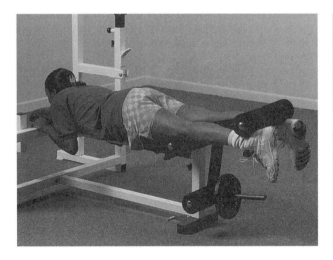
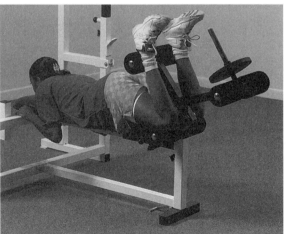

LEG EXTENSION

This works the quadriceps. Sit on the bench, with your instep under the padded bar. Extend your legs to elevate the weight. Return to starting position.

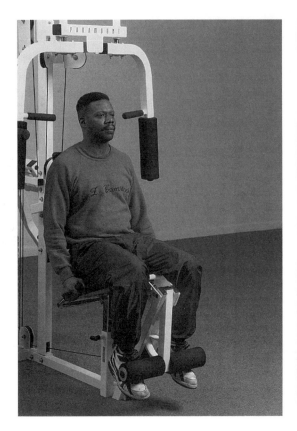 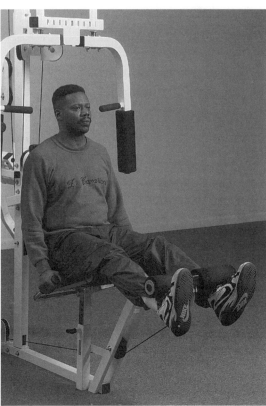

Isokinetics

Isokinetic devices, as well as variable and accommodating resistance machines, are available in health and fitness clubs, in recreation centers, in schools and colleges, and even in private homes. The good ones allow you to exert near-maximum force as the device moves through a full range of motion. You can vary the speed and resistance to suit specific training needs. Low-cost home devices can be used in a variety of ways. Least expensive of all is isokinetic exercise with a friend (counterforce). Your partner provides resistance throughout the range of motion; for example, as you attempt forearm flexion your partner provides resistance (see the following exercises). You can do fast, medium, or slow isokinetics, depending on the goal of your training. But recent studies indicate that moderately fast training against resistance is more likely to develop strength and power.

Follow the program on an alternating day schedule. Select the program to suit your needs, not those of the club. If you need medium or fast contractions for your sport, do them. Also, if they say to do one set, take their advice for the first 8 weeks. But when your strength plateaus, as it will with one set, progress to two and then three sets. Fitness clubs like slow contractions that save wear and tear on the machines, and they advise one set not because it is the best way to train—but because it avoids long waits to use the apparatus.

ARM FLEXION

As partner 1 tries to lift his arms, partner 2 resists the movement. Partner 2 should allow movement to progress slowly (range of motion in 3 seconds). Do three sets of eight repetitions.

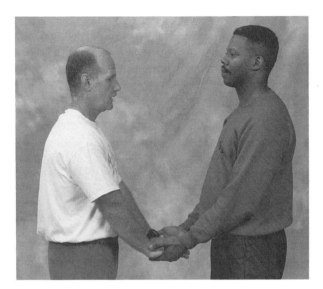
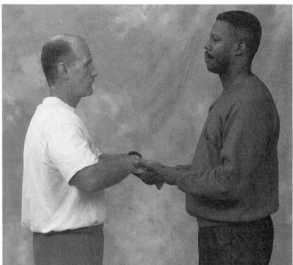

ARM EXTENSION

As partner 1 tries to extend arms down, partner 2 resists the movement. Partner 2 should allow movement to progress slowly (range of motion in 3 seconds). Do three sets of eight repetitions.

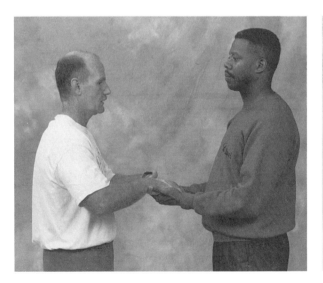
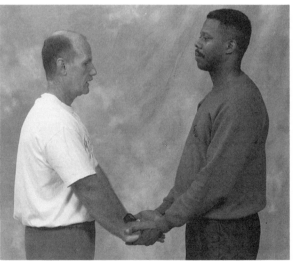

PUSH-UP

As partner 1 does a conventional push-up, partner 2 provides resistance. Do three sets of eight repetitions. Switch places between sets to allow time to rest.

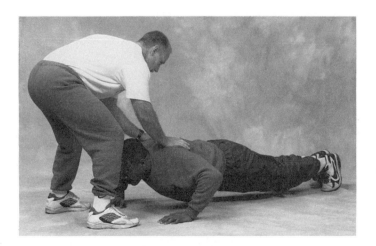

LEG FLEXION

As partner 1 tries to flex his leg, partner 2 resists the movement. Partner 2 should allow movement to progress slowly through range of motion in 3 seconds. Switch legs and repeat. Do three sets of eight repetitions each. Switch positions between sets; watch out for leg cramps.

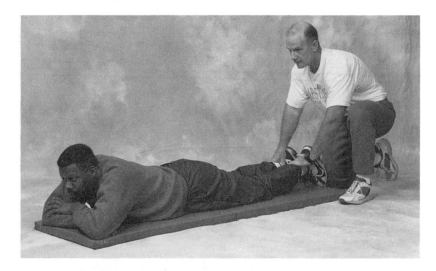

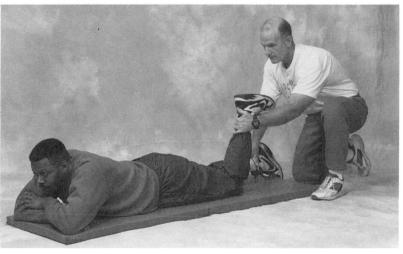

LEG EXTENSION

As partner 1 tries to extend her leg, partner 2 resists the movement. Partner 2 should allow movement to progress slowly through range of motion in 3 seconds. Switch legs and repeat. Do three sets of eight repetitions each. Switch positions between sets.

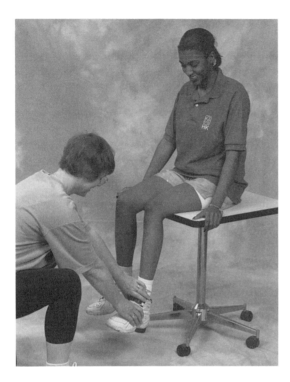 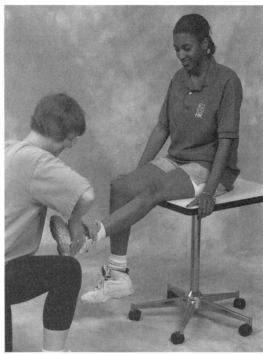

Low Back Health

More than 30 million Americans are afflicted with low back pain, and an estimated 24 million (80%) of these problems are due to improper posture, weak muscles, or inadequate flexibility. Weak abdominal muscles cannot counter the forward tilt of the pelvis, which can displace the vertebrae and cause pain. Lack of flexibility in back and hamstring muscles has also been associated with low back pain, which has been called a hypokinetic disease, one that results from a lack (hypo) of movement (kinetic).

Back care specialists continue to explore new approaches to low back health, including greater use of back extension exercises to maintain trunk flexibility and to strengthen extensor muscles. Several companies are marketing sophisticated back testing devices that allow measurement of flexion and extension strength and flexibility. And back extension devices are beginning to appear in health clubs. If you have a low back problem ask your physician or physical therapist about these and other approaches to the prevention, diagnosis, and treatment of low back disorders. If you decide to improve the strength of back extensor muscles, avoid hyperextension. Finally, when you do have a problem, consider the results of a recent study of patients with acute low back pain. The outcomes of treatment, recovery from pain, and return to function and work were similar whether the care came from primary care physicians, chiropractors, or orthopedic surgeons. However, the care from the primary care practitioners was the least expensive (Carey, Garrett, Jackman, et al., 1995).

Low Back Fitness Tests

The simple tests that follow, developed at the Sun Valley Health Institute, will help identify areas that need additional attention. Take the tests again after several months to monitor your progress.

Curl-Up

Lie on your back, and bend your knees to a 90-degree angle. Using one of the following arm positions, slowly curl up to a sitting position; don't swing your arms or allow your feet to come off the floor. If successful, try a more difficult position (higher number); if not, try an easier one (lower number). Your score is the highest number achieved.

1. Arms at side, unable to curl up without aid of partner
2. Arms at side, hands pull back of thighs
3. Arms at side
4. Arms folded across chest
5. Hands behind neck
6. Arms extended overhead, fingers intertwined, with arms pressing against ears

This test indicates abdominal muscle strength and flexibility of back muscles. If you can't do number 5, you need more than a maintenance program. Do repetitions of 3 and 4 to achieve 5.

Leg Lift

This test evaluates the strength of the lower abdominal muscles. Lie on your back, head on floor, legs straight, hands under the hollow of your back. Flatten your back, then attempt to raise both feet 10 inches and hold the position for 10 seconds.

1. Unable to lift both legs
2. Back raises immediately
3. Back raises after several seconds
4. Able to hold back flat

If you can't do number 4, you need more abdominal tone. Use the basket hang and other exercises to improve abdominal tone.

Sit and Reach

This is a test of lower back flexibility. Sit with legs flat on the floor. With one hand over the other and toes pointing to the ceiling, reach forward and try to touch your toes or beyond. Hold for several counts. Score as follows after several warm-up trials.

1. Well short of toes (more than 3 inches short)
2. Touch toes (or come within 2 inches)
3. Touch well beyond toes (more than 3 inches beyond)

Although extreme flexibility isn't necessary for a healthy back, the lower back and leg muscles need adequate flexibility. A 2 is adequate; with practice you may be able to score a 3.

Hip Flexion

Lie on your back on the floor with your legs straight and flat. Keep your head on the floor throughout the test. Bend your right leg, and pull your knee to your chest. Test both sides, and score as follows.

1. Knee to chest but left leg completely off floor
2. Knee to chest but left leg lifts somewhat
3. Knee completely to chest with left leg flat on floor

Tight hip flexors may cause an exaggerated lumbar curve, which predisposes the back to injury. Do this test and other stretching exercises to improve flexibility of the hip flexors. In time you should be able to score a 3.

Low Back Exercises

Many cases of low back pain can be prevented by assuming good posture and adhering to a regular program of flexibility and abdominal exercises. It also helps to maintain weight control and a trim waistline. To avoid injury to the lower back, use your legs instead of your back when lifting heavy objects, and avoid carrying heavy objects above the level of the elbows. Other suggestions for prevention of low back problems include:

Many cases of low back pain can be prevented by assuming good posture and adhering to a regular program of flexibility and abdominal exercises.

- Sleep with the knees somewhat flexed; avoid lying flat on your back or stomach. Use a firm mattress, or sleep with a piece of plywood under the mattress.
- Sit with one or both knees above your hips; cross your legs or use a footrest.
- Keep your knees bent while driving. If your car seat doesn't provide lumbar support, use a cushion.
- When standing, place one foot on a stool, especially while ironing, washing dishes, or working at a counter or workbench.
- Reduce stress. Tense muscles and psychological stress may also contribute to the problem. If you think that stress is affecting your back, try some relaxation techniques or sign up for a stress management class.
- Remain fit. A well-designed total fitness program, including aerobic and muscular fitness, will provide a balanced approach to low back health. You'll get abdominal muscle training and flexibility, along with substantial stress reduction.
- When low back pain does arise, remember that the best treatment is not bed rest but rather a return to normal activity as soon as possible (Malmivaara et al., 1995).

Daily practice of the following exercises will help prevent or improve lower back problems (Williams, 1974).

KNEE TO CHEST

With knees bent and arms above your head, move one knee as far as possible toward your chest while straightening the other. Return to the starting position and repeat, switching leg positions. Relax and repeat.

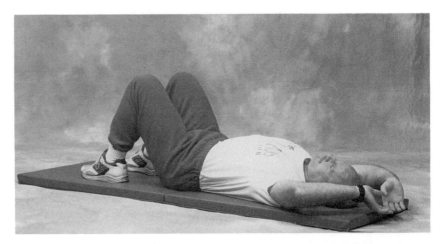

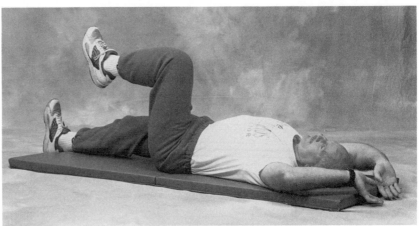

FLAT BACK

Bend your knees, with your feet flat on the floor and arms above your head. Tighten the muscles of your lower abdomen and buttocks at the same time, keeping your back flat on the floor. Hold 10 seconds, and relax; repeat.

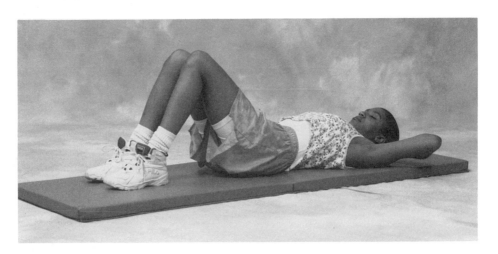

DOUBLE KNEE PULL

Starting in the same position, with your arms at your side, draw your knees to your chest, and clasp your hands around your knees. Keeping your shoulders flat against the floor, pull your knees tightly against your chest, hold 10 seconds, and relax; repeat. Repeat and touch your forehead to your knees.

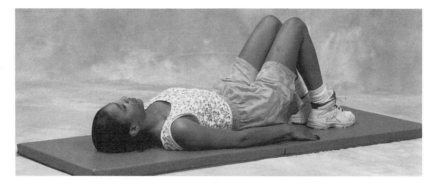

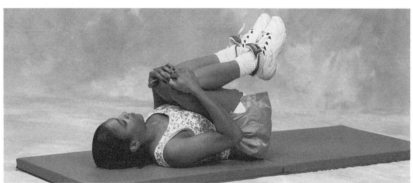

CURL-UP

Bend your knees with your feet flat on the floor; lift one leg and rest the ankle on the knee of the opposite leg. Lock your hands behind your head. Raise your head and shoulders from the floor. With chin to chest and with back rounded, curl up as far as possible, trying to touch your elbow to the opposite knee. Be sure to pull with the stomach muscles. Lower slowly. Do 5 to 10 repetitions; increase until you can do 20.

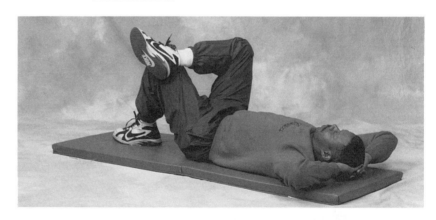

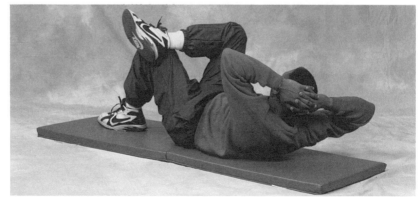

ANGRY CAT

Kneel and place your hands on the floor. Lower your head, and contract your stomach and buttock muscles; arch your lower back; hold 5 seconds, and relax.

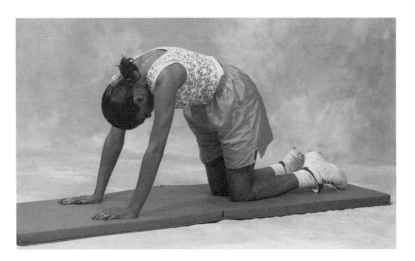

SEATED BACK STRETCH

With your knees bent, bend forward at the waist to bring your head between your knees; pull your stomach in as you curl forward. Keep your weight back on your hips. Release your stomach muscles, and reach to stretch your lower back. Come up slowly. Relax, repeat.

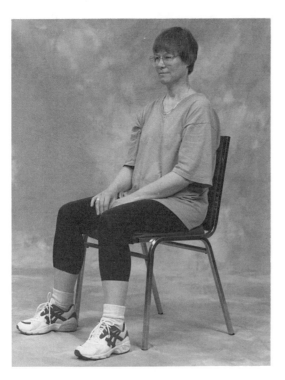
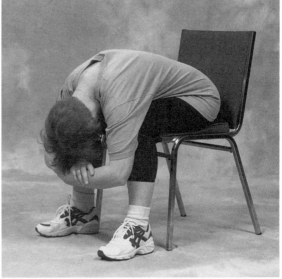

Summary

This chapter has provided prescriptions and guidelines for the development of muscular strength and endurance. I've suggested ways to train, shown what progress you can expect and how to maintain muscular fitness, and described what happens when training stops. Also provided were prescriptions for speed and power. Be certain to precede this dynamic training with at least 8 weeks of sport-specific buildup (strength, progressively faster running, throwing, jumping) to avoid excessive soreness or injury. An important part of the chapter dealt with the issue of low back health and the essential contributions of muscular fitness exercises.

In addition to the obvious benefits of strength and endurance to appearance and performance, other important reasons for muscular fitness include avoidance of crippling osteoporosis and lifelong maintenance of mobility. Avoidance of osteoporosis, the weakening of bone via the loss of bone minerals, requires regular weight-bearing activity, such as walking or jogging, as well as moderate resistance exercises for the upper body. Normal household tasks, such as lifting, vacuuming, mowing grass, and shoveling snow, will help avoid the problem. But research shows that best results are achieved by a combination of weight-bearing and resistance exercises, along with a diet that includes adequate calcium and vitamin D (exposure to sunlight is a natural way to form vitamin D). Excessive endurance training, fat loss, and low calcium intake contribute to osteoporosis in young female athletes. So, moderate activity is the sensible approach to prevention. Postmenopausal women may need high-intensity strength training to preserve bone density and improve muscle strength and balance (Nelson et al., 1994). And they will need to consider hormonal replacement therapy to ensure calcium uptake and utilization if they are to avoid crippling fractures of the hip, upper spine, and other bones.

Finally, mobility is preserved by living the active life, including engaging in aerobic and muscular activities. It can be restored by becoming active, regardless of one's age. Studies of senior citizens and frail elderly people indicate that resistance training improves strength as well as performance of activities of daily living, including getting out of a chair, walking, climbing stairs, and carrying groceries. If you can't perform these activities, you will be relegated to family care or a nursing home. Start now to maintain or improve your muscular fitness.

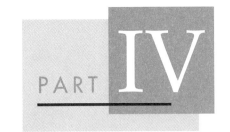

Activity and Weight Control

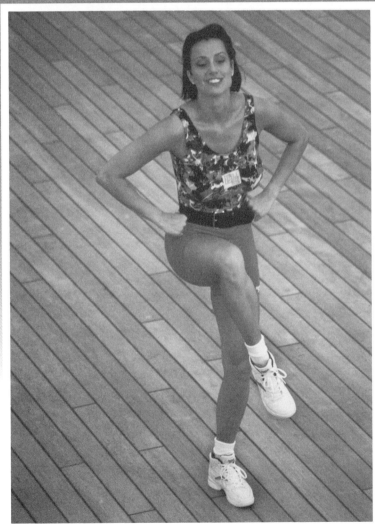

© W. Lynn Seldon

Ours is a nation of paradoxes. We boast more dieters, diet books, diet foods, and diet centers than any other place on earth, and yet we have become the fattest nation on earth. The reason for this is simple: the diets themselves. The more we diet, the fatter we get!

Part IV reviews basics of good nutrition, deals with the importance of activity in weight control, and discusses the contributions of fitness to fat metabolism and weight control. I'll show how diet alone is a recipe for failure, and how the active life provides a positive approach to weight control, while allowing enjoyment of your favorite foods. These ideas are not new; they appeared in my first book, published in 1974. But in the two decades that followed, overweight and obesity—and their consequences—have been, so to speak, expanding.

This section will provide a plan to help you gain control of your weight, then show you how the active life will keep you there. But you don't want to just lose weight; you want to lose fat. The active life and fitness help you attain that goal by making muscle cells efficient users of fat. Diet leads to the loss of muscle, the furnace in which fat is burned. Activity conserves muscle while it burns fat, and fitness increases muscle tissue while further enhancing its ability to consume fat. All this and more in Part IV.

CHAPTER 11

Nutrition and Health

"One must eat to live, and not live to eat."

Molière

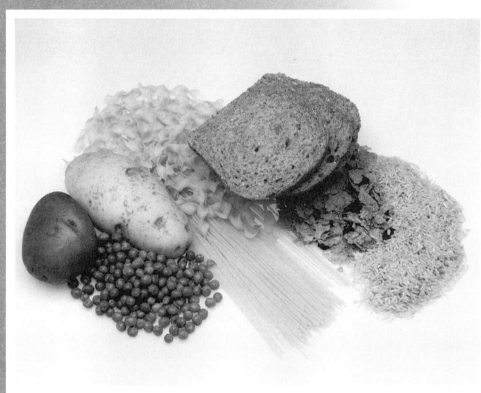

As more people work longer hours, less time is available for the selection and preparation of food, leading to an increasing reliance on prepared food, fast food, and eating out, and a loss of control over the food we eat. We select the item but have little influence over its preparation. As a consequence, we eat more fat, more saturated and hydrogenated fat, and more salt, and run the risk of getting shortchanged in other areas of nutrition.

THIS CHAPTER WILL HELP YOU

- understand the basics of good nutrition,
- identify sources of energy and their contribution to performance and health,
- consider your need for vitamin and mineral supplementation,
- understand the relationship between diet and health, and
- select foods that are good for your health.

Energy

Energy from the sun grows plants that are eaten by animals. Our sources of energy—carbohydrate, fat, and protein—are derived from plants and animals. Using enzyme catalysts aligned in metabolic pathways, we convert these energy sources into molecules of ATP (adenosine triphosphate), the high-energy compound responsible for muscular contractions and many other cellular functions. The pathways control the combustion of the fuels that we burn, and we measure energy needs with a unit for measuring heat, the calorie.

You always expend some energy, even when asleep. If you stay in bed for 24 hours and do nothing at all, you will expend about 1,600 calories (for a 154-pound, or 70-kilogram, body). This energy is used by heart and respiratory muscles, for normal cellular metabolism, and for the maintenance of body temperature. Heavy thinking does little to raise energy needs, but as soon as you begin to move, energy expenditure increases dramatically. Caloric expenditure can go from 1.2 calories per minute at rest to more than 20 calories per minute during vigorous effort. Physical activity has the greatest effect on energy needs. Walking burns about 5 calories per minute, jogging burns about 10, while running burns more than 15.

THE CALORIE

A calorie is the amount of heat required to raise 1 cubic centimeter of water 1 degree Celsius. The kilocalorie is 1,000 calories, or the heat required to raise 1 kilogram of water 1 degree Celsius. As I noted in chapter 1, throughout this book, when I talk about calories, I refer to the kilocalorie, the standard measurement in nutrition and exercise.

ON A DAILY BASIS:

_____ How many servings of fruits and vegetables do you eat?

_____ How many calories do you consume?

_____ What percentage of your caloric intake comes from fat . . . protein . . . or carbohydrate?

_____ What percentage of each should you get?

_____ What percentage of your fat intake comes from saturated fat?

_____ Do you meet your vitamin and mineral needs?

_____ Do you eat out, order in, or eat prepared foods?

_____ Do you eat rich sauces, fatty meats, or dessert?

You can evaluate your responses later in this chapter, with information from the section on food choices.

Carbohydrate

Throughout the world carbohydrate provides the major source of energy. It is available in simple and complex forms. Simple sugars such as glucose, fructose, and sucrose (refined sugar composed of molecules of glucose and fructose) contain energy but few nutrients. Complex carbohydrates found in potatoes, corn, beans, rice, and whole-grained products (bread, pasta) come with important nutrients and fiber. Unfortunately, the average American gets half of his or her dietary carbohydrate from concentrated or refined simple sugars, packed with so-called empty calories that have little or no nutritive value. Fresh fruits contain simple sugars, but they also provide important nutrients.

Digestion of complex starch molecules begins in the mouth where an enzyme (salivary amylase) reduces complex carbohydrates to simple sugars. It is temporarily halted in the stomach when the enzyme is inactivated by gastric secretions. In the small intestine, starches are further digested with the help of another enzyme (pancreatic amylase). Final breakdown to simple sugar form is completed by enzymes secreted by the wall of the intestine. Glucose and other simple sugar molecules are then absorbed into the bloodstream. The absorption is rather complete; most of the sugar you eat gets into the blood, and complex carbohydrates, such as potatoes, can enter the blood as quickly as table sugar (Jenkins, Taylor, & Wolever, 1982).

After a meal, absorbed sugars are taken up by the blood, heart, skeletal muscle, and liver, in that order. When blood sugar levels are restored, heart and skeletal muscles accept glucose. The constantly working heart uses it for energy, while the skeletal muscle can store glucose as glycogen, for use when energy is needed. The liver accepts the simple sugars from the blood and converts them to gylcogen. When sufficient gylcogen has been stored in the liver (about 80 to 100 grams), the leftover glucose suppresses fat oxidation and is itself used for energy. Thus, an excess intake of carbohydrate does not become a supply of "quick energy"; it is oxidized, thereby conserving fat (Swinburn & Ravussin, 1993). The glucose stored in the liver is readily available when needed, but muscle glycogen can be used directly only by the muscle in which it is stored. Blood glucose also can be used by nerves, muscles, or other tissues in need of energy.

THE GLYCEMIC INDEX

The rate of carbohydrate digestion and its effect on the rise of blood glucose is described by the glycemic index. Foods that digest rapidly and cause a pronounced rise in blood sugar have a high glycemic index, while those digested and absorbed more slowly, because of fiber or fat, have a low index. As you might expect, foods with a high index include sugar and honey, as well as corn, white bread, refined cereals, and baked potatoes. Moderate-index foods include pasta, whole-grain breads, rice, oatmeal, bran, and peas; low-index foods include beans, lentils, and fruits (apples, peaches, grapefruit). High-index foods lead to a greater rise in insulin, the hormone responsible for lowering blood glucose (Fosterpowell & Miller, 1995). Individuals with *insulin resistance*, a condition associated with overweight, hypertension, low HDL-cholesterol, and elevated triglycerides and blood glucose, are wise to select low-index foods. High-index foods prompt an insulin surge from the pancreas, stimulating body cells to store glucose. Over time the cells become less sensitive to insulin, eventually leading to adult-onset diabetes. Insulin resistance is linked to heart disease, obesity, age, and inactivity. Weight loss and regular moderate activity reduce insulin resistance.

Since carbohydrates are important for muscular contractions, and since they are not stored in large quantities, we should consume a sizable percentage of the day's calories from complex carbohydrates and fruit. The "Performance Diet" recommended for active people and athletes suggests 60 to 65% of the calories from carbohydrates, up from the 45% typically consumed (see table 11.1).

As I've noted, carbohydrate is stored in muscles and the liver as granules of glycogen, a compound consisting of many linked molecules of glucose. We use this stored carbohydrate at the start of exercise, and its contribution increases as exercise intensity increases. During prolonged exercise, when muscle glycogen stores become depleted, we draw on blood glucose supplied from the liver stores. When that limited supply runs out, we *bonk*—a term coined by cyclists to describe the utter fatigue, confusion, and lack of coordination that results when blood glucose falls below the level required by the nervous system. To avoid bonking, distance athletes drink beverages containing 4 to 10% carbohydrate.

TABLE 11.1   The Performance Diet

Component	Performance diet (% of total calories)	Typical diet (% of total calories)
Carbohydrate	60-65	45-50
Fat	20-25	35-40
Protein	15	10-15

Lactate is not just a metabolic by-product, but rather a metabolic intermediate that can shuttle energy from muscle to liver or from muscle to muscle.

LACTATE

Skeletal muscle may convert glucose to lactate, which diffuses from the muscle and travels to the liver for reconversion to glucose, or travels to another muscle for use as a source of energy. In other words, lactate is not just a metabolic by-product, but rather a metabolic intermediate that can shuttle energy from muscle to liver or from muscle to muscle (Brooks, 1988).

Fat

Fat is the most efficient way to store energy, with 9.3 calories per gram versus the 4.1 and 4.3 for carbohydrate and protein respectively. Dietary fat is broken down and absorbed in the small intestine. It then travels via the lymphatics, a system of tiny vessels and nodes that transport and filter cellular drainage. The fat is eventually dumped into the circulation for transport in clumps (chylomicrons) to cells for energy or to adipose tissue for storage. However, dietary fat intake isn't the only way to acquire this source of energy; excess carbohydrate or protein can be converted to fat and stored in adipose tissue. We have many ways to acquire fat, but only one good way to remove it: physical activity.

Fat isn't all bad. It is an essential component of cell walls, vital insulation in the nervous system, a precursor for important compounds such as hormones, and a shock absorber for internal organs. And fat can be a most efficient fuel for sustained physical activity, especially in muscles that have undergone endurance training. Furthermore, fat enhances the taste of food and helps fill us up. So, we don't need to eliminate dietary fat, just limit the intake. Excess dietary fat is a major cause of overweight and obesity and a contributor to heart disease, hypertension, diabetes, some cancers, and other illnesses. And a recent study indicates that a high fat intake is inversely related to physical activity, suggesting a behavioral link between the two (Simoes et al., 1995).

Fat comes in several forms, including triglycerides and cholesterol. Triglyceride fat is composed of three fatty acids and glycerol. The fatty acids can be saturated (with a hydrogen molecule filling each binding site on a carbon molecule), or unsaturated, with one or more double bonds (see figure 11.1).

Monounsaturated fatty acids have one double bond, while the polyunsaturated have two or more. The double bonds of unsaturated fatty acids may be

FAT INTAKE

If you eat 2,000 calories a day and get 25% of your calories from fat—as recommended by the performance diet—you'll get 500 calories from fat. Divide 500 by 9.3 calories per gram of fat (500/9.3) and you get 54 grams, the amount of fat you can eat each day (far less than the 86 grams you'd eat when fat constitutes 40% of your caloric intake).

The fatty acid may be saturated, meaning they have single bonds, such as stearic acid;

$$
\begin{array}{c}
\text{H\ H\ H\ H\ H\ H\ H\ H\ H\ H\ H\ H\ H\ H\ H\ H\ H}\\
\text{HC - C - C - C - C - C - C - C - C - C - C - C - C - C - C - C - COOH}\\
\text{H\ H\ H\ H\ H\ H\ H\ H\ H\ H\ H\ H\ H\ H\ H\ H}
\end{array}
\qquad \text{Stearic Acid}
$$

they may be monounsaturated, meaning they have one double bond, such as oleic acid;

$$
\begin{array}{c}
\text{H\ H\ H\ H\ H\ H\ H\ H\ H\quad H\ H\ H\ H\ H\ H\ H\ H}\\
\text{HC - C - C - C - C - C - C - C - C = C - C - C - C - C - C - C - C - COOH}\\
\text{H\ H\ H\ H\ H\ H\ H\qquad\quad H\ H\ H\ H\ H\ H}
\end{array}
\qquad \text{Oleic Acid}
$$

or they may be polyunsaturated, meaning they have two or more double bonds, such as linoleic acid.

$$
\begin{array}{c}
\text{H\ H\ H\ H\ H\ H\quad H\ H\ H\quad H\ H\ H\ H\ H\ H\ H\ H}\\
\text{HC - C - C - C - C = C - C - C = C - C - C - C - C - C - C - C - COOH}\\
\text{H\ H\ H\ H\ H\qquad\quad H\qquad\quad H\ H\ H\ H\ H\ H}
\end{array}
\qquad \text{Linoleic Acid}
$$

Figure 11.1   Fatty acids: saturated, monounsaturated, and polyunsaturated.

more susceptible to oxidation. Therefore, unsaturated fats are recommended rather than saturated fats, which facilitate cholesterol synthesis. Saturated fats are found in meat and dairy products. Watch out also for the tropical oils, palm and coconut, which are believed to be more atherogenic, or likely to clog arteries, as are a variety of otherwise healthful oils when they are hydrogenated (e.g., soybean oil). Hydrogenation eliminates double bonds and creates unhealthy trans-fatty acids. Read labels! The performance diet recommends 25% of the day's calories from fat, with no more than one-third from saturated (or hydrogenated) fats. This is substantially less than the 35 to 40% currently being consumed.

Cholesterol can be eaten in the diet or synthesized in the liver. Once in the blood it joins with clumps of fat and very low-density lipoprotein (VLDL). Over a period of 2 to 6 hours, enzymes remove much of the triglyceride, leaving low-density lipoprotein (LDL) cholesterol, which the liver removes over a period of 2 to 5 days. Because of its small size and high concentration of cholesterol, it finds its way into the walls of coronary arteries and contributes to the development of the atherosclerotic plaque. Thus, LDL cholesterol is believed to be a major culprit in the development of coronary artery disease. As LDL levels rise, so does the risk of heart disease (see table 11.2).

High-density lipoprotein cholesterol (HDL) seems to carry cholesterol away from arterial walls to the liver, where it can be removed from the body. This "good" cholesterol has been found to be inversely related to heart disease risk: As HDL goes up, the risk of CAD goes down! The longitudinal Framingham study of an entire community found HDL to be the single best predictor of heart disease risk. Cholesterol, by itself, doesn't provide enough information; you need total cholesterol, LDL cholesterol, and HDL cholesterol to assess heart disease risk. And the total cholesterol/HDL ratio may be one of the best ways to assess risk (see table 11.3).

I'll say more about the effects of activity and fitness on triglycerides, cholesterol, and heart disease risk in chapter 13.

TABLE 11.2   Cholesterol Evaluation

	Desirable	Borderline-high	High risk
Cholesterol	<200	200-239	>240 mg/dl*
LDL-C	<130	130-159	>160
HDL-C	>60	59-35	<35

*Milligrams per deciliter (per tenth of a liter); to convert to International System units (millimoles per liter) multiply by 0.0259.

TABLE 11.3   Total Cholesterol/HDL Ratio

Risk ratio	Male*	Female
0.5	3.43	3.27
1.0	4.97	4.44
2.0	9.55	7.05
3.0	23.4	11.0

*250/50 = 5, an average risk for a male.

Protein

When we ingest animal or plant protein, the large molecules are cleaved into amino acids and absorbed. The amino acids are building blocks used to construct cell walls, muscle tissue, hormones, enzymes, and a variety of other molecules. The blood carries large proteins: globulin for antibody formation, albumin for buffering and osmosis, fibrinogen for clotting, and hemoglobin for oxygen transport. Fitness training builds proteins—enzymes for aerobic training and contractile proteins (actin and myosin) for strength training. So, it should be no surprise to learn the importance of protein to the active life.

The performance diet recommends 15% of daily caloric intake in the form of protein. Moderately active adults can get by with 10%, but those who are very active or training should have more. Fifteen percent of 2,000 calories is 300 calories (300/4.3 = 70 grams; 1 gram per kilogram for a person who weighs 70 kilograms, or 154 pounds). However, more important than quantity is the quality of protein. Quality protein is high in essential amino acids, those that cannot be synthesized in the body. These essential amino acids are an important part of the macronutrients, major food sources that must be available for optimal function. When essential amino acids are missing, the body is unable to construct proteins that require them. Although animal protein is a better source of essential amino acids (as well as iron and vitamin B12), proper combinations of plant protein can meet nutritional needs. If you plan to become a vegetarian, be ready to eat a variety of grains, beans, and leafy vegetables.

Moderately active adults can get by with consuming 10% of daily calories from protein, but those who are very active or training should have more.

PROTEIN NEEDS?

A recent review of protein needs for athletes concludes that endurance athletes will benefit from dietary intakes of 1.2 to 1.4 grams of protein per kilogram of body weight, and strength athletes need 1.4 to 1.8 grams (Lemon, 1995). These values are well above the recommended daily allowance or RDA (1989) of 0.8 grams per kilogram but are attainable with the performance diet recommended in this chapter. If you participate in endurance and strength training you'll need 1.4 grams of protein per kilogram of body weight. Simply multiply 1.4 by your body weight in kilograms (1 kilogram equals 2.2 pounds) to get your daily requirement.

For example, if you weigh 154 pounds, divide 154 by 2.2 to get your weight in kilograms (70 kilograms). Then multiply 70 by 1.4 grams to get your daily protein needs (98 grams). Since each gram of protein yields 4.3 calories, you'll need about 98 grams, or 420 calories, of energy from protein.

If your diet fails to meet the requirement, raise your intake of good-quality protein (lean meats, skinned poultry, fish, beans) (see table 11.4).

Protein isn't a major source of energy at rest or during exercise, seldom amounting to more than 5 to 10% of energy needs, but when one trains hard while dieting to lose weight, the body senses starvation and begins to use tissue protein for energy. To avoid the loss of muscle tissue and to achieve the benefits of training, ensure adequate protein and energy intake. The best bet is to lose weight slowly or not at all during vigorous training. Even with adequate protein, rapid weight loss while training risks the loss of the muscles you are trying so hard to improve.

Excess intake of protein, which is often accompanied with fat (eggs, meat, fish, poultry, dairy products), leads to the storage of energy in the form of fat.

TABLE 11.4   Protein in Common Foods

Food	Portion	Protein (g)
Beans	1/2 cup	6-8
Beef	1/4 lb	20-28
Cheese	1 ounce	7
Chicken	3-1/2 ounces	24-30
Chili	1 cup	20
Corn	1/2 cup	3
Fish	4 ounces	25-30
Hamburger	1/4 lb	20
Milk	1 cup	9
Peanut butter	1 tablespoon	4
Pizza	1 slice	10

Follow the performance diet and you will have all the protein you need, especially since a high-carbohydrate intake spares or conserves tissue protein.

Nutrients

Sometimes called micronutrients because only small amounts are needed, vitamins and minerals play essential roles in metabolism and other important functions.

Vitamins

Why are vitamins, which do not supply energy and are needed only in minute quantities, considered essential for life? In many cases the answer lies in the structure of enzymes, which are essential for cellular metabolism. Enzymes are composed of a large protein portion and a coenzyme. The shape of the protein molecule dictates the role of the enzyme, while the coenzyme is the active portion that performs a specific task. For example, vitamin B1 (thiamin) is a coenzyme that removes carbon dioxide in a metabolic pathway. Without the vitamin coenzyme, the metabolic pathway grinds to a halt, usually with the toxic buildup of intermediary compounds. Lack of vitamin B1 leads to beriberi, a vitamin deficiency disease characterized by weakness, wasting, nerve damage, even heart failure. Fortunately, the small amount of vitamins needed is readily available in a variety of foods in a well-balanced diet. Doses far in excess of daily requirements (megadoses) do not improve function or performance, and they may be toxic.

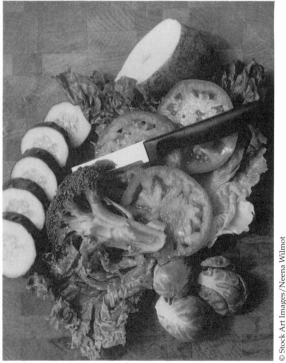

© Stock Art Images/Neena Wilmot

Vitamins in food have been proven more effective than vitamin supplements.

Fat-Soluble Vitamins

Vitamins are classified according to their solubility. The fat-soluble vitamins A, D, E, and K have widely different functions (see table 11.5). These vitamins are ingested with fats in the diet. Amounts in excess of daily needs are stored in body tissue, and megadoses can become toxic. Since they are stored, deficiencies are less likely, except in very low-fat diets.

Water-Soluble Vitamins

B complex vitamins and vitamin C are water-soluble. Excess water-soluble vitamins are washed away in the urine, making deficiencies more likely. Table 11.5 lists the vitamins, some good food sources, and their roles in nutrition.

Vitamins and Health

It is clear that vitamins perform many functions that are essential for life and health. Recent studies indicate that some vitamins are important to the optimal function of the immune system.

To help maintain a healthy immune system, the well-balanced diet should include:

- Beta-carotene—(carrots, sweet potatoes) stimulates natural killer cells, immune system cells that fight infections
- Vitamin B6—(potatoes, nuts, spinach) promotes proliferation of white cells
- Folacin—(peas, salmon, romaine lettuce) increases white cell activity
- Vitamin C—(citrus fruits, broccoli, peppers) enhances the immune response
- Vitamin E—(whole grains, wheat germ, vegetable oils) stimulates the immune response

The minerals selenium and zinc also aid the immune response: Selenium (tuna, eggs, whole grains) promotes action against toxic bacteria; and zinc (eggs, whole grains, oysters) promotes wound healing. Vitamins beta-carotene, C, and E, the so-called *antioxidant vitamins*, have been found to reduce muscle damage and even to reduce the risk of heart disease, cancer, and eye disease. Intense exercise produces compounds called *free radicals*. These highly reactive compounds can damage muscle tissue, especially in untrained individuals who have limited antioxidant capabilities. While we have natural antioxidant protection, the supply is limited. The antioxidant vitamins have been shown to react with the free radicals and reduce their ability to do microscopic damage (Kanter, 1995).

In regard to heart disease, the antioxidant vitamins may prevent the oxidative deterioration of lipid in cell membranes, a step in the artery-clogging process of atherosclerosis. When LDL is oxidized, it turns rancid and becomes part of the growing plaque in the wall of the artery. Dietary antioxidants have been associated with a lower risk of heart disease. However, vitamin supplements have not been as effective. Vitamins in food come with other vitamins, minerals, and trace nutrients that may enhance the effect of the nutrient. Vitamin supplements are not a satisfactory replacement for a well-balanced diet, but moderate supplements of vitamins C, E, beta-carotene, and selenium do offer a margin of safety. Also, regular activity and fitness training have been shown to increase the body's ability to deal with free radicals.

TABLE 11.5   Vitamins and Minerals: Functions and Sources

Nutrient	Important functions	Sources
Fat-soluble vitamins		
Vit A	Vision, immune function	Milk products
Beta-carotene	Cell growth, antioxidant	Fruits, vegetables
Vit D	Bones, teeth	Sunlight, eggs, fish, milk products
Vit E	Antioxidant	Vegetable oils, nuts, greens
Vit K	Blood clotting	Greens, cereals, fruits, milk products, meats
Water-soluble vitamins		
Vit B_1 (thiamin)	Energy production	Pork, grains, beans
Vit B_2 (riboflavin)	Energy production	Milk, eggs, fish, meat, greens
Niacin	Energy production	Nuts, fish, poultry, grains
Vit B_6 (pyridoxine)	Energy production, protein metabolism	Meats, grains, vegetables, fruits
Folate	Red and white blood cells, RNA, DNA, amino acids	Vegetables, beans, nuts, grains, meat, fruit
Vit B_{12}	Blood cells, RNA, DNA, energy production	Meats, milk products, eggs
Biotin	Fat and amino acid metabolism, glycogen synthesis	Beans, vegetables, meats
Vit C (ascorbic acid)	Wound healing, connective tissue, antioxidant, immune function	Citrus fruits, vegetables
Minerals		
Calcium	Bones, teeth, blood clotting, muscle contraction	Milk products, vegetables, legumes
Chloride	Digestion, extracellular fluids	Salt in food
Chromium	Energy metabolism	Legumes, grains, meats, vegetable oils
Copper	Iron metabolism	Meats, water
Fluorine	Bones, teeth	Water, seafood, tea
Iodine	Thyroid hormone	Fish, milk products, vegetables, iodized salt
Magnesium	Protein synthesis	Grains, greens
Phosphorus	Bones, teeth, acid-base balance	Milk products, meats, poultry, fish, grains
Potassium	Nerve transmission, fluid and acid-base balance	Greens, bananas, meats, milk products, potatoes, coffee
Selenium	Antioxidant	Seafood, meats, grains
Sodium	Nerve function, fluid and acid-base balance	Salt
Sulphur	Liver function	Dietary protein
Zinc	Enzyme activity	Meat, poultry, fish, milk products, grains, fruits, vegetables

Vitamins and Performance

Athletes are a gullible bunch, inclined to try anything to improve performance. And there are plenty of "snake oil salesmen" willing to sell a food or drug guaranteed to enhance performance. Vitamin supplements are frequently marketed to this gullible audience, and to millions of others in search of health. Unfortunately, much of the money spent on vitamin megadoses is washed away in the urine, without any noticeable effect on performance. Vitamin supplements will not improve the performance or health of people on an already adequate diet.

> During periods when vigorous training is combined with weight loss, it's probably a good idea to take a supplement containing the recommended daily allowance.

However, in recent years I have come to believe that supplementation may sometimes be prudent. Highly active individuals and athletes need more vitamins when they burn more energy. This increased need should be met with the increased intake of food calories to meet energy and nutrient requirements, but during periods when vigorous training is combined with weight loss, it's probably a good idea to take a supplement containing the recommended daily allowance. And since certain vitamins enhance the immune response, supplementation may help reduce the risk of illness that often accompanies exhaustion and overtraining. Finally, the antioxidant vitamins could also reduce the likelihood of muscle damage during intense activity. That being said, I still recommend vitamins in food over those contained in pills. And I do not endorse megadoses of fat or water-soluble vitamins.

Minerals

Ever wonder why the body needs iron, zinc, magnesium, and even chromium, while it definitely doesn't need lead? Minerals are important for enzyme and cellular activity and some hormones, for bones, for muscle and nerve activity, and for acid-base balance. Some are required in small daily amounts (less than

DIET AND PERFORMANCE

Rick was the top runner on the university track team, with a mile time approaching 4 minutes. The coach expected big things from this elite athlete, but that is not what happened. Instead, as training progressed, his performance began to deteriorate. By mid-season he was struggling to approach 4:20, and things got worse. Eventually he was forced to rest and seek medical advice. The team physician was perplexed, since Rick wasn't sick or injured, yet his vitality was gone and he exhibited signs of chronic fatigue and overtraining. As the coach and the physician continued their search for the problem, they turned to a specialist in sports nutrition. A computerized dietary analysis helped identify the cause of Rick's problem—his vegetarian diet. Several months before the season, he decided to try vegetarianism. Since meat and animal products are important sources of essential amino acids, vitamins, and minerals, his abrupt dietary shift was unwise, especially for an athlete. A vegetarian diet is good for your health and it can sustain training and performance, but only if you are willing to study and spend extra time shopping and preparing nutritious meals.

100 milligrams), while we need more of others. Minerals are available in many food sources, but concentrations are higher in animal tissues and products (as shown in table 11.5).

Minerals, like vitamins, are readily available in a well-balanced diet, one drawn from a variety of food sources. Problems arise when one decides to eliminate a major nutrient source, such as meat.

Iron

Iron is particularly important for active individuals, both male and female. Much of the iron absorbed in the blood goes into the production of hemoglobin, the compound in red blood cells that carries oxygen from the lungs to the working muscles. Iron is also used in muscle myoglobin to transport and store oxygen, and in important oxidative (aerobic) enzymes. Individuals who are deficient in iron risk anemia and poor endurance. Since only 10 to 20% of the iron in food is absorbed into the bloodstream, athletes must take in 10 times the amount needed. Lean meat is a rich source of iron, and the iron in meat is more readily absorbed than that from other sources.

Females lose blood and iron during menstruation, and all active individuals are subject to iron loss and reduced absorption during hard training. Meats, dates, raisins, beans, prunes, and apricots are good sources of iron. If you are concerned about your iron status, consult a physician and nutrition specialist before you supplement with more than the RDA, since high levels of iron have been associated with increased risk of heart disease. And don't rely on a simple hemoglobin measurement to establish anemia. Get an iron profile before you turn to supplementation.

Calcium

Calcium is a major component of bones and teeth. It is also involved in muscle contraction, nerve transmission, blood clotting, and enzyme activity. In regard to the active life, calcium is most important because of its relationship to osteoporosis, the loss of bone density that predisposes bones to fractures. Bone is a tissue that responds to stress. Calcium intake and weight-bearing exercise help keep bones strong and help to slow the inevitable loss of bone density with age. After menopause, when estrogen levels decline, bone density is lost at a more rapid rate. Use of estrogen replacement therapy to slow bone loss must be balanced against other effects of estrogen, such as an increased risk of breast cancer.

Young women face a dilemma caused in part by exercise. Too much strenuous training, combined with weight loss, inadequate calcium intake, and stress, sometimes interferes with the normal menstrual cycle in female athletes. These changes seem to diminish estrogen's protective effect on bones, leading to reduced bone density and risk of stress fractures. Reduced training, weight gain, and increased calcium intake will stop the loss of bone, but we still don't know if young women ever recover from early bone loss.

Zinc

Zinc has received recent attention because of its role in growth, tissue repair, enzyme reactions, and red cell formation. It is readily available in whole-grain products.

Minerals are essential to health and performance, but supplementation beyond what is called for in the RDA is unnecessary and could cause side effects. Excesses of some minerals pose no threat, while others can cause problems including diarrhea (magnesium, zinc), high blood pressure (sodium), and cirrhosis (iron). If you are concerned that your diet may be deficient, consider a supplement that provides the recommended daily allowance for vitamins and minerals, including trace minerals. This may be especially important for those who lose weight during training in an effort to enhance performance. But remember, supplements are not an adequate substitute for good nutrition.

Fluids

In addition to energy and nutrients, the body needs an ample supply of water. More than half of body weight is contributed by water, which is found in the cells and in extracellular fluids such as blood, lymph, saliva, tears, glands, and the gastrointestinal tract. Water serves to transport energy, gases, waste products, hormones, antibodies, and heat. In the blood it is also involved in the regulation of the acid-base balance. It lubricates surfaces and membranes and, via perspiration, serves as a main avenue for temperature regulation.

An inactive individual needs about 2.5 liters daily to replace water lost in urine, feces, skin, and exhalation from the lungs. During activity in a hot environment, sweat loss can average 1 liter per hour for many hours, and can tem-

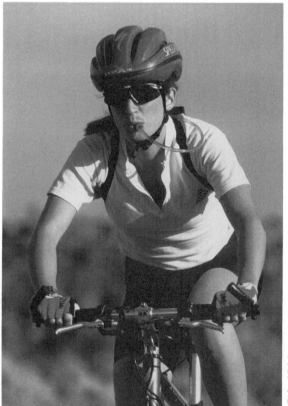

Failure to replace fluids will impair performance and raise the risk of heat disorders.

porarily exceed a rate of 2 liters per hour. Failure to replace this fluid will lead to impaired performance, dehydration, and heat stress disorders, ranging from cramps to heat exhaustion to life-threatening heat stroke.

Water constitutes 55 to 60% of adult body weight. Thirst, activated by excess sodium or water loss, helps us maintain body fluid levels. Several hormones, such as antidiuretic hormone, or ADH, assist in the maintenance of fluids and electrolytes (sodium, potassium, calcium chloride). The kidneys get rid of excess fluids. In other words, the body knows how much water it needs, and you should not attempt to lose water as a means of weight reduction.

You should not attempt to lose water as a means of weight reduction.

It is true that each liter of fluid weighs about 2 pounds, and that dehydration can lead to impressive, albeit short-term weight loss. But the loss is water, not fat; you need the water, and the body will do all it can to get it back. Water and electrolyte loss during dehydration can cause diminished muscular strength and endurance. The loss of blood volume reduces cardiac output and endurance. Every responsible sports medicine organization cautions against dehydration weight loss. It compromises athletic performance and health.

So, don't exercise in a rubber suit, sauna, or steam room in order to lose weight. Sweat is a crucial part of the temperature-regulating mechanism. Sweat must be allowed to evaporate in order to cause evaporative heat loss and help you avoid heat stress. When you do lose weight via sweat loss you should replace it as soon as possible. For example, if you lose 4 pounds of weight during a run or bike ride, you'll need to replace it with 2 quarts of fluid.

I'll discuss fluid replacement in chapter 17, where I'll deal with heat stress, with fluid intake before, during, and after activity, and with carbohydrate/electrolyte drinks and their effect on performance.

Food Choices

The U.S. Departments of Agriculture and Health and Human Services have compiled a guide to daily food choices (see figure 11.2). The guidelines are consistent with the performance diet, providing more than 60% of the calories from carbohydrate and about 25% from fat.

A study of Mediterranean people with low rates of chronic disease and high life expectancies led researchers to recommend a variation of the food guide pyramid. The Mediterranean diet emphasizes daily intake of complex carbohydrates, fruits, vegetables, olive oil, yogurt, and cheese; reduces intake of fish, poultry, eggs, and sweets to a few times per week; and limits red meat consumption to a few times per month. The study also recommended regular physical activity and daily but moderate intake of wine.

If your health risk is high, consider the Mediterranean diet. If not, utilize the food guide pyramid, but realize you'll need to increase food intake to fuel more vigorous or prolonged activity, and consume somewhat more protein to meet the needs of aerobic and strength training.

By now it is becoming clear that your diet is a necessary part of weight control and the active lifestyle. But is diet related to health for other reasons? Diet has been implicated as a major factor in obesity; heart disease; cancer; diabetes; digestive problems such as diverticulitis, irritable colon, and gallstones; and other problems such as dental caries, hernia, and hemorrhoids. A low-fat diet is prescribed for those at risk for heart disease. But how does diet influence cancer and other problems?

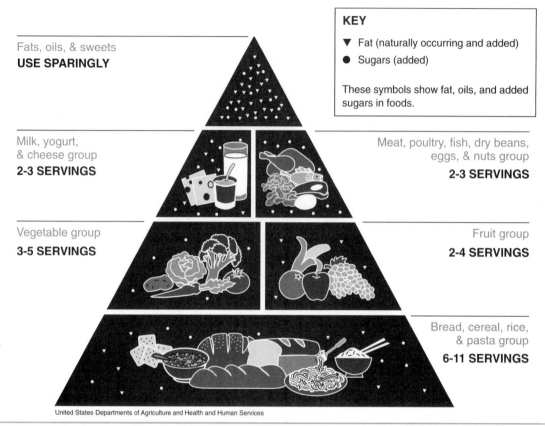

Figure 11.2   The food guide pyramid.

Anticancer Diet

The anticancer diet recently proposed by the National Academy of Sciences endorses the reduction of fat in the diet. The committee advice includes:

- Eat less fat, fatty meats, and dairy products.
- Eat few salt-cured, pickled, or smoked foods.
- Eat more whole-grain products, including fiber-rich foods.
- Eat more fruits and vegetables, including those in the cabbage family and those high in vitamins A and C.
- Drink alcohol in moderation, if at all.
- Keep caloric intake low.

Remember, fat is a factor in cancer and heart disease, and aside from dieting, exercise is the best way to eliminate excess fat from the body.

Dietary Fiber

Fiber, roughage, bulk, and bran all refer to the portion of plants that is indigestible. Why consume an indigestible material? In addition to its long-standing reputation for maintaining regularity, fiber has other advantages. Insoluble fiber (wheat bran, beans) holds water, increases bulk, and increases the rate at which stool and cancerous toxins are removed. Soluble fiber, such as oat bran, apples, and citrus fruits, forms a gel that slows absorption of carbohydrate and

Epidemiologic
studies show that
people on a low-
fiber diet have a
higher incidence
of heart disease
and cancer.

binds cholesterol for removal from the body. It may also produce a chemical that slows the rate of cholesterol production.

Epidemiologic studies show that people on a low-fiber diet have a higher incidence of heart disease and cancer. The average American consumes about one-third of the 25 to 35 grams of fiber recommended by the National Cancer Institute, and the majority regularly ignore fresh fruits and vegetables. If fiber isn't part of your daily regime, begin now to add bran cereals, fruits, vegetables, beans, and whole-grain bread products (bread, pasta) to your diet. Read labels, and try to seek a balance between soluble and insoluble fiber. Finally, consider that when fiber is combined with a low-fat diet, you'll be able to eat freely, with little concern for weight gain.

Health Foods

Companies spend millions to convince us that fitness and health can be achieved by eating their products. While sound nutrition is absolutely essential to health and fitness, nothing you eat will improve your fitness if you are already on an adequate diet. The only way to achieve fitness is via regular exercise; you can't get there just by eating.

Concerns about the quality of our food supply—of the use of hormones, pesticides, dyes, and other chemicals—have led to an increase of so-called natural or organic foods as an alternative source of nutrition. To the extent that these chemical additives may be harmful to health, especially over extended periods of time, natural food sources could be safer than those with no additives. However, the nutritional value of a food or vitamin is not related to the manner of growth. Foods grown with chemical fertilizers are just as nutritious as those grown with organic fertilizers. What matters is the active amount of the essential ingredient, such as a vitamin, and how that contributes to the recommended daily allowance. So, purchase more expensive health foods if you are concerned about the effect of synthetic hormones and chemicals on your health, but don't expect to get super nutrition for your money. Table 11.6 summarizes the recommended daily allowances (RDA) of proteins, vitamins, and minerals according to age and sex.

Interest in health and weight control has led to the development of so-called lite foods and beverages. The products are usually lo-cal versions of the original, such as lite beer, lite or no-calorie soft drinks, and lite crackers and cheese. The products must contain at least one-third fewer calories than the original. While eating these products will not make you lose weight, it can help reduce your caloric intake, so long as you don't eat more of them than you would of the regular style. Since lite foods usually cost as much or more than the regular version, it shows that we will pay more for less—fewer calories, or less sodium or caffeine. Sometimes the products utilize undesirable substitutes (coconut, palm, or cottonseed oil) or hydrogenated oils such as otherwise healthy soybean oil. The new fat substitute Olestra, recently approved by the FDA, may reduce vitamin absorption or cause diarrhea. Read the label to be certain you are getting what you paid for.

A variation of the lite meal is the diet platter at the restaurant. People select these choices because they believe they are more nutritious and have fewer calories and less fat. However, a salad isn't particularly high in nutritive value, and if gobs of high-fat salad dressing are used, it could be a bad food choice (1 tablespoon of dressing can contain 100 calories and 8 grams of fat, and the ladle used to pour the dressing usually holds lots more than 1 tablespoon).

TABLE 11.6   Food and Nutrition Board, National Academy of Sciences-National Research Council Recommended Dietary Allowances,[a] Revised 1989

Category	Age (years) or condition	(kg)[b]	(lb)	(cm)	(in.)	Protein (g)	Vit. A (μg RE)[c]	Vit. D (μg)[d]	Vit. E (mg α-TE)[e]	Vit. K (μg)	Vit. C (mg)	Thiamin (mg)
Infants	0.0-0.5	6	13	60	24	13	375	7.5	3	5	30	0.3
	0.5-1.0	9	20	71	28	14	375	10	4	10	35	0.4
Children	1-3	13	29	90	35	16	400	10	6	15	40	0.7
	4-6	20	44	112	44	24	500	10	7	20	45	0.9
	7-10	28	62	132	52	28	700	10	7	30	45	1.0
Males	11-14	45	99	157	62	45	1,000	10	10	45	50	1.3
	15-18	66	145	176	69	59	1,000	10	10	65	60	1.5
	19-24	72	160	177	70	58	1,000	10	10	70	60	1.5
	25-50	79	174	176	70	63	1,000	5	10	80	60	1.5
	51+	77	170	173	68	63	1,000	5	10	80	60	1.2
Females	11-14	46	101	157	62	46	800	10	8	45	50	1.1
	15-18	55	120	163	64	44	800	10	8	55	60	1.1
	19-24	58	128	164	65	46	800	10	8	60	60	1.1
	25-50	63	138	163	64	50	800	5	8	65	60	1.1
	51+	65	143	160	63	50	800	5	8	65	60	1.0
Pregnant						60	800	10	10	65	70	1.5
Lactating, 1st 6 months						65	1,300	10	12	65	95	1.6
2nd 6 months						62	1,200	10	11	65	90	1.6

[a]The allowances, expressed as average daily intakes over time, are intended to provide for individual variations among most normal persons as they live in the United States under usual environmental stresses. Diets should be based on a variety of common foods in order to provide other nutrients for which human requirements have been less well defined.

[b]Weights and heights are actual medians for the U.S. population of the designated age. The use of these figures does not imply that the height-to-weight ratios are ideal.

Responsible restaurants are now labeling menus to indicate better choices for those concerned with fat intake. Look for food that is nutritious but low in fat. Avoid fried foods, those with cream sauces or butter, and high-calorie desserts. Ask for dressings and other sauces on the side. Request a dry muffin or toast. Eating out is difficult for people on weight-loss or low-fat diets, but things are improving as some restaurant owners realize what the customer wants. Of course, many fast-food outlets continue to promote high-calorie, high-fat food choices (see table 11.7).

Summary

This chapter has provided a thumbnail sketch of nutrition as well as suggestions for improving health and performance. While much more could be written on the subject, the basics here form the framework for a safe and sensible eating plan. Minor adjustments in the diet will lower your daily intake of fat. Reduce fat further if your family history or risk factors indicate the need. Select

TABLE 11.6   *(continued)*

Riboflavin (mg)	Niacin (mg NE)[f]	Vit. B$_6$ (mg)	Folate (µg)	Vit. B$_{12}$ (µg)	Calcium (mg)	Phosphorus (mg)	Magnesium (mg)	Iron (mg)	Zinc (mg)	Iodine (µg)	Selenium (µg)
0.4	5	0.3	25	0.3	400	300	40	6	5	40	10
0.5	6	0.6	35	0.5	600	500	60	10	5	50	15
0.8	9	1.0	50	0.7	800	800	80	10	10	70	20
1.1	12	1.1	75	1.0	800	800	120	10	10	90	20
1.2	13	1.4	100	1.4	800	800	170	10	10	120	30
1.5	17	1.7	150	2.0	1,200	1,200	270	12	15	150	40
1.8	20	2.0	200	2.0	1,200	1,200	400	12	15	150	50
1.7	19	2.0	200	2.0	1,200	1,200	350	10	15	150	70
1.7	19	2.0	200	2.0	800	800	350	10	15	150	70
1.4	15	2.0	200	2.0	800	800	350	10	15	150	70
1.3	15	1.4	150	2.0	1,200	1,200	280	15	12	150	45
1.3	15	1.5	180	2.0	1,200	1,200	300	15	12	150	50
1.3	15	1.6	180	2.0	1,200	1,200	280	15	12	150	55
1.3	15	1.6	180	2.0	800	800	280	15	12	150	55
1.2	13	1.6	180	2.0	800	800	280	10	12	150	55
1.6	17	2.2	400	2.2	1,200	1,200	320	30	15	175	65
1.8	20	2.1	280	2.6	1,200	1,200	355	15	19	200	75
1.7	20	2.1	260	2.6	1,200	1,200	340	15	16	200	75

[c]Retinol equivalents. 1 retinol equivalent = 1 µg retinol or 6 µg β-carotene.

[d]As cholecalciferol. 10 µg cholecalciferol = 400 IU of vitamin D.

[e]α-Tocopherol equivalents. 1 mg d-α tocopherol = 1 α-TE.

[f]1 NE (niacin equivalent) is equal to 1 mg of niacin or 60 mg of dietary tryptophan.

foods from a variety of sources to ensure the availability of essential amino acids, vitamins, and minerals. Use a daily vitamin/mineral supplement with the recommended daily allowances (RDA) during heavy training or weight loss, or if you are concerned about your diet. It's that simple.

Before we move on, let me make a confession. I've been using a daily vitamin/mineral supplement for many years. My justification? I exercise regularly, train often, and always strive to maintain or sometimes lose weight, in spite of a prodigious appetite. At times I engage in strenuous or even exhausting activities, such as hiking, biking, or ski trips, for which I may be inadequately prepared. The RDA supplement is a hedge against less-than-perfect nutrition. There's more. For the last few years I have further supplemented my diet with modest amounts of the antioxidants, vitamins C (500 milligrams), E (400 International Units), and beta-carotene (15 milligrams every other day). These were added in response to studies that showed a lower risk of heart disease, reduced muscle damage, and improved immune function with the antioxidants. I take any reasonable step to minimize my familial risk of heart disease. The bonus is the effect of the antioxidants on the immune system: During the period of supplementation I have been blessed with consistent good health. In the next chapters you'll learn how to gain lasting control of your weight.

TABLE 11.7   Caloric Values for Fast Food

	Energy (cal)	Protein (g)	Fat (g)	Carbohydrate (g)
McDonald's				
2 hamburgers, fries, shakes	1,030	40	37	135
Big Mac, fries, shake	1,100	40	41	143
Big Mac	550	21	32	45
Quarter Pounder	420	25	19	37
Hamburger	260	14	9	30
French fries	180	3	10	20
Chocolate shake	315	9	8	51
Burger King				
Whopper, fries, shake	1,200	40	47	147
Whopper	630	29	35	50
Whopper, Jr.	285	16	15	21
Double hamburger	325	24	15	24
Hamburger	230	14	10	21
French fries	220	2	12	10
Chocolate shake	365	8	8	65
Pizza Hut				
10-in. Supreme (cheese, tomato sauce, sausage, pepperoni, mushrooms, etc.)	1,200	72	35	152
10-in. pizza (cheese)	1,025	65	23	140
Kentucky Fried Chicken				
3-piece dinner (chicken, potatoes, roll, slaw)	1,000	55	55	71
Dairy Queen				
4-ounce serving soft ice cream	180	5	6	27
Arby's				
Sliced beef sandwich, 2 potato patties, slaw, shake	1,200	27	40	166

To convert grams to calories multiply:

Protein (g) $\times$ 4.3

Fat (g) $\times$ 9.3

Carbohydrate (g) $\times$ 4.1

CHAPTER 12

Energy and Activity

"Fortunate, indeed, is the man who takes exactly the right measure of himself, and holds a just balance between what he can acquire and what he can use, be it great or be it small!"

Peter Latham

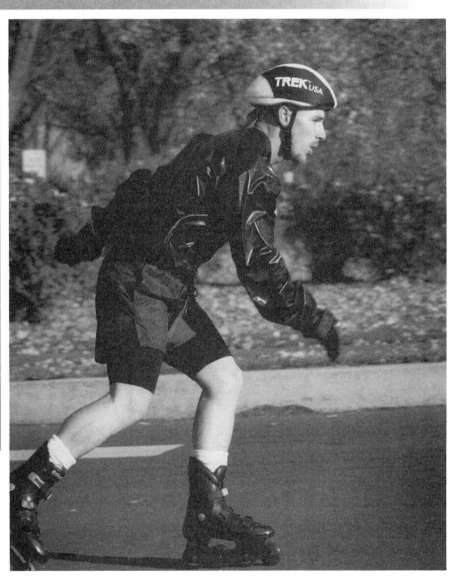

Ages ago, when the food supply was not so predictable and humans couldn't count on three meals a day plus snacks, their bodies learned how to store energy in the form of fat. Our bodies still store energy, even though the food supply now makes the practice unnecessary most of the time. This ability to store energy, coupled with a plentiful food supply, has created a problem for more than one-third of the population. We put calories in the energy account but seldom draw enough out, so our energy balance grows and grows. This chapter is about energy intake and energy expenditure and the consequences of taking in more than we expend.

THIS CHAPTER WILL HELP YOU

- calculate your energy balance: caloric intake versus caloric expenditure,

- understand the causes and consequences of overweight and obesity, and

- establish sensible body weight and body fat goals.

Energy Intake

In chapter 11, I explained how energy is consumed in the form of carbohydrate, fat, and protein. Once it is ingested and stored, energy remains until it is utilized.

Carbohydrate is stored in the liver and muscles in clumps of glucose molecules known as glycogen. The liver supply is a reserve that helps to maintain the blood glucose level, which is the essential energy source for the brain and nervous tissue. Muscle glycogen is the fuel we use to power high-intensity contractions; when the supply is depleted we are unable to sustain those contractions.

Fat is stored in adipose tissue, around organs (visceral fat), and in the muscles. Muscular fat can be used as energy for contractions. Moreover, fat can be mobilized from adipose tissue storage and transported via the circulation to fuel working muscles. The amino acids from the protein you eat are used to con-

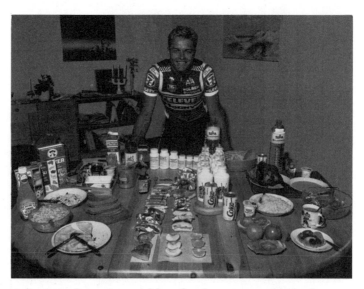

Caloric intake isn't a problem for the active individual.

struct proteins in your body. A small portion of the energy used for activity (5 to 10%) comes from tissue protein.

How is the energy or caloric value of food determined? Nutrition researchers use a calorimeter to measure the energy content of foods. A small amount of food is placed in a chamber and burned in the presence of oxygen. The heat liberated in the process indicates the energy content. When a gram of carbohydrate is ignited, the energy yield is 4.1 calories per gram. When fat is tested, more than twice as much energy is released (see table 12.1).

TABLE 12.1   Caloric Equivalents of Foods

Food	Energy (cal/g)[a]	Oxygen (L/g)	Caloric equivalent (cal/L)
Fat	9.3	1.98	4.696
Carbohydrate	4.1	0.81	5.061
Protein	4.3	0.97	4.432

The alcohol in alcoholic beverages has a high caloric value, 7.1 cal/g. The calories are "empty" and provide no nutritional value. Moreover, because alcohol diminishes appetite and interferes with digestion by inflammation of the stomach, pancreas, and intestine, alcohol often leads to malnutrition. Alcohol also interferes with vitamin activation by the liver and causes liver damage (Lieber, 1976).

[a]Cal (kilocalories) refers to the amount of heat energy required to raise the temperature of 1 kg of water 1°C.

Reprinted from Sharkey 1974.

Energy Expenditure

Walking involves an expenditure of about 5 calories per minute, jogging burns 10 or more, and running can expend 15 to 20 calories per minute.

You always expend some energy, even when asleep. If you stay in bed for 24 hours and do nothing at all, you will expend about 1,600 calories (for a 154-pound, or 70-kilogram, body). This is your basal metabolism. Energy expenditure can go from 1.2 calories per minute during rest to more than 20 calories per minute during vigorous activity. Additional energy is also needed when you eat, to power the processes of digestion and absorption. But it is physical activity that has the greatest effect on energy expenditure. Walking involves an expenditure of about 5 calories per minute, jogging burns 10 or more, and running can expend 15 to 20 calories per minute (see figure 12.1).

In the fasted state, 12 hours after your last food intake, fat, including plasma free fatty acids (plasma FFA) and muscle triglyceride, is the predominant source of energy at light and moderate levels of exercise intensity. At higher levels of intensity, carbohydrate—in the form of muscle glycogen and blood glucose—becomes the major fuel. The contribution of carbohydrate is somewhat higher following a high-carbohydrate meal. The relative contribution of each fuel changes throughout several hours of continuous exercise. For example, at 75% of maximal oxygen uptake, or $\dot{V}O_2$max, the contribution of muscle glycogen drops from 45% to near zero upon depletion of the supply, while energy derived from muscle triglyceride declines from 25% to 10%. The role of blood glucose increases from 5% to 40% as muscle glycogen is depleted. But when the liver glycogen supply declines, the blood glucose falls precipitously. The contribution of fat from adipose tissue (plasma FFA) increases throughout prolonged exercise, rising from 25% to 50% after several hours (Coyle, 1995).

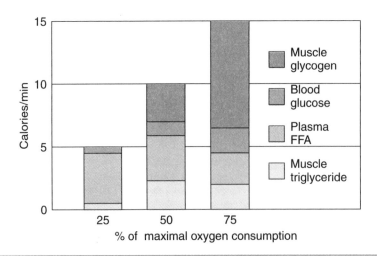

Figure 12.1   Sources of energy. Approximate contribution of energy sources at three levels of exercise. Plasma free fatty acids (FFA) are transported via the blood to the muscles.

Your energy expenditure depends on the size of your body. The greater the body weight, the higher the caloric expenditure. The caloric expenditure tables in this book are based on a body weight of about 70 kilograms (154 pounds). If you weigh 7 kilograms more (15 pounds), add 10%; if you weigh 7 kilograms less, subtract 10%; and so forth. For example, if you weigh 124 pounds and the caloric cost of slow jogging is 10 calories per minute, subtract 20%, or 2 calories, to find the calories burned when you jog (8 calories per minute).

Exercise and Weight Control

Some types of exercise are better than others for weight control. As discussed, we shift from fat to carbohydrate metabolism as exercise becomes more vigorous. If you desire to burn off excess fat, consider moderate exercise (see table 12.2). Since extremely vigorous activity cannot be sustained for very long, the total caloric expenditure may not be great. Also, fat utilization increases over time, with more fat being burned after 30 minutes of exercise. Moderate activity can be continued for hours without undue fatigue, thereby allowing significant fat metabolism and caloric expenditure.

TABLE 12.2   Physical Activity and Caloric Expenditure

Work intensity	Pulse rate	Expenditure (cal/min)	Examples
Light	Below 120	Under 5	Golf, bowling, walking, volleyball, most work
Moderate[a]	120-150	5 to 10	Jogging, tennis, bike riding, aerobic dance, basketball, hiking, racquetball, strenuous work
Heavy	Above 150	Above 10	Running; fast swimming; other brief, intense efforts

[a]Preferred for weight control benefits

Reprinted from Sharkey 1974.

Incidentally, while we are on the subject of fat metabolism, ₊
exercise for weight control may be in the morning, before breakfast.
has shown that you are more likely to burn fat in the morning, after a₊
night fast. So, if you are interested in fat metabolism and weight control, ₊
morning exercise. However, if it doesn't suit your biological clock, don't despair. Exercise always burns calories, so it always contributes to weight control.

Measuring Energy Expenditure

In the early part of this century, scientists found a way to measure human energy expenditure. Subjects were placed in a double-walled chamber very much
like a calorimeter; heat generated in normal activities, such as sitting or standing, eventually increased the temperature of the water layer surrounding the
chamber, indicating the caloric (heat) expenditure. However, this method was
far too expensive, time-consuming, and cumbersome for the measurement of
vigorous activity. Drawing on their knowledge concerning the oxygen requirements of metabolism, researchers developed indirect methods of calorimetry.
Since each liter of oxygen utilized by the body is equivalent to about 5 calories,
why not just measure the oxygen used during exercise? The closed-circuit
method of indirect calorimetry still is used in hospitals for resting or basal metabolic studies. The oxygen intake is the amount that is removed from a large
oxygen tank. The exhaled air, which contains some oxygen, is returned to the
tank after the carbon dioxide has been removed, hence the term closed circuit.
The open-circuit method, where the subject breathes readily available atmospheric air, is best suited for vigorous exercise. The subject breathes in atmospheric air, which contains 20.93% oxygen, and the exhaled air is collected for
analysis. The oxygen consumed and carbon dioxide produced during the activity are analyzed along with the total volume of exhaled air. Oxygen consumption per minute is simply:

$$(\text{Atmospheric Oxygen} - \text{Exhaled Oxygen}) \times \text{Volume Exhaled Air}$$
$$(20.93\% - 17.93\%) \times 33.3 \text{ liters} = 1.0 \text{ liter oxygen per minute}$$

One liter of oxygen equals about 5 calories per minute, the energy cost of a
brisk walk. Jogging requires 2 liters per minute, or about 10 calories (see figure 12.2).

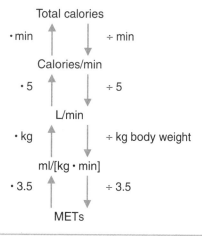

Figure 12.2 Metabolic conversions. It is easy to convert from total calories to
calories per minute (cal/min) to oxygen equivalents in liters (L/min) or milliliters
(ml/[kg · min]) to metabolic equivalents (METs). To convert from one unit to
another, simply carry out the calculation in the direction indicated by the arrow.
For example, if you use 1 L of oxygen per minute (1 L/min) in a brisk walk, you'll
burn 5 cal/min (1 L × 5 = 5 cal/min) and 300 cal/hr (5 × 60).

Energy Balance

Energy balance refers to energy intake, or the calories consumed in the diet, and energy expenditure, or the calories burned in the course of all daily activities (see figure 12.3). If intake exceeds expenditure, the excess will be stored as fat. Since the 1960s, Americans have reduced total dietary fat intake from 40% of daily calories to about 34%. Unfortunately, we've increased total caloric intake about 250 calories each day, and worst of all, we've reduced our level of physical activity.

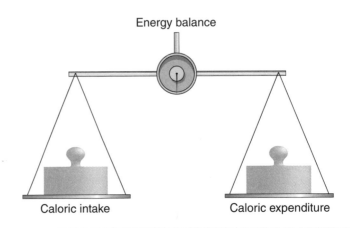

Figure 12.3   Energy balance.

One pound of body fat has the energy equivalent of 3,500 calories. Thus, about 3,500 calories must be expended (oxidized or burned) to remove 1 pound of stored fat. Conversely, 3,500 calories of excess dietary intake will lead to an additional pound of body weight. For example, the daily activity of a young man whose body weight is around 70 kilograms (154 pounds) consists of light office work. He does not engage in any physical activity, so his daily caloric needs approximate 2,400 calories. If he eats a sweet roll for an additional 250 calories every day, what will happen to him over the course of 1 year?

$$250 \text{ calories} \times 30 \text{ days per month} = 7,500 \text{ calories} \times 12$$
$$= 90,000 \text{ calories per year}$$

That 90,000 calories he has gained divided by 3,500 calories per pound equates to 25.7 pounds of added weight. No wonder 33% of the population is overweight. Our friend has upset his energy balance to the tune of more than 2 pounds per month, or 25.7 pounds a year. If he does nothing about his diet or exercise, he could gain 257 pounds in 10 years! Of course, the reverse is also true: If he gives up 250 calories each day, he could lose more than 25 pounds per year. One purpose of this book is to teach you how to have your cake and eat it too, how to use diet and exercise to achieve control of your weight.

Caloric Intake

The determination of daily caloric intake is the first step toward the calculation of the energy balance. Table 12.3 includes comprehensive calorie charts organized according to general categories (e.g., vegetables, meat). Calories contained in each portion are given. Remember:

- 3 teaspoons = 1 tablespoon
- 2 tablespoons = 1 fluid ounce
- 16 tablespoons = 1 cup
- 1 cup = 8 fluid ounces, or one-half pint
- 4 cups = 1 quart
- 1 pound = 16 ounces

Determine your daily caloric intake by keeping an accurate account of everything you eat and drink. The most accurate picture comes when you keep records for several days. Record the type of food or drink and the amount actually consumed. Then use table 12.3 to determine your caloric intake. For example: Breakfast consists of a 1-cup bowl of cornflakes (100 calories) with one-half cup of nonfat milk (40), sugar (25), and a sliced banana (94), plus two pieces of toast (110) with butter (20) and jelly (50), and black coffee (1). Total caloric intake is 440 calories. Do the same for all meals, snacks, beverages . . . everything. Add up the day's total, and that is your caloric intake. If it regularly exceeds your daily caloric expenditure you will gain weight. See figure 12.4 (page 235) for a sample worksheet.

Carry a small notepad with you so you can jot down any food, drink, or snack consumed. At the end of the day sit down with the calorie charts and figure your daily intake. Many computer programs are available to simplify the calculations and provide information on the nutritional value of your diet. You should attempt to assess your caloric intake for at least several days; it is a most educational experience.

Table 12.3 also includes the grams of fat contained in each portion of food or beverage. This should help you avoid unwanted fat if you decide to pursue a low-fat diet, which works to reduce body weight as well as cholesterol. Each gram of fat contains 9.3 calories. If your goal is to reduce fat intake from the typical 40% of calories, try to stay within the following targets:

For a daily calorie intake of 2,000 calories:

40% fat = 86 grams of fat
(40% × 2,000 calories = 800 calories / 9.3 calories per gram = 86 grams)
30% fat = 65 grams
20% fat = 43 grams
10% fat = 22 grams

TABLE 12.3   Caloric Content of Foods

Food	Portion	Fat[a] (grams)	Calories
Beverages, alcoholic			
Beer	12 ounces	0	150
Beer, light	12 ounces	0	100
Brandy	1 ounce	0	70
Eggnog	1 cup	19	335
Highball	1 cup	0	165
Port, vermouth, muscatel	1/2 cup	0	155
Rum	1 jigger (1-1/2 ounces)	0	140
Whiskey	1 jigger (1-1/2 ounces)	0	130
Wine, white, rosé	1/2 cup	0	85-105

(continued)

TABLE 12.3   (*continued*)

Food	Portion	Fat[a] (grams)	Calories
Beverages, nonalcoholic			
Carbonated soft drinks	1 cup	0	80
Chocolate milk	1 cup	10.5	200
Cocoa	1 cup	11	175
Coffee, black	1 cup	0	1
with cream and sugar (1 teaspoon each)	1 cup	3	45
Tea	1 cup	0	1
Cereals, cereal products			
Bread			
Boston, enriched, brown	2 large slices	1.2	200
corn or muffins, enriched	2	6	220
raisin, enriched	2 slices	1.5	130
rye, American	2 slices	0.6	110
white, enriched	2 slices	1.5	120
whole wheat	2 slices	1.5	110
Bread, rolls, sweet, unenriched	1	3	320
Cornflakes	1 cup	0.1	100
Crackers, graham	2	1.0	60
saltines	2	1.5	50
soda	10 oyster	1.3	40
Macaroni, cooked	1/2 cup	0.3	70
Noodles, cooked	1 cup	2.0	150
Oatflakes, cooked	1 cup	1.0	75
Pancakes, wheat	2 cakes	6.0	150
Popcorn, popped	1 cup	0.8	60
Pretzels	Handful	1.0	110
Rice, cooked	1/2 cup	0.1	100
Spaghetti with tomato sauce	1 cup	7.0	220
Tapioca, cooked	1/2 cup	4.0	130
Waffles, baked (frozen or mix)	1 waffle	4-8	225
Wheat germ	1 ounce	3.5	120
Confections			
Chocolate	1 ounce	16	150
Fudge	1 piece	5	120
Honey	1 tablespoon	0	65
Jams	1 tablespoon	0	55
Jellies	1 tablespoon	0	50
Molasses	1 tablespoon	0	50
Syrup (chiefly corn syrup)	1 tablespoon	0	60
Sugar, maple	1 tablespoon	0	55
cane or beet	1 tablespoon	0	50

TABLE 12.3

Food	Portion	Fat[a] (grams)	Calories
Dairy products, eggs			
Cheese, cheddar	1 ounce	9.5	115
cottage	1/2 cup	5	100
cream	2 tablespoons	10	100
Limburger	1 ounce	8	100
Parmesan	1 ounce	8.5	110
Roquefort	1 ounce	8	105
Swiss	1 ounce	8	105
Cream, light	1 tablespoon	3	30
heavy or whipping	1 tablespoon	5.5	50
Eggs, whole	1 medium	5	75
Egg white, raw	1 medium	0	15
Egg yolk, raw	1 medium	5	60
Milk, pasteurized, whole	1 cup	8.5	165
buttermilk, cultured	1 cup	0.4	80
canned, evaporated, unsweetened	1/2 cup	10.0	140
condensed, sweetened	1/2 cup	14	480
nonfat	1 cup	0.4	80
Ice cream	1/2 cup	9-13	155-225
Sherbet	1/2 cup	2-3	135
Yogurt, low fat	1 cup	2.0	61
regular	1 cup	8.5	152
Fats, oils			
Butter	1 tablespoon	4.0	35
Mayonnaise	1 tablespoon	11.0	100
Olive oil	1 tablespoon	12.0	125
Peanut butter	1 tablespoon	8.0	85
Fruit, fruit juices			
Apples	1	0.8	60-90
Apple juice, fresh	1 cup	0	120
Applesauce, sweetened	1/2 cup	0	80
Apricots	1 medium	0	18
Avocados, fresh	1/2	18	190
Bananas	1 (about 6 in.)	0	94
Blackberries, fresh	1/2 cup	0.6	40
Blueberries, fresh	1/2 cup	0.4	45
Cantaloupe, fresh	1/2	0.2	40
Cherries, canned, sweetened	1/2 cup	0.2	100
Cranberry sauce	2 tablespoons	0	60
Dates, dried, pitted	5	0.2	100

(continued)

TABLE 12.3   (*continued*)

Food	Portion	Fat[a] (grams)	Calories
Fruit cocktail, canned	1/2 cup	0.2	90
Grapes, fresh	20	0.8	45
Grape juice	1/2 cup	0	80
Grapefruit	1/2 (4-1/4 in. dia.)	0.1	75
Grapefruit juice, fresh	1/2 cup	0.2	45
Lemons, fresh	1 (2 in.)	0	30
Olives, green or ripe	5 large	2.5/4.0	20/35
Oranges, fresh	1 (3 in.)	0.1	70
Orange juice, fresh	1/2 cup	0.3	55
Peaches, fresh	1 (2-1/2 in.)	0.1	45
canned, sweetened	2 halves	0.2	85
Pears	1 (2-1/2 in.)	0.7	95
Pineapple, canned, sweetened	1/2 cup	0.2	100
Pineapple juice, canned	1/2 cup	0.1	60
Plums	1 (2 in.)	0.1	30
Prunes, dried, uncooked	4 large	0.3	110
Raisins, dried	1/4 cup	0.1	100
Raspberries, fresh	1/2 cup	0.5	50
Strawberries, fresh	10 large	0.5	35
frozen, sweetened	1/2 cup	0.2	125
Sorbet	1/2 cup	0.2	110
Meat, poultry (raw unless otherwise stated)			
Bacon, medium fat, cooked	2 strips	9.0	100
Beef (medium fat), hamburger, cooked	1/4 lb	15	225
rib roast, cooked	3 ounces	33	335
sirloin, cooked	3 ounces	27	330
canned, corned	4 ounces	11	240
liver, fried	3 ounces	9.0	200
Chicken, fried	1/4 lb	9.0	275
roasted	1/4 lb	3.0	170
liver	3 ounces	15.0	235
Ham, baked	3 ounces	19	250
canned, spiced	3 ounces	21	245
Lamb (medium fat), leg roast	3 ounces	6.0	160
rib chop	1	15.0	230
Pork (see also bacon and ham), medium fat	3 ounces	24	310
loin or chops	1	24.5	300
Turkey, light and dark	3 ounces	3.5-7.0	150/170
Veal	3 ounces	9.5	180
Venison	3 ounces	2.5	120

TABLE 12.3

Food	Portion	Fat[a] (grams)	Calories
Nuts			
Almonds	15	8.0	100
Brazil nuts	5	12.0	100
Cashews, roasted or cooked	10	14.0	200
Peanuts, roasted	30	14.0	165
Pecans	1 tablespoon	5	52
Walnuts	2 tablespoons	10	95
Seafood (raw unless otherwise stated)			
Clams	1/4 lb	0.8	80
Cod	4 ounces	6.0	180
Crab, canned or cooked	1/2 cup	2.0	100
Flounder	1/4 lb	7.0	180
Frog legs, fried	4 legs	28.0	418
Haddock	1/4 lb	7.0	180
Halibut	1/4 lb	8.0	200
Lobster	1 (3/4 lb)	5.0	300
Oysters	5-8 medium	2.0	80
Salmon, Pacific, cooked	1/4 lb	7.0	180
canned	1/2 cup	7.0	190
Sardines, canned in oil	5 medium	9.0	180
Scallops, fried	4 ounces	10.0	200
Shrimp, canned	3 ounces	0.9	100
Shrimp, fried	3 ounces	9.5	190
Trout	1/4 lb (brook/lake)	10-13	210-290
Soup			
Broth	1 cup	0	25
Bean	1 cup	6.0	170
Beef	1 cup	4.0	115
with vegetables	1 cup	2.0	90
Chicken noodle	1 cup	2.0	68
Pea	1 cup	3.0	140
Tomato	1 cup	2.5	100
Vegetable	1 cup	2.0	90
Vegetables			
Asparagus, canned	1/2 cup	0.4	25
Beans, kidney	1/2 cup	0.5	120
lima, fresh	1/2 cup	0.4	90
snap, fresh	1/2 cup	0.4	35
wax, canned	1/2 cup	0.2	20

(continued)

TABLE 12.3   (*continued*)

Food	Portion	Fat[a] (grams)	Calories
Beets (beetroots), peeled, fresh	1/2 cup	0.1	35
Broccoli, fresh	1/2 cup	0.2	30
Brussels sprouts, fresh	1/2 cup	0.3	30
Cabbage, fresh	wedge	0.2	25
Carrots, canned	1/2 cup	0.2	30
fresh	1 carrot (6 in.)	0.1	20
Cauliflower, fresh	1 cup	0.2	25
Celery	2 stalks	0.1	17
Corn, fresh, with butter	1 ear	2.0	90
canned	1/2 cup	0.6	70
Cucumbers	1 (7-1/2 in.)	0.2	20
Eggplant, fresh	1/2 cup	0.2	25
Kale, fresh	1/2 cup	0.4	20
Lentils	1/2 cup	—	110
Lettuce, headed, fresh	1/4 head	0.1	15
Mushrooms	1/2 cup	0.1	10
Onions	1 (2-1/2 in.)	0.1	40
Peas, green, fresh	1/2 cup	0.2	55
canned	1/2 cup	0.4	70
Peppers, green, fresh	1 large	0.1	24
Potatoes, raw	1 medium	0.2	90
French fried	20 pieces	12	220
Radishes, fresh	4 small	—	10
Rhubarb, fresh	1/2 cup	—	10
Spinach, canned	1/2 cup	0.2	25
Sweet potatoes, fresh	1 small	0.6	150
candied	1 medium	3.5	180
Tomatoes, fresh	1 medium	0.2	25
canned	1/2 cup	0.2	25
Tomato juice, canned	1/2 cup	0.2	35
Miscellaneous			
Gelatin dessert	1/2 cup	0	60
Pie	1 slice	16-18	300-400
Pecan pie	1 slice	31.5	580
Potato chips	7-10	8.0	110
Salad dressing (French, Thousand Island)	1 tablespoon	6-8	60-100
Tomato catsup	2 tablespoons	0.1	40
Yeast, compressed, baker's	1 cake	0.1	20

[a]1 g of fat contains 9.3 calories

Caloric Intake

(Use calorie charts in table 12.3.)

Date _____   Weight _____

	FOOD	PORTION	INTAKE (cal)
Breakfast			
Lunch			
Dinner			
Desserts			
Snacks			
Drinks			
Other			

Total caloric intake   _____

Total caloric expenditure (figure 12.5)   _____

Energy balance (+ or -) _____

Cal/day

Figure 12.4   Caloric intake record.

Caloric Expenditure

For the next few days, keep an inventory of your activity. Simply list your activity (exercise, work, household chores) and the time spent for each (see figure 12.5). Don't omit anything, even sleeping. This exercise is most educational; it shows you when calories are burned and provides insight about how you can increase caloric expenditures in your normal routine.

Then estimate the caloric expenditure by referring to figure 12.4 and the instructions here. I've provided two ways to estimate your caloric expenditure, one short and one long. The short method is an estimate based on 4 simple steps. The long method requires that you keep records of your daily activities, such as sleep, dressing, cooking, work, and all physical activity, including walking, stair climbing, fitness, and recreation.

When intake and expenditure have been determined, you will be able to assess your energy balance, and you'll have a clear idea of what you can do to reduce caloric intake and increase caloric expenditure.

Short Method

Follow steps 1 through 4:

1. Calculate basal energy expenditure using table 12.4.
2. Add increases in caloric expenditure using table 12.5.
3. Adjust total for age: subtract 4% of caloric expenditure for each decade (10 years) over 25 years of age.
4. Add calories expended in nonwork (recreational) activities.

Caloric Expenditure Log
(Use energy expenditure tables in this chapter)

Activity	Time (min)	Expenditure rate (cal/min)	Total expenditure (cal)
Sleep	_____	_____	_____
Nonwork and household			
_____	_____	_____	_____
_____	_____	_____	_____
_____	_____	_____	_____
Work			
_____	_____	_____	_____
_____	_____	_____	_____
_____	_____	_____	_____
Recreation and sport			
_____	_____	_____	_____
_____	_____	_____	_____
_____	_____	_____	_____
	24 hr	Day's total =	_____

Examples	Time (min)	Expenditure rate (cal/min)	Total expenditure (cal)
Sleep	480	1.2	576
Nonwork			
Personal toilet	10	2.0	20
Cook breakfast	10	1.5	15
Cook dinner	60	1.5	90
Work			
Walk to work and return	20	5.0	100
Work (standard activity)	400	2.6	1,040
Rest breaks	80	1.5	120
Lunch	30	1.5	45
Jogging	30	10.0	300
		TOTAL	2,306

Figure 12.5 Caloric expenditure log.

TABLE 12.4   Basal Energy Expenditure for Men and Women

Men		Women	
Weight	Energy expenditure[a] (cal)	Weight	Energy expenditure[b] (cal)
140	1,550	100	1,225
160	1,640	120	1,320
180	1,730	140	1,400
200	1,815	160	1,485
220	1,900	180	1,575

[a]5 ft 10 in. tall (add 20 cal for each inch taller; if shorter subtract 20 cal).

[b]5 ft 6 in. tall (add 20 cal for each inch taller; if shorter subtract 20 cal).

Basal energy = calories expended in 24 hr of complete bed rest.

Use the caloric expenditure charts in figure 12.6 to calculate minutes of activity and cost in calories per minute.

Example: A 45-year-old construction worker, 5 feet 10 inches tall, weighing 200 pounds

$$
\begin{aligned}
\text{Basal} \;=\;& 1{,}815 \text{ calories} + 100\% \\
=\;& 3{,}630 \text{ calories} - 8\% \text{ (age)} \\
=\;& 3{,}340 \text{ calories} + 30 \text{ minutes of table tennis with his} \\
& \text{son (30 minutes} \times 5 \text{ calories per minute)} \\
=\;& 150 \text{ calories} \\
\text{Total} \;=\;& 3{,}490 \text{ calories per day}
\end{aligned}
$$

TABLE 12.5   Approximate Increases in Caloric Expenditure for Selected Activities

Activity	Percent above basal
Bed rest (eating and reading)	10
Quiet sitting (reading, knitting)	30
Light activity (office work)	40-60
Moderate activity (housekeeping)	60-80
Heavy occupational activity (construction)	100

Long Method

You calculated your daily caloric expenditure using the short method. This section provides the information for a minute-by-minute estimation of caloric expenditure that allows the computation of a 24-hour total. You may be interested in comparing the two methods to see if they agree. If so, begin by making a list of your daily activities. Then proceed to determine the cost of each activity in calories per minute. Finally, get the total for each activity and the total for the day. Figure 12.6 shows how this can be done.

Form for Assessment of Energy Expenditure and Energy Balance

Activity	Kcal/min	Min	Totals
Sleeping	_____ ×	_____ =	_____
Working	_____ ×	_____ =	_____
Eating	_____ ×	_____ =	_____
Personal	_____ ×	_____ =	_____
Play or sport	_____ ×	_____ =	_____
Relaxation (e.g., TV)			
_____	_____ ×	_____ =	_____
_____	_____ ×	_____ =	_____
_____	_____ ×	_____ =	_____
_____	_____ ×	_____ =	_____
		24 hr	cal/day

Example

Activity	Kcal/min	Min	Totals
Sleeping	1.2 ×	480 =	576
Working	2.6 ×	480 =	1,248
Reading	1.3 ×	120 =	156
Writing	2.6 ×	60 =	156
Eating	1.5 ×	60 =	90
Personal	2.5 ×	60 =	150
Walking, moderate pace	5.0 ×	60 =	300
Talking	1.3 ×	60 =	78
Tennis	7.0 ×	60 =	420
		24 hr	3,174 cal/day

Figure 12.6 Form for assessment of energy expenditure and energy balance.

Table 12.6, which shows caloric expenditure, also serves as a useful guide to *exercise intensity*, because intensity is directly related to calories expended per minute. Also, the caloric expenditure charts can guide you to appropriate weight-control activities. You can readily see that walking burns more calories than recreational volleyball, that slow running (jogging) requires more energy than calisthenics. Finally, a glance at the caloric expenditure charts will tell you how long you must exercise to accomplish a 100-, 200-, or 300-calorie workout.

Adjust the total for your body size: Add 10% for each 15 pounds above 150 pounds. Subtract 10% for each 15 pounds under 150.

Your energy balance can now be calculated:

Caloric intake = ___ calories—Caloric expenditure = ___ calories

If intake exceeds expenditure (regularly) you have a positive energy balance. The excess will be stored as fat.

TABLE 12.6   Caloric Expenditure During Various Activities

Activity	Cal/min[a]
Sleeping	1.2
Resting in bed	1.3
Sitting, normally	1.3
Sitting, reading	1.3
Lying, quietly	1.3
Sitting, eating	1.5
Sitting, playing cards	1.5
Standing, normally	1.5
Classwork, lecture (listening)	1.7
Conversing	1.8
Personal toilet	2.0
Sitting, writing	2.6
Standing, light activity	2.6
Washing and dressing	2.6
Washing and shaving	2.6
Driving a car	2.8
Washing clothes	3.1
Walking indoors	3.1
Shining shoes	3.2
Making bed	3.4
Dressing	3.4
Showering	3.4
Driving motorcycle	3.4
Metalworking	3.5
House painting	3.5
Cleaning windows	3.7
Carpentry	3.8
Farming chores	3.8

(continued)

TABLE 12.6   *(continued)*

Activity	Cal/min[a]
Sweeping floors	3.9
Plastering walls	4.1
Repairing trucks and automobiles	4.2
Ironing clothes	4.2
Farming, planting, hoeing, raking	4.7
Mixing cement	4.7
Mopping floors	4.9
Repaving roads	5.0
Gardening, weeding	5.6
Stacking lumber	5.8
Sawing with chain saw	6.2
Working with stone, masonry	6.3
Working with pick and shovel	6.7
Farming, haying, plowing with horse	6.7
Shoveling (miners)	6.8
Shoveling snow	7.5
Walking down stairs	7.1
Chopping wood	7.5
Sawing with crosscut saw	7.5-10.5
Tree felling (ax)	8.4-12.7
Gardening, digging	8.6
Walking up stairs	10.0-18.0
Playing pool or billiards	1.8
Canoeing, 2.5 mph-4.0 mph	3.0-7.0
Playing volleyball, recreational to competitive	3.5-8.0
Golfing, foursome to twosome	3.7-5.0
Pitching horseshoes	3.8
Playing baseball (except pitcher)	4.7
Playing Ping-Pong or table tennis	4.9-7.0
Practicing calisthenics	5.0
Rowing, pleasure to vigorous	5.0-15.0
Cycling, easy to hard	5.0-15.0
Skating, recreational to vigorous	5.0-15.0
Practicing archery	5.2
Playing badminton, recreational to competitive	5.2-10.0
Playing basketball, half or full court (more for fast break)	6.0-9.0
Bowling (while active)	7.0
Playing tennis, recreational to competitive	7.0-11.0
Waterskiing	8.0

TABLE 12.6

Activity	Cal/min[a]
Playing soccer	9.0
Snowshoeing (2.5 mph)	9.0
Slide board	9.0-13.0
Playing handball or squash	10.0
Mountain climbing	10.0-15.0
Skipping rope	10.0-15.0
Practicing judo or karate	13.0
Playing football (while active)	13.3
Wrestling	14.4
Skiing	
Moderate to steep	8.0-20.0
Downhill racing	16.5
Cross-country; 3-10 mph	9.0-20.0
Swimming	
Leisurely	6.0
Crawl, 25-50 yd/min	6.0-12.5
Butterfly, 50 yd/min	14.0
Backstroke, 25-50 yd/min	6.0-12.5
Breaststroke, 25-50 yd/min	6.0-12.5
Sidestroke, 40 yd/min	11.0
Dancing	
Modern, moderate to vigorous	4.2-5.7
Ballroom, waltz to rumba	5.7-7.0
Square	7.7
Walking	
Road or field (3.5 mph)	5.6-7.0
Snow, hard to soft (2.5-3.5 mph)	10.0-20.0
Uphill, 15% grade (3.5 mph)	8.0-11.0-15.0
Downhill, 5-10% grade (2.5 mph)	3.5-3.7
15-20% grade (2.5 mph)	3.7-4.3
Hiking, 40-lb pack (3.0 mph)	6.8
Running	
12-min mile (5 mph)	10.0
8-min mile (7.5 mph)	15.0
6-min mile (10 mph)	20.0
5-min mile (12 mph)	25.0

[a]Depends on efficiency and body size. Add 10% for each 15 lb over 150; subtract 10% for each 15 lb under 150. Use activity pulse rate to confirm the caloric expenditure (see figure 13.1, page 263).

Overweight and Obesity

In horse racing, the favorite often is "handicapped" to provide a better contest. If a few pounds are added, the favorite may become an also-ran. Excess weight can affect performance in the human race as well; few of us realize how much. Excess weight will prove a burden physically, socially, psychologically, and economically. It may be the largest health problem shared by the majority of Americans. Yet it is a symptom, not a disease, and it is among the least complicated of all health problems.

What are the medical consequences of overweight and obesity? The death rate for this group is higher than it is among persons of normal weight, especially in the younger age groups. There is a higher incidence of atherosclerotic heart disease, hypertension, some cancers, diabetes, and cirrhosis of the liver. Accidents and surgical complications are more prevalent, as are complications of pregnancy. When the excess weight is removed, these problems are reduced or eliminated.

Overweight

You may say, "I'm not overweight; I weigh the same as I did my senior year of high school." However, your *weight* may be the same, but what about your ratio of lean to fat tissue? Isn't it possible that you have lost muscle and gained some fat? Has your waist measurement remained the same? The standard method of determining overweight is by comparison with the *desirable* body weight (see table 12.7). Desirable weights are those associated with the longest life span for individuals of a certain skeleton size. (Incidentally, since overweight is associated with heart disease, diabetes, and hypertension, insurance companies often charge a higher premium for individuals judged to be 20% or more above desirable weight.)

Excess pounds of fat *or* muscle can make you overweight, but extra fat poses more of a burden, since the muscles can do useful work and take less space for equal weight (muscle is denser than fat). But even excess muscle seems unnecessary for the adult, unless it is needed for occupational reasons. Also, there are disturbing indications of increased risk of high blood pressure and heart disease among muscular men with excess fat, such as inactive former football players.

Obesity

Obese people eat more fat and engage in less physical activity than nonobese people.

Obesity is an excessive accumulation of fat beyond what is considered normal for the age, sex, and body type. Obesity is a case of being overfat, not just overweight. It is possible to be underweight and still be obese, such as when an individual has excess fat and poorly developed muscles. Obesity can be defined as more than 20% above desirable weight, or as more than 20% fat for men or 30% fat for women. These levels are arbitrary, and some experts prefer lower or higher levels, but by this definition one-third of the adult population is obese (see table 12.8).

TABLE 12.7   Desirable Weights for Men and Women*

Height (without shoes)	Weight (lbs) (without clothes)	
	Women	Men
5'0"	103-115	—
5'1"	106-118	111-122
5'2"	109-122	114-126
5'3"	112-126	117-129
5'4"	116-131	120-132
5'5"	120-135	123-136
5'6"	124-139	127-140
5'7"	128-143	131-145
5'8"	132-147	135-149
5'9"	136-151	139-153
5'10"	140-155	143-158
5'11"	—	147-163
6'0"	—	151-168
6'1"	—	155-173
6'2"	—	160-178
6'3"	—	165-183

*Age 25 and above.

These guidelines, issued by the Metropolitan Life Insurance Company in 1959, are recommended over more recent editions, which provide false reassurance to a large fraction of individuals who are not defined as overweight, but who are at a substantially increased risk of heart disease.

TABLE 12.8   Average (Not Desirable or Ideal) Values for Body Fat According to Age and Gender

Age	Men (%)	Women (%)
15	12.0	21.2
17	12.0	28.9
18-22	12.5	25.7
23-29	14.0	29.0
30-40	16.5	30.0
40-50	21.0	32.0
Minimum	5-7	11-12
Obese	>20	>30

Measuring Body Fat

College-aged men average 12.5 to 15% fat; college women average about 25%. The standard method for determining percentage of body fat is underwater weighing. The nude subject is weighed both in air and while submerged in water. After appropriate adjustments are made for the air in the lungs and gas in the gastrointestinal tract, body density is determined.

$$\frac{\text{Weight in air}}{\text{Weight in air} - \text{Weight in water}}$$

Since fat is less dense than bone or muscle, it is possible to calculate the percentage of body fat. As the weight of the submerged body goes up, the percentage of body fat goes down, and vice versa. Thus it is that lean people sink and fat people float; fat weighs less than muscle per unit of volume. A less accurate but serviceable method for the estimation of percentage of body fat utilizes skinfold calipers. The skinfold calculation of body fat is based on the relationship of subcutaneous (under the skin) fat to total body fat. Note that as much as one-third of the body's fat may be stored under the skin, and the rest is around internal organs, around nerves as insulation, and in all cells, including muscle. To perform the skinfold measurement, grasp skinfolds between the thumb and forefinger, then apply calipers about one-half inch from the fingers. The calipers go in about as deep as the fold is wide (e.g., if the fold is one-half inch, go in one-half inch with the calipers). Take the measurement, release, repeat the measurement, and continue until your measure is consistent. Use chest, abdomen, and thigh skinfolds for males, and triceps, thigh, and suprailium for females (see figure 12.7). Several carefully selected skinfolds provide an estimate of body fat (use figure 12.8 to calculate your percentage).

If skinfold calipers are not available, simply pinch the skin on the back of the upper arm (midway between shoulder and elbow). If the width of the fold, exclusive of muscle tissue, exceeds 10 millimeters (more than three-eighths of an inch), the accumulated fat could indicate a need for weight control (see table 12.9)

Alternative methods used to determine body fat range from girth or other body measurements to expensive laboratory techniques. Many health clubs use a bioelectric impedance technique, which estimates fat from body water

TABLE 12.9   Minimum Thickness of Triceps Indicating Obesity

Age	Male (mm)	Female (mm)
5	12	14
10	16	20
15	16	24
20	16	28
25	20	29
30-50	23	30

Obesity is defined as more than 20% fat for men; more than 30% fat for women.

Adapted from Seltzer and Mayer 1965.

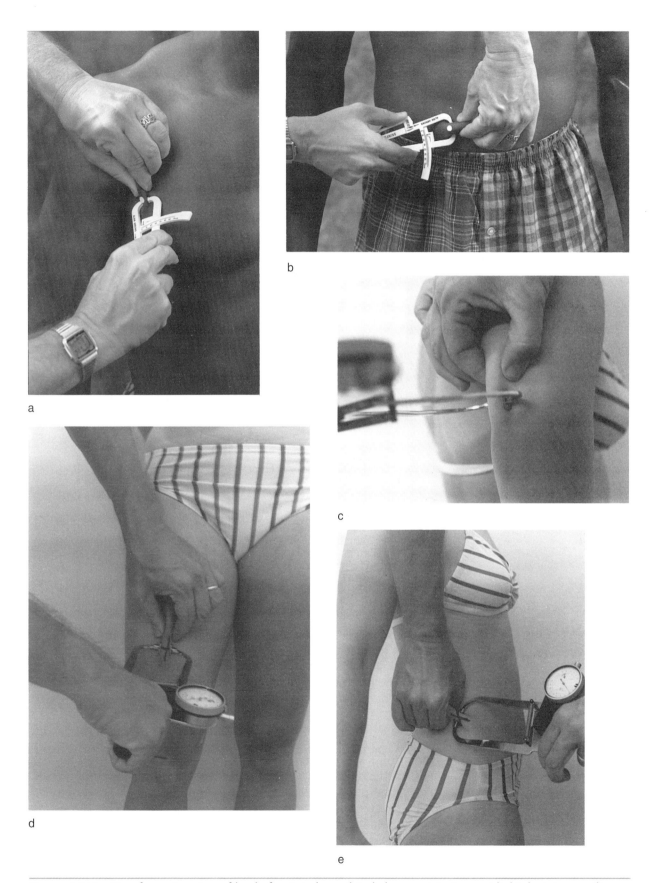

Figure 12.7   Sites for estimation of body fat; (a) chest; (b) abdomen; (c) triceps; (d) thigh; (e) suprailium.

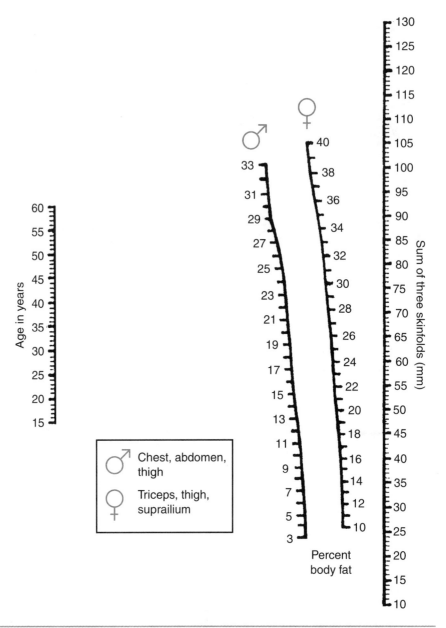

Figure 12.8 A nomogram for the estimate of percent body fat for both male and female populations, using age and the sum of three skinfolds. Use a straight edge to draw a line from your age to the sum of the three skinfolds, and read your percent fat from the appropriate scale.
Reprinted from Baun, Baun, and Raven 1981.

content. This technique, based on the fixed amount of water in fat, requires strict adherence to hydration standards to achieve acceptable accuracy. Scientists use the Potassium-40 emitted from lean tissue to measure total body fat. New methods of estimating fat, such as bioelectric impedance, are often compared with underwater weighing to see if they are accurate. However, recent studies indicate that underwater weighing itself is subject to errors, especially with younger and older subjects and with those at the extremes of leanness and fatness. Age-related differences in body water and bone density can throw off this method, as can dehydration. So, studies are under way to improve the

GETTING FAT

Excess caloric intake starts the process. Fat intake, though, poses more of a problem, since it has 9.3 calories per gram, while carbohydrate and protein have 4.1 and 4.3 respectively. Moreover, the fat is similar to the composition of our adipose tissue and easier to store. Obese people eat more fat and engage in less physical activity (Rising, Harper, Fontvielle, et al., 1994), thereby contributing to the problem. Some researchers believe that fat cells may continue to increase in size and number in severely obese individuals with increasing food intake, creating an even greater urge to eat. Rising obesity increases levels of the enzyme lipoprotein lipase (LPL), which helps fat cells take on more fat. Excess fat seems to inhibit the action of insulin, the hormone that helps glucose get into cells, leading to feelings of weakness and hunger that cause one to eat more. And the cycle continues.

equations used to calculate body fat from underwater weighing. Until then, skinfolds, girth measurements, or the body mass index (figures 12.9 and 12.10) can guide your weight control efforts.

The body mass index (BMI) provides a simple way to assess body composition. All you need is your body weight in pounds and your height in inches. Then consult figure 12.10 to get your score. You should strive to remain at or near the desirable category. The BMI is determined by the formula: BMI = weight in kilograms divided by height in meters squared.

Causes of Overweight and Obesity

Why are 80 million Americans overweight to the point of obesity? Is it merely because their caloric intake exceeds expenditure? To a large extent the answer is yes! While Americans have lowered the proportion of fat in their diets, they have simultaneously increased carbohydrate and caloric intake and decreased their level of physical activity. However, scientists continue to study other possible contributions to the epidemic of obesity.

Heredity Versus Environment

When we see obese parents with obese offspring, we are likely to think the problem "runs in the family." Obesity is more common in offspring when both parents are obese. (The child has an 80% risk of obesity.) Studies of identical twins reared in different environments also indicate that obesity has a genetic root. However, the pattern and extent of that relationship have not been well defined.

Much of the obesity we see in families could be due as much to the environment as to a genetic cause. Overweight people eat more and exercise less, and the same may be true of their children. However, in a study of identical and fraternal twins (Stunkard, Foch, & Hrubec, 1986), the authors found a high heritability for weight and body mass index (weight in kilograms divided by

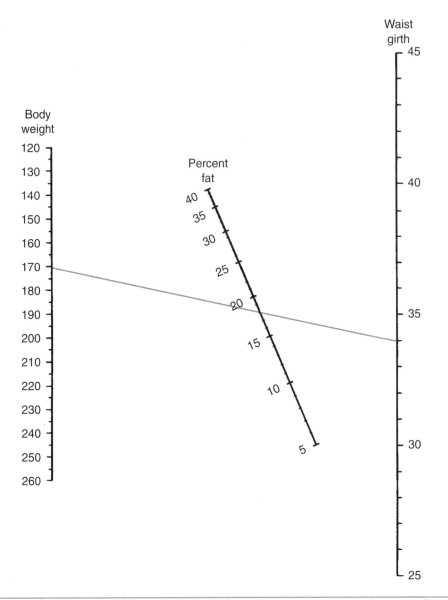

Figure 12.9 Girth measurements. Various body dimensions have been used to predict the lean body weight and percent fat. For men only, the girth at the waist seems to be a good predictor of body fat. For this method simply measure the girth of the waist at the level of the navel, then use a straight edge and go from waist girth to body weight to estimate percent fat. For other tape measure methods to estimate body fat consult McArdle, Katch, and Katch (1994).
Reprinted from Sharkey 1977.

height in meters squared) and concluded that body weight and obesity are under strong genetic control, and that childhood family environment by itself has little effect. Recent discovery of genes partially responsible for obesity supports this reasoning.

Does that mean that energy balance is meaningless? No, it doesn't. In spite of the genetic influence, the basic cause of overweight and obesity remains a positive energy balance due to excess caloric intake, inadequate caloric expenditure, or both. Then, what else causes this tendency to store fat?

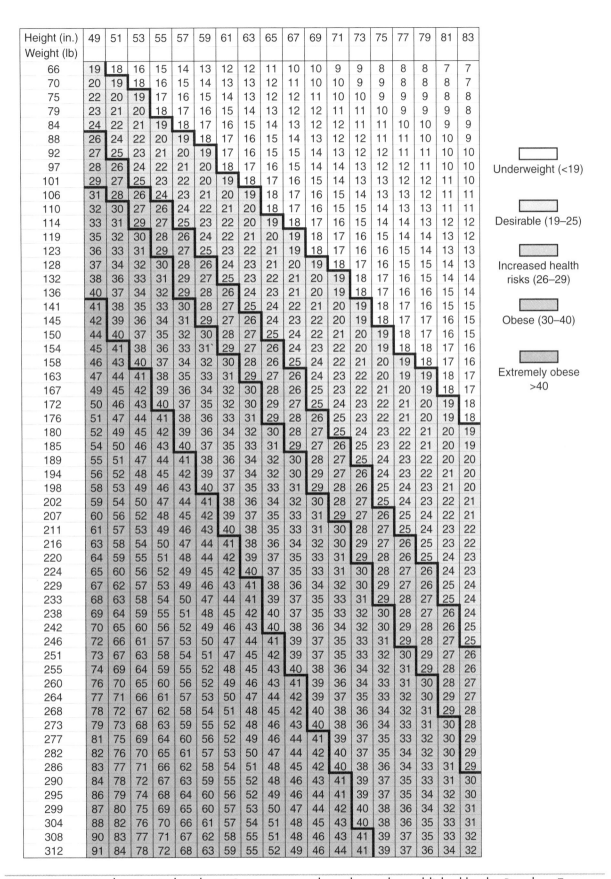

Figure 12.10 Body mass index chart. Categories are based on value published by the Panel on Energy, Obesity, and Body Weight Standards, 1987, *American Journal of Clinical Nutrition*, **45**, p. 1,035.

Glandular Causes

The endocrine glands secrete hormones that exert considerable influence on metabolism. For many years the glands were blamed for overweight and obesity. One authority (Gwinup, 1970) has said: "With the exception of diabetes, glandular disease is associated with obesity in less than one case out of a thousand. Even in the presence of such a disease, the individual is obese because energy acquisition has exceeded energy expenditure." Obese individuals have a significantly higher incidence of diabetes than those of normal or desirable weight, but it is not clear whether obesity is a cause or result of diabetes. After weight reduction, individuals with non-insulin-dependent diabetes mellitus (NIDDM) need less insulin to control their blood sugar. In fact, overeating, particularly on a high-fat diet, may lead to obesity and non-insulin-dependent diabetes, according to scientific evidence.

Diabetes is characterized by a deficiency of the hormone insulin, which is needed to get blood sugar into cells, including fat cells. When sugar doesn't reach the cells, energy is low and the appetite is stimulated, so the diabetic individual eats more. There is a growing awareness that a high-fat diet may increase insulin resistance, thereby requiring more insulin to do the same job. After a while, years perhaps, the pancreatic cells responsible for the production of insulin may fatigue, thereby producing a bona fide case of diabetes.

Prior to the discovery of insulin in 1921, diet and exercise were the only treatments available to persons with diabetes. Nowadays, diet and insulin injections have become the standard treatment to control this metabolic malfunction of insulin production and sugar utilization. Since muscular activity increases the transport of glucose into muscle cells, even in the absence of insulin, and since muscular activity is effective in the reduction of body weight and the risk of heart disease (diabetes and heart disease frequently are associated), it seems logical that attention has returned to the use of exercise in the treatment and control of diabetes. Moderate physical activity reduces insulin resistance and requirements for normal as well as diabetic subjects. Regular participation in aerobic activity often reduces reliance on insulin. When aerobic activity is coupled with a low-fat diet and significant weight loss, the need for insulin can be further reduced.

Fat Cells

In recent years, researchers have studied the growth and development of fat cells. Excess calories are stored in fat cells in the form of triglyceride. Some individuals have more fat cells, causing them to store fat more readily. With the development of methods to determine fat cell size and number, researchers have been able to follow the development of obesity. It appears that fat cells are able to increase in size or number, and that the increase can be stimulated by overfeeding. Traditionally, a chubby baby has been considered a healthy baby, but overfeeding during the first few years of life will stimulate the development of larger and more numerous fat cells (three times more). These cells remain for life and may exert an influence on the appetite when they are not filled. This early onset of hypercellularity generally leads to the most severe form of obesity. While the risk is always there, another period of intense concern comes at or around the time of puberty, when overfeeding can lead to increases in fat cell number and size.

Adult-onset obesity is characterized by enlarged fat cells. The number of fat cells, however, does not seem subject to significant change. The pattern of obesity is a significant factor in determining health risk; obesity that begins in childhood and continues into the adult years is a greater risk than adult-onset obesity. The location of stored fat also predicts health risk; pot bellies are associated with a higher risk of heart disease, while pear shapes are not. Since men tend to accumulate fat in their bellies, that may be a factor in their higher risk of heart disease. Studies are now under way to determine why some cells take in more fat, and why that is related to heart disease.

Pot bellies are associated with a higher risk of heart disease.

WAIST-TO-HIP RATIO

Unfortunately the fat of pot bellies, located around the visceral organs, can't be measured with skinfold calipers, since it lies below abdominal muscles. Researchers are looking closely at the waist-to-hip girth ratio (WHR) to determine why this visceral fat carries a greater risk of heart disease, hypertension, stroke, and some cancers. To calculate your ratio, simply measure the waist at the level of the navel, and the hips at the greatest circumference of the buttocks, and divide the waist by the hip measurement (measure to the nearest quarter-inch). Early results suggest that WHR values above 0.85 to 0.9 for men or 0.75 to 0.8 for women exceed safe limits (see figure 12.11).

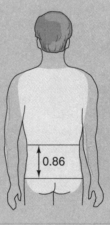

Figure 12.11   Waist-to-hip ratio (e.g., 32/37 = 0.86).

Why is visceral fat of the pot belly a risk? One reason may be that fat stored in and around the viscera has a direct circulatory route to the liver. Fat cells in that region are likely to send free fatty acids directly to the liver, where they can be used to synthesize additional cholesterol, and increase the risk of heart disease. Whatever the reason for the relationship, we know that exercise is the best way to reduce the amount of metabolically active visceral fat. We also know that insulin resistance, stress hormones (cortisol and epinephrine), alcohol, and cigarette smoking tend to increase the WHR.

Metabolic Rate

Studies on obese infants, adolescents, and adults all agree that fat people are more fuel-efficient; their bodies burn calories more sparingly than bodies of normal weight subjects. The lower metabolic rate or energy expenditure makes weight loss more difficult. Perhaps this helps explain how heredity may influence overweight and obesity. Why is the metabolic rate lower? One line of reasoning points to a lethargic or less active sympathetic nervous system. This portion of the autonomic nervous system secretes epinephrine (adrenalin) to speed up the heart rate and other responses during stress or exercise. Epinephrine also prompts the release of fatty acids from fat cells. Less sympathetic activity means less epinephrine, and less epinephrine means a lower metabolic rate and less fat utilization.

Other lines of research, as listed here, tend to lift some of the blame for excess fat from the shoulders of the obese.

• **Brown fat thermogenesis:**   Brown fat, a form of fat that uses excess food to make heat, may be deficient in some obese individuals. Normally, brown fat serves to keep extra calories from being stored as fat. Studies on lean and obese humans will shed more light on this potential contributor to obesity.

• **Lipoprotein lipase:**   Lipoprotein lipase (LPL) is an enzyme in adipose tissue (also found in muscle). Its activity has been found to increase in the fat cells of obese individuals who lose weight, leading researchers to wonder if it might be a reason why previously overfat individuals usually regain lost weight. The effect of exercise on muscle LPL will be discussed in chapter 13.

• **Sodium pump enzyme:**   Sodium-potassium ATPase is an enzyme involved in pumping sodium out of cells. Some researchers have found reduced activity in the cells of obese animals, and they postulate that the deficiency could reduce overall energy expenditure. The findings on obese humans are inconclusive.

If one or several of these lines of research are confirmed on human subjects, we will be better able to understand why so many millions are overweight or obese. It is too early to tell if metabolic problems result in obesity or if overeating is the cause (Bray, 1983). What is clear is that weight loss via dieting is associated with a reduction in 24-hour energy expenditure, and that this reduction makes it more difficult to maintain a body weight that is different from the usual weight (Leibel, Rosenbaum, & Hirsch, 1995). The implications of this finding will be dealt with in chapter 13. Just remember: Regardless of genetic, glandular, psychological, or other complications or causes, overweight and obesity are problems of energy balance. Too many calories are taken in, too few are expended, or both.

Other Causes

There may be a few other causes of overweight as well.

• **Psychological causes.**   Overweight can stem from an underlying emotional problem. Eating may be a defense mechanism, a retreat from reality, or a defiant gesture used to get attention or sympathy. All of us have used food as a crutch when we were bored or lonely, and all of us have eating habits that border on overfeeding—doughnuts during coffee break, chips with TV, or late-night snacks. Eating and drinking are complex social behaviors, and failure to participate may be viewed as a social rebuff. The psychological and social causes of overeating are beyond the scope of this book, but eating behaviors are not. Chapter 14 will deal with ways to alter eating behavior.

While some obese individuals suffer anxiety and depression, it isn't clear if these reactions are a consequence of the excess weight, of social and psychological treatment by others, or of problems related to dieting. In other words, emotional problems associated with obesity may be a cause or a result of excess weight, and some may be a consequence of the treatment, *dieting*.

• **Lack of activity.** Even the most voracious eater would have difficulty gaining weight if he or she ran 10 miles a day. The evidence suggests that overweight children are less active than their thinner counterparts. Trained observers plotted the movements of fat and thin children while they engaged in games such as volleyball. The thin children ranged all over the court, while the heavyweights literally held down their positions (Mayer & Bullen, 1974).

You may be wondering, "What comes first, inactivity or fat?" The earlier section on fat cells implicates fat intake, but we do know that people reduce their activity and range of movement as they become larger, not wishing to call attention to their size. However, when adult-onset obesity follows an active youth, the individual is likely to be less inhibited and more active than one who became obese as a child. But whatever the case, inactivity leads to weight gain, which leads to further inactivity, which leads to more weight gain, and so on. The problem is to break this painful cycle, and to restore normal levels of activity and food intake.

Dieting is a major cause of overweight and obesity.

• **Dieting!** Surprised? How can dieting lead to overweight or obesity? When animals or humans gain weight, diet, gain weight, diet, etc.— a process called weight cycling—the body becomes more fuel-efficient, and metabolic rate declines. Thereafter, more dieting or exercise is required to reduce excess weight. Weight loss slows, and weight is regained three times faster during the second cycle. Eventually, weight is maintained on a reduced caloric intake that inhibits weight loss and promotes regain (Brownell, Greenwood, Stellar, & Shrager, 1986). In other words, the "yo-yo" approach to weight control leads to weight *gain*, not loss.

One reason for the yo-yo effect is the loss of muscle protein with each round of dieting. Muscle is *metabolically active*; it is the furnace that burns unwanted calories. Lose muscle, and you have less ability to burn calories, at rest or during exercise. Every time you diet to lose weight, lean tissue is lost; so, you must decrease caloric intake to avoid subsequent weight gain. Return to past eating habits, and you increase weight and fat above previous levels. Exercise is the only way to minimize the loss of lean tissue while dieting. In fact, do enough exercise, and you can reverse the drop in metabolic rate and increase lean tissue, thereby easing the problem of weight control.

OPRAH!

When popular television personality Oprah Winfrey used a commercial diet program to lose weight, it was big news. But it was even bigger news when she gained it all back within a few months. Today, Oprah maintains her weight and her appearance the sensible way, with regular activity. She runs a phenomenal 8 miles a day and recently completed the Chicago Marathon!

Ideal Body Weight

Is there such a thing as an ideal body weight or body fat? Should one strive to reduce body fat to the minimum? The minimum amount of fat consistent with good health and nutrition probably is around 5 to 7% for young men and 11 to 12% for young women. Healthy high school wrestlers and male distance runners sometimes have a bit less than 5%, and female distance runners have had a temporary low of 7%. This does not suggest that all men and women should attempt to achieve these levels; I offer them only to indicate a minimum level consistent with health and performance. Studies show that for health reasons, weight should not regularly fall more than 10% below desirable weight. The upper limit consistent with good health is 20% above the desirable weight. Somewhere between these boundaries (minus 10% to plus 20% of desirable weight) lies a level that is best for you. The level you choose will relate to your current activity and interests. If you are training for a long-distance race or bike ride, you'll want to minimize your "handicap." If you've been burdened with a large number of fat cells, you may be doing well to keep the level below 20%. Data indicates that those who weigh less than the desirable body weight for their height and frame live longer than those who weigh more. Since desirable weights are based on average body fat values, it would seem advisable to maintain body weight and fat values at or below desirable weight or average fat levels, respectively. But in the absence of heart disease, hypertension, or diabetes, there is little health difference between the extremes of 5% and 20% fat for men, or 12% and 30% fat for women.

IDEAL WEIGHT?

New findings strongly suggest that U.S. weight guidelines are too lax, encouraging obesity in both men and women. The researchers found that 40% of all heart attacks in middle-aged women are due to over-weight, a figure similar to that found in men. Women of average (not desirable) weight had a 50% higher risk of heart attack than those 15% below the average U.S. weight. Also, gaining more than 10 pounds in early to middle adult life increased the risk (Manson et al., 1995). Based on this study, ideal weights can be estimated as follows:

Women
100 pounds for 5 feet (60 inches)
plus 5 pounds for each additional inch
e.g., For a woman 5 feet, 6 inches tall:
$100 + (5 \times 6) = 130$ pounds

Men
106 pounds for 5 feet
plus 6 pounds for each additional inch
e.g., For a man 5 feet, 6 inches tall:
$106 + (6 \times 6) = 142$ pounds

Estimated weights are plus or minus 10%.

Gender-Specific Fat

Some of the fat differences between males and females are due to gender-specific fat. Female hormones dictate different patterns of fat deposition, including breasts, which are largely fat. However, only a portion of the difference, perhaps an extra 6%, is due to gender-specific fat; the rest is probably due to lack of activity or excess caloric intake, or both. But that is changing as more women undertake the active life. Active college-age women average 18 to 22% fat, and female endurance athletes are often in the 12-to-17% range (Sharkey, 1984).

Age and Body Fat

With each decade above age 25, the body loses about 4% of its metabolically active cells.

With each decade above age 25, the body loses about 4% of its metabolically active cells. If the diet remains relatively unchanged during a 10-year period, weight will be gained, since the total energy expenditure has declined. This means that the adult should either exercise more or eat less in order to maintain a desirable weight. Individuals who can claim that their weight has not changed since college should be congratulated. However, they should also know that the loss of metabolically active cells with age usually means a decline in lean body weight. Therefore, the maintenance of body weight usually indicates an *increase* in the percentage of body fat. Body weight alone is not sufficient evidence that you are winning the battle of the bulge.

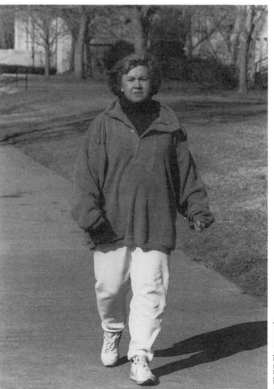

Exercise is the only way to minimize the loss of lean tissue while dieting.

Seasonal Fluctuation

Body weight and body fat values fluctuate from season to season and year to year. Typically, the lean body weight (body weight minus fat weight) does not change that rapidly. The lean body weight consists mainly of muscles, bones, and organs. Thus, seasonal changes in body weight can be attributed to differences in the amount of fat being stored in adipose tissue. Total body fat storage often is higher during the winter months, when subcutaneous fat serves as insulation against the cold. In the summer, the weight and fat often decline in response to an increase in energy expenditure and a decrease in appetite (stimulated in part by the increase in daylight).

Summary

It seems clear that overweight and obesity have a genetic link, and that individuals who inherit the tendency are more metabolically efficient (they use less energy). Thus, someone can become overweight even though he or she may eat little more than those who remain thin. But how much can be attributed to heredity and how much to a positive energy balance, eating more calories than you burn? Obesity researcher Claude Bouchard has estimated that 35 to 40% of the variance in body weight among individuals of similar stature can be attributed to genetic causes, leaving 60 to 65% as your personal responsibility (Malina & Bouchard, 1991). Of course it is possible to become overweight in the absence of a genetic influence by eating too much and exercising too little. Earlier we talked about energy balance and caloric intake and expenditure. Recent research suggests that we may need to refine that equation and focus specifically on *fat balance*. Unlike carbohydrate and protein stores, fat stores are not controlled, and their capacity for expansion is enormous (Swinburn & Ravussin, 1993). Obesity can be seen as a long-standing positive fat balance, the consequence of a high fat diet. The message, therefore, is simple: Lower dietary fat intake.

Calorie-burning exercise is the other side of the fat balance equation; it burns fat while preserving lean tissue, something that dieting alone cannot do. Chapter 13 will tell you how to incorporate activity into a sensible program of weight control and show how improved aerobic and muscular fitness can magnify the benefits of regular moderate activity.

Activity, Diet, and Weight Control

"A journey of a thousand miles must begin with a single step."

Lao-tzu

"The swiftest traveler is he that goes afoot."

Henry David Thoreau

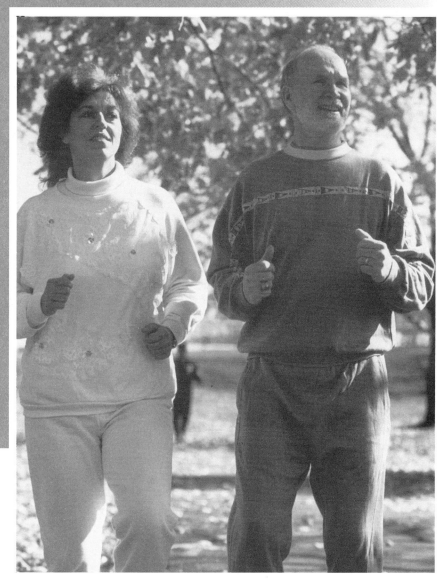

Weight control is a lifelong journey. The best time to start is when you are young; the next best time is today. Physical activity is the positive approach to weight control. When you decide to do something about your weight, you are committing to a course of action. No other approach is so physiologically sound, so definite, so enjoyable. It is more psychologically rewarding to act than it is to avoid. When you walk a mile after dinner you relax, improve your digestion, enhance your vitality, and, incidentally, burn fat and calories. After the walk you feel better both physically and emotionally. Problems loom large when you sit and brood, but how quickly they shrink when you undertake a plan of action!

Dieting carries negative connotations of avoidance, deprivation, and punishment. Dieting creates false hopes, contributes to stress, ruins the disposition, causes fatigue, and often leads to increases in body weight and fat. The ups and downs of frequent dieting (weight cycling, or yoyo dieting) increase the risk of psychopathology, life dissatisfaction, binge eating, and morbidity and mortality (Brownell & Rodin, 1994).

The most exciting part of this chapter deals with the extra benefits you obtain with improved fitness, benefits that exceed the effects of activity. This material, while not new, is only beginning to come to the attention of public health and fitness professionals. In my estimation, it provides the most convincing case for activity and fitness and their relationship to health.

THIS CHAPTER WILL HELP YOU

- understand why activity is superior to dieting as a means of weight control,
- determine the effects of activity on the appetite, and
- understand the extra weight control and fat metabolism benefits associated with improved fitness.

Activity and Weight Control

The only way to remove stored fat is to burn it off. By now you know that exercise increases caloric expenditure and that the rate of expenditure is related to both the intensity and duration of activity. As exercise becomes more intense, the duration of participation becomes limited. While we may be able to expend as many as 125 calories in one all-out mile run, we can jog at a comfortable pace for 3 miles and triple the caloric expenditure without becoming exhausted. This explains why moderate activity instead of high-intensity effort is recommended for weight control.

Caloric expenditure can remain elevated for 30 minutes or more after vigorous exercise.

The effects of exercise do not stop when the exercise ceases. Caloric expenditure can remain elevated for 30 minutes or more after vigorous exercise. Long-duration effort such as a distance run will elevate body temperature and call forth hormones to mobilize energy and increase metabolism. When the exercise stops, there is a recovery period when caloric expenditure remains elevated above resting levels. This post-exercise increase in energy expenditure is usually neglected when the caloric benefits of exercise are tabulated.

Activity Versus Dieting

Many people claim that dieting is better than exercise for controlling weight. They point out, quite correctly, that it is easier to reduce caloric intake by refusing a piece of cake (250 calories) than it is to burn off the cake after it is eaten (2 miles at 120 calories per mile). But let's return to the question "Is dieting a better method of weight control?" The answer has been available for more than 25 years.

Oscai and Holloszy (1969) compared the effects of dieting and exercise on the body composition of laboratory rats. The experiment was controlled so that both groups lost the same amount of weight. Following 18 weeks of either food restriction (dieting) or swimming (exercise), carcass analysis was performed. Table 13.1 displays the amounts of fat, protein, and water lost by the groups.

TABLE 13.1   Exercise Versus Dietary Weight Loss

Body component	Weight lost (%)	
	Exercise	Diet
Fat	78	62
Protein	5	11
Minerals	1	1
Water	16	26

Adapted from Oscai and Holloszy 1969.

A control group of sedentary, freely eating animals gained weight during the study. Their weight gain consisted of 87% fat and 10% water.

It appears (see table 13.1) that exercise is a more effective way than dieting to lose fat. Furthermore, the study provided vivid evidence of the "protein-conserving" effects of exercise. Notice also the amount of water lost through caloric restriction. This water loss is a common occurrence among dieters and accounts for the early success of most fad diets, and for the eventual failure of the overall goal, fat loss. Can the results of this animal study be generalized to human subjects?

Six months of dieting were compared with a similar period of dieting and exercise in a study involving 16 obese patients. The exercise group achieved greater fat loss, and the exercise produced other benefits, including a lower resting heart rate and improved heart rate recovery after exercise (Kenrick, Ball, & Canary, 1972). And when 25 women created a 500-calorie-per-day deficit by dieting, exercise, or a combination, the results were the same no matter what method was used. All the women lost the same amount of weight, but those in the dieting group lost less fat and more lean tissue. The authors of the study, Drs. Zuti and Golding (1976), recommended that those interested in losing weight combine dieting and exercise to ensure a greater fat loss and a conservation of lean tissue. A recent study of 24 obese women confirms the superiority of diet and exercise for the reduction of adipose tissue and preservation of lean tissue and skeletal muscle, as compared with diet alone (Ross, Pedwell, & Rissanen, 1995).

These studies clearly indicate the need for activity in a program of weight control. Dieting or caloric restriction can lead to the loss of weight, but the loss is accompanied by a greater loss of protein (lean tissue) and water. When lean tissue is lost the body becomes less able to burn calories, and more fat weight is eventually gained. A dietary weight loss leads to a disproportionate decline in metabolic rate and almost certain weight gain (Leibel, Rosenbaum, & Hirsch, 1995). Complicating the loss of lean tissue to burn fat is a possible resetting of the metabolic thermostat, making weight gain likely with even less caloric intake. Weight loss with exercise maximizes the removal of fat, minimizes the loss of protein, and helps maintain the metabolic rate. Exercise and dieting combine to provide a positive attack on both causes of overweight: excess caloric intake and inadequate caloric expenditure.

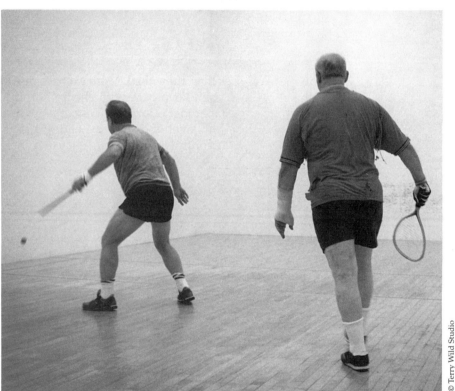

© Terry Wild Studio

Weight loss with exercise maximizes the removal of fat.

METABOLIC RATE

A recent study indicates an added benefit of exercise in relation to weight control and diet. Several weeks of severe caloric restriction imposed by dieting led to the usual loss of lean tissue and decrease in metabolic rate. The drop in metabolic rate makes it difficult for dieters to maintain a lower body weight, since the more efficient body burns 10 to 15% fewer calories daily. However, on the bright side, just 2 weeks of exercise restored the metabolic rate to pre-diet levels. Moreover, the exercise reduced the loss of protein and increased the utilization of fat as the source of energy (Móle, Stern, Schultz, Bernauer, & Holcomb, 1989).

Activity and Appetite

In the past, the use of activity to achieve energy balance and weight control drew criticism. Detractors claimed exercise would increase the appetite as the body attempted to keep pace with energy needs. Many assume that the desire for food signifies a real need for nourishment, but it doesn't. Appetite is a psychological desire that is influenced by several factors. The control center for food intake, the *appestat*, is located in the hypothalamus, an area of the brain that functions like a thermostat to turn on eating behavior, then turn it off when the desire or hunger has been satisfied. Unfortunately, it takes many minutes for the food you eat to reach the bloodstream, where the appestat can sense that you've satisfied the need. It is possible to tuck away several hundred extra calories before the appestat gets the message.

Physiological factors such as low blood sugar, hormones, cold temperatures, hunger pangs from an empty stomach, and unfilled fat cells can stimulate the appestat. Physical activity also stimulates eating behavior, but the increased caloric intake serves only to maintain body weight. Sedentary individuals take in more calories than they need. More exercise results in more food intake, but the appetite doesn't keep pace with energy output. Regular activity seems to help the appestat adjust caloric intake to energy needs. The appestat is rather imprecise at a low level of energy expenditure, but for regularly active individuals, appetite control is much more related to energy needs (Mayer & Bullen, 1974). And at the high end of the activity scale, where endurance athletes burn 4,000 to 6,000 calories daily in running, cycling, or swimming, the appetite usually underestimates energy needs.

Psychological factors such as the smell, sight, or taste of food can evoke the desire to eat. Habit and emotional factors also condition eating behavior. We eat to celebrate, to prolong feelings of excitement. Appetite is a complex phenomenon, subject to many influences, reflecting more than the need for nourishment. The appestat frequently overestimates energy needs. Weight control becomes possible when you realize that your eyes are bigger than your stomach, and your potential for energy intake is greater than your regular energy expenditure.

Premeal or Postmeal Exercise

Years ago, when the American diet was first implicated as a culprit in the heart disease epidemic, researchers roamed the world studying the relationship between diet and the incidence of heart disease. They found that diet alone did not account for the presence or absence of the problem; other factors such as a lack of tension and stress or physical activity confounded the relationship. Since then, several researchers have focused on the effect of pre- or postmeal exercise on postprandial lipemia (lipemia is the presence of fat in the blood). Studies conducted at the University of Florida have shown that exercise before or after a meal is effective in reducing the magnitude and duration of postprandial lipemia (Zauner, Burt, & Mapes, 1968). Mild exercise proved to be as effective as strenuous effort in this regard.

Lipemia long has been associated with atherosclerosis, reduced myocardial blood flow, and accelerated blood clotting. Thus, anything that reduces the level of fat in the blood seems prudent and advisable. Vigorous premeal exercise can inhibit the appetite and increase the metabolism of fat, even fat ingested after the exercise. The metabolic rate remains somewhat elevated after exercise, and the ingested fat is used quickly to restore energy burned during exercise. Mild postmeal effort such as a walk after dinner also serves to reduce lipemia. Both premeal and postmeal exercise increase caloric expenditure and fat metabolism, lead to improved fitness, and contribute to health and weight control.

And, while we're on the subject of meals and blood lipids, you should know that the number of meals you eat has an influence on blood fat levels. Spread the same number of calories over more meals (e.g., go from three to six) and cholesterol levels will be lower. Presumably we are able to handle fat better in smaller doses. Conversely, if you avoid meals in an effort to lose weight, your metabolic rate will decline and your cholesterol level will climb. And your temporary weight loss may be followed by a rapid gain.

Spread the same number of calories over more meals and cholesterol levels will be lower.

Fitness and Fat

The effects of activity on weight control and energy balance are well established. When the exercise is systematic and progressive, it leads to an improvement in aerobic fitness. This section deals with the extra benefits associated with improved fitness, benefits that provide dramatic evidence of the role fitness plays in health and the prevention of heart disease. These benefits include:

- Increased caloric expenditure
- Increased fat mobilization
- Increased fat utilization
- Reduced blood lipids
- Increased lean tissue (muscle)

Caloric Expenditure

Unfit individuals tire quickly during exercise and are limited in their ability to expend calories. As fitness improves, caloric expenditure increases with increases in the intensity, duration, and frequency of exercise and because of the inevitable participation in more vigorous activities. The fit individual does more with less fatigue. Thus, increased fitness contributes to energy expenditure and weight control.

I studied the effects of training on individuals' perception of effort and fatigue (Docktor & Sharkey, 1971). As fitness improved, more work could be performed at the same heart rate and level of perceived exertion. Work levels once perceived as difficult became less so, and formerly tiring exertion could be managed with ease. After training, a given task could be accomplished with a lower heart rate as well as a lower level of perceived exertion. Thus, the subjects were able to burn more energy without experiencing a greater sense of fatigue.

Further proof of the value of fitness to caloric expenditure is found in the relationship of caloric expenditure to heart rate. Caloric expenditure is related directly to the heart rate, but the relationship is also influenced by level of fitness. For people in low fitness categories, a high heart rate (pulse rate) does not indicate an extremely high caloric expenditure (see figure 13.1). For those in high categories, the same heart rate (HR) indicates a much higher energy expenditure:

140 HR for the very poor fitness level = 6 to 7 calories per minute expended

140 HR for the very good fitness level = 12 calories per minute expended

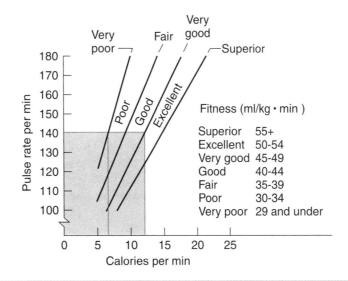

Figure 13.1 Predicting calories burned during physical activity from pulse rate.
Adapted from Sharkey 1974.

You can use figure 13.1 to estimate your caloric expenditure in any activity. After several minutes of participation, stop and immediately take your pulse at wrist, throat (use gentle contact), or temple for 15 seconds. Multiply by 4 to get your rate per minute. Then use the line corresponding to your fitness level to estimate your caloric expenditure per minute. Also notice how caloric expenditure will improve (at the same heart rate) as your fitness improves. This should convince you that fitness provides extra benefits to those who persevere.

As for perceived exertion, it too is related to heart rate. Since training allows you to do a certain effort, such as jog at a 10-minute-per-mile pace, at a lower heart rate, your perception of effort will also be lower.

Fat Mobilization

Fat is stored in fat cells in the form of triglyceride (three molecules of fatty acid and one glycerol). Triglyceride is too large to pass through the wall of the fat cell into the circulation. So, when energy is needed, the triglyceride is broken down, and the fatty acid molecules pass into the blood for transport to the working muscles. It is the hormone epinephrine that stimulates a receptor in the fat cell membrane and activates the enzyme lipase. Lipase splits the triglyceride molecule, and the fatty acids are free to enter the circulation.

As exercise becomes more intense we produce lactic acid. The point at which lactic acid begins to accumulate in the blood, the lactate (anaerobic) threshold, indicates when lactate production exceeds removal, and when a significant shift from fat to carbohydrate metabolism is taking place. You will recall that the anaerobic threshold is related to activity and fitness. It may be below 50% of the maximal oxygen uptake for an unfit individual and above 80% for one who is highly trained. But what does that have to do with fat?

Researchers discovered years ago that lactic acid seemed to inhibit the mobilization of free fatty acids (FFAs) from adipose tissue. The lactic acid blocked the action of epinephrine, thereby reducing the availability of fat for muscle metabolism (Issekutz & Miller, 1962). One of the best documented effects of training is that more work can be accomplished before lactic acid levels rise.

The same workload that, before training, leads to lactic acid production, can be accomplished with little increase in lactic acid after training. This may be due to a decrease in lactic acid production or an increase in lactic acid clearance, or both. Whatever the case, improved aerobic fitness allows more work to be accomplished aerobically; the lactate threshold is raised, and more fat can be made available for use as an energy source.

A more recent study of trained subjects illustrates that FFA mobilization and utilization are not affected by moderate levels of lactic acid (Vega deJesus & Siconolfi, 1988). The fit subjects were able to mobilize fat at the lactate threshold (4 millimoles lactic acid), which defines the highest level of exercise intensity that can be sustained during prolonged exertion. These findings help to explain the tremendous increase in endurance associated with training. Fat is the most abundant energy source (50 times more abundant than carbohydrate). Improved fitness allows greater access to that immense storehouse of energy.

Fat Utilization

Studies have shown that trained animals and humans are capable of extracting a greater percentage of their energy from FFA during submaximal exercise.

The mobilization of fat does not ensure its metabolism. How does training influence the utilization of FFA as a source of energy for muscular contractions? Studies have shown that trained animals and humans are capable of extracting a greater percentage of their energy from FFA during submaximal exercise. How does fitness, then, influence fat utilization?

Lipoprotein Lipase

Earlier we talked about LPL in adipose tissue. In muscle the LPL helps grab circulating fat from the blood and use it for energy. Muscle LPL activity increases with endurance training and enhances the muscle's ability to use fat as a fuel (Nikkila, Taskinen, Rehunen, & Harkonen, 1978).

Fat Oxidation

Convincing proof of the effect of training on FFA utilization was provided by Móle, Oscai, and Holloszy (1971). They found the ability of rat muscle to oxidize the fatty acid palmitate was doubled following 12 weeks of treadmill training. The authors suggested that the shift to fat metabolism was

LACTIC ACID

Lactic acid is produced when the breakdown of muscle glycogen (to three carbon pyruvic acid molecules) exceeds the ability of the mitochondria to process this metabolite. So, the pyruvic acid picks up hydrogen, becomes lactic acid, and begins to accumulate in the muscle and blood. Lactate can be used by the heart and skeletal muscle as a source of energy, and it can be oxidized in the liver. However, when production exceeds removal, the level in muscle increases. The rising level of acid in the muscle reduces force by interfering with muscle contractions, and decreases endurance by lowering the efficiency of aerobic enzymes.

key in the development of endurance fitness and an important mechanism serving to spare carbohydrate stores and prevent low blood sugar during prolonged exertion. Thus, the physically fit individual is able to derive a greater percentage of energy requirements from fat than the unfit subject can. At a given workload, the fit subject may obtain as much as 90% of his or her energy from fat. Free fatty acids are used during all forms of muscular activity except for all-out bursts of effort such as the 100-yard dash. Training even seems to improve the ability of the heart muscle to oxidize the fat (Keul, 1971).

Improved fitness increases the availability of fat via mobilization of free fatty acids, as well as an increase in enzyme activity. Both contribute to the rate of FFA utilization.

Blood Lipids

The blood lipids, triglyceride and cholesterol, have been associated with the incidence and severity of coronary heart disease. Both also seem to be related to other risk factors, including diet, body weight, and lack of exercise. Recent findings suggest that the lipids are also influenced by fitness training.

Triglycerides

Dietary fat intake shows up in the blood as chylomicrons, large clumps of triglycerides. Most of the triglycerides are removed from the plasma in the capillaries adjacent to muscle and adipose tissue. Any remains are cleared from the circulation by the liver.

Serum triglyceride levels can be reduced by dieting or through participation in regular physical activity. The reduction due to exercise occurs several hours afterwards and lasts for about 2 days. With regular exercise, further reductions occur until the individual reaches a plateau consistent with his or her exercise, diet, and other factors, such as inherited blood lipid patterns.

Earlier in this chapter the influence of exercise on postmeal fat in blood was established. Research supports the hypothesis that regular exercise enhances the removal and utilization of triglycerides by muscle cells, rather than allowing their deposit in adipose tissue or removal by the liver, possibly to synthesize more cholesterol. Sedentary rats were trained for 12 weeks on a treadmill. Following the training, the muscles were analyzed for the activity of lipoprotein lipase (LPL), the enzyme responsible for the uptake of plasma triglyceride fatty acids (TGFA) from plasma chylomicrons and other sources in the blood. The researcher reasoned that any increase in the uptake of TGFA by skeletal muscle during exercise would be accompanied by an increase in LPL activity. The results of the study confirmed the hypothesis. Regular endurance training led to a two- to fourfold increase in the LPL activity, indicating that training

CHYLOMICRONS

Chylomicrons are responsible for the milky appearance of blood plasma following a meal (postprandial lipemia). In addition to 80 to 95% triglyceride, they contain 2 to 7% cholesterol, 3 to 6% phospholipid, and 1 to 2% protein.

increases the capacity of the muscle fibers to take up and oxidize fatty acids originating in plasma triglycerides (Borensztajn, 1975).

Since the fat is used before it can be deposited in adipose tissue, these findings have tremendous significance in the area of weight control. The implications for cardiovascular health are even more exciting, as is the realization that these benefits are associated with an entirely natural, enjoyable, and satisfying experience: aerobic fitness training.

Cholesterol

Cholesterol ingested in the diet is absorbed in the small intestine, finds its way into the lymph system, and then is dumped into the blood. There it joins with cholesterol produced by the body in the chylomicrons and in very low-density lipoprotein particles (VLDL). Once in the plasma, the VLDL are attacked by the same enzymes that act on the chylomicrons. Much of the triglyceride is removed (within 2 to 6 hours). The VLDL is degraded to low-density lipoprotein (LDL), which is removed by the liver over a period of 2 to 5 days. Because of the smaller size of the LDL particle and its high concentration of cholesterol, the LDL particle seems to be involved directly in the development of coronary artery disease. The LDL particles find their way into coronary arteries and contribute to the growth of atherosclerotic plaques. Thus, LDL is believed to be a major culprit in the development of coronary artery disease.

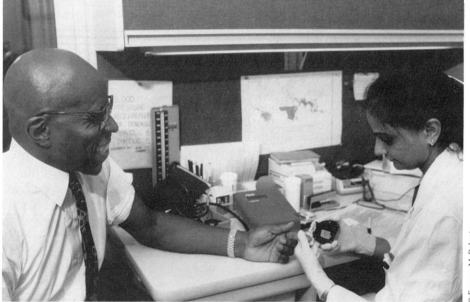

© Frances M. Roberts

A blood test can help you determine your total cholesterol/HDL ratio.

Until the mid-'70s, diet, weight loss, and drugs were believed to be the major weapons in the fight against cholesterol. Studies on the effect of exercise on cholesterol typically reported a modest reduction, but only when the exercise was vigorous and of long duration (3 or more miles of running per day). But remember that cholesterol is transported in the blood in several ways. A single measure of serum cholesterol does not indicate how the cholesterol is distributed among the several lipoprotein fractions, nor does it indicate the effects of exercise.

Dr. Wood and his associates (1975) at the Stanford Heart Disease Prevention Program compared the lipoprotein patterns of sedentary and active middle-aged men (35 to 59 years old). The active group consisted of joggers who averaged at least 15 miles per week for the preceding year. As expected, the triglycerides were "strikingly" lower for the active group, while total cholesterol was only "modestly" reduced. However, when the lipoprotein pattern was analyzed, the joggers exhibited a significantly lower level of dangerous LDL and an elevated level of high-density lipoprotein (HDL). These findings were astounding, since there is a direct relationship between LDL and heart disease, and an inverse relationship between HDL and heart disease (as HDL goes up, the incidence of heart disease goes down). HDL seems to carry cholesterol away from the tissues for removal by the liver. Dr. Wood noted that the lipoprotein pattern could be mistaken for that of the typical young woman, who carries the lowest risk of heart disease in the entire adult population.

I don't want to bore you with an overly complicated discussion of blood lipids and lipoproteins, but I do want you to realize the inadequacy of *total cholesterol* as an indicator of the effects of exercise and fitness on blood lipids and health. For those who doubt the validity of comparison groups (sedentary vs. active) as an indicator of the effects of activity on blood lipids, I offer the following. When researchers (Lopez, Vial, Balart, & Arroyave, 1974) studied the effects of 7 weeks of training on the serum lipids and lipoproteins in 13 young medical students, as expected, triglycerides were reduced (from 110 milligrams to 80). Furthermore, they found a marked reduction of beta lipoprotein cholesterol (cholesterol in LDL and VLDL), a concomitant increase in alpha lipoprotein cholesterol (HDL), and no changes in body weight to confuse the results. Studies in our lab (Sharkey, Simpson, Washburn, & Confessore, 1980) agree with those reported by Dr. Wood and many others. They clearly indicate how training helps shift cholesterol from the dangerous LDL to the favorable HDL, why total cholesterol fails to indicate all the effects of exercise, and how activity and fitness help prevent the development or progression of atherosclerosis and heart disease.

How's that for an extra benefit of fitness? Not only does fitness allow increased caloric expenditure and enhanced fat mobilization and utilization, but it also allows you to have a direct effect on the blood lipids and reduce the risk of heart disease. In my view, this may be the most important benefit of exercise and fitness. If all this doesn't convince you to become active and improve your aerobic fitness . . . I'll just keep trying.

One final word to keep your interest. There is a growing belief among researchers in this area that it may be possible to lower serum cholesterol levels enough to actually reverse the process of atherosclerosis, to remove fatty buildup from the lining of the coronary arteries. If it proves to be true that diet and exercise, perhaps with the help of drug therapy, can accomplish this reversal, it will be possible to cure, not just treat, many cases of the nation's number one killer.

It may be possible to lower serum cholesterol levels enough to actually reverse the process of atherosclerosis, to remove fatty buildup from the lining of the coronary arteries.

Lean Tissue

Finally, let me remind you that muscle is the furnace that burns fat. While dieting leads to a loss of muscle, a lower metabolic rate, and a reduced ability to exercise and burn fat, fitness training has the capacity to maintain or increase muscle mass. Aerobic training such as running leads to a small increase in lean body weight. Training with more resistance, such as in cycling, can cause more noticeable changes in muscle. And, of course, muscular fitness (resistance) training leads to impressive changes in muscle mass. Fortunately, muscle lost in dieting can be rapidly reclaimed with activity and training.

While aerobic exercise doesn't have a great effect on the resting metabolic rate, resistance training has been shown to increase strength and metabolic rate and maintain metabolically active tissue in older adults (Campbell, Crim, Young, & Evans, 1994). Moreover, resistance training has been shown to lower visceral fat, the fat associated with a higher risk of heart disease (Treuth et al., 1995).

Activity and Diet

When exercise and diet are combined, you can eat more and still achieve a 1,000-calorie deficit (2 pounds per week weight loss). Exercise tones muscles, improving your appearance as you lose weight, conserves protein, and increases the utilization of fat. The combination of exercise and sensible caloric intake should be a way of life. Let's see how diet and exercise can be combined in a program of weight loss and weight control.

An analysis of body composition and fitness indicates that John is 20 pounds overweight and in the poor fitness category. He achieves energy balance when his caloric intake equals his typical daily expenditure, 2,500 calories. How should he proceed? John should reduce his caloric intake by 500 calories per day and begin exercising (see table 13.2).

TABLE 13.2   Sample Weight Loss Program

20 lb × 3,500 cal/lb = 70,000 cal overweight			Cal	Total cal
Weeks 1 & 2	Exercise = 200 cal/day × 7 days	=	1,400	
	Diet = 500 cal/day × 14 days	=	7,000	
			8,400	8,400
Weeks 3 & 4	Exercise = 250 cal/day × 14 days	=	3,500	
	Diet = 500 cal/day × 14 days	=	7,000	
			10,500	18,900
Weeks 5 & 6	Exercise = 300 cal/day × 14 days	=	4,200	
	Diet = 500 cal/day × 14 days	=	7,000	
			11,200	30,100
Weeks 7 & 8	Exercise = 350 cal/day × 14 days	=	4,900	
	Diet = 500 cal/day × 14 days	=	7,000	
			11,900	42,000
Weeks 9 & 10	Exercise = 400 cal/day × 14 days	=	5,600	
	Diet = 500 cal/day × 14 days	=	7,000	
			12,600	54,600
Weeks 11 & 12	Exercise = 450 cal/day × 14 days	=	6,300	
	Diet = 500 cal/day × 14 days	=	7,000	
			13,300	67,900

After 12 weeks = 67,900 cal lost.

Weeks 13 & 14–forget the diet. Exercise just 150 cal/day (14 days × 150 cal = 2,100 cal). 67,900 + 2,100 = 70,000 cal, or 20 lb.

Now that he has achieved his goal, John has several choices:

- Continue his exercise habits and eat as he chooses,
- Continue activity and the reduced-fat diet,
- Return to sedentary habits and restrict caloric intake . . . for life, or
- Return to a sedentary lifestyle and a high-fat diet and regain all the weight he has lost . . . and more.

If he chooses to remain active (400 calories of exercise daily), he will be able to eat the foods he enjoys and to splurge occasionally on extravagant foods. He should still consider a reduction of fat in the diet, but it is possible that with sufficient exercise (e.g., running 4 to 5 miles daily) he will be able to eat whatever he wishes with no adverse effect on his health or weight. However, only a cholesterol test will confirm that possibility.

Summary

Exercise is clearly beneficial as a means of losing weight and keeping it off. Given recent studies showing its association with maintenance, it would be difficult to argue that any factor is more important than exercise (Brownell, 1995). Activity is the positive way to achieve weight control, without the loss of lean tissue. Dieting is a negative approach that uses deprivation to achieve results. It is not surprising that dieting by itself is seldom successful in the long run. Most weight-loss diets end in failure, with more weight and fat than before the dieting began. Activities such as walking, jogging, or cycling may seem slow ways to lose weight, but they work. If your activity burns 250 extra calories each day, you'll burn in excess of 1,500 calories a week. In the course of a year you'll lose more than 20 pounds. Calories do count, and you should learn how to count them. Turn to chapter 14 for a sensible and effective approach to achieve energy balance and take the first step in your lifelong quest for a trim, healthy body.

Weight-Control Programs

"When the stomach is full, it is easy to talk of fasting."

St. Jerome

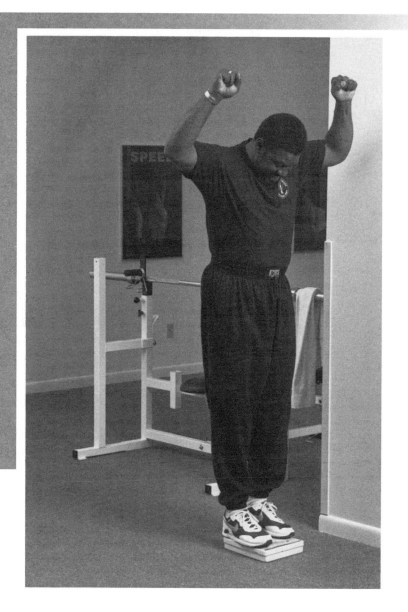

This chapter outlines activity, food selection, and eating behaviors that provide a three-pronged approach to lifelong weight control. If you are slightly overweight, simply increase daily activity to achieve your goal. Twenty minutes of brisk walking each day (at 6 calories per minute) will result in 1 pound of weight loss each month. If your problem is moderate, use activity and food selection to gain control. Eliminate empty calories, substitute low-fat for high-fat foods, and eat moderate portions. This alone should help you lose another pound each month. Activity and diet can help you lose 4 or more pounds a month, but you should never attempt to lose more than 2 pounds per week or 8 per month. Finally, if your problem is significant and long-standing, you should add a behavioral approach to your program. Proper use of any one of the three—activity, food choices, and eating behavior—will help you lose weight, but if you are interested in long-term weight loss, if your weight-control problem is significant, if you want to gain complete and lasting control, consider combining the benefits of all three approaches.

THIS CHAPTER WILL HELP YOU

- implement the weight-control program suited to your needs,
- utilize the essentials of behavior therapy, and
- lose, maintain, or gain weight.

The Weight-Control Program

If you want to approach weight control systematically, you should determine your energy balance (caloric intake minus caloric expenditure), as explained in the following pages.

Caloric Expenditure

In chapter 12, I asked you to keep an inventory of your activities, listing each activity (exercise, work, household chores) and the time spent for it (figure 12.5, page 236). You then estimated your daily caloric expenditure by referring to the tables in the chapter. That exercise is most educational; it shows you when calories are burned and provides insight into how you might increase caloric expenditures in your normal routine.

Bear in mind that energy expenditure values in the tables are based on the oxygen cost and caloric expenditure of various activities, and that these values sometimes underestimate the actual caloric expenditure. For example, a study of the energy cost of running was conducted on a laboratory treadmill using highly trained endurance runners as subjects. The values obtained underestimate your cost of running for the following reasons:

- The treadmill is perfectly flat (unlike the road or trail you use).
- The air in the lab is still (whereas, outside even on a calm day, the moving body must overcome some wind resistance).
- Trained runners are up to 10% more efficient than untrained runners.
- The lab values didn't consider the post-exercise period, when energy is used to replace stores of energy consumed during the run. Post-exercise oxygen consumption may be elevated for up to an hour after a long, hard run.

Some estimates of the calories expended during running may be 10% too low for many runners, especially when the post-exercise energy expenditure is considered. Over a period of weeks, an error of that size renders a serious disservice to exercise and its role in weight control.

Caloric Intake

In chapter 12, I encouraged you to calculate your daily caloric intake by keeping records of all the food you eat, including snacks (figure 12.4, page 235). You then tallied the calories per serving, per meal, and each day from the calorie tables in the chapter. You'll want to refer to those results in order to calculate your energy balance. Of course, you could utilize one of the excellent computer programs that calculate caloric intake, calories from carbohydrate, fat, and protein, and vitamin and mineral intake from food. Consult a dietitian or health educator about a computerized dietary analysis. In any case you'll have to estimate portion size to get a good idea of your caloric intake. Don't overlook any source of calories, including the sugar in your coffee. You may be surprised to learn how many calories you consume in snacks or large helpings.

Energy Balance

For best results you should calculate energy intake and expenditure for several days and average the results. Using the averages, figure your energy balance by subtracting caloric intake from expenditure. If intake regularly exceeds expenditure you will gain weight. A mere 100 calories of extra intake daily will lead to more than 10 pounds of extra weight in 1 year:

$$100 \text{ calories} \times 365 \text{ days}$$
$$= 36{,}500 \text{ calories} / 3{,}500 \text{ calories per pound of fat}$$
$$= 10.4 \text{ pounds}$$

A mere 100 calories of extra intake daily will lead to more than 10 pounds of extra weight in 1 year.

You gained excess weight when your energy intake exceeded your expenditure, leading to a positive energy balance. Now you must reverse the process. When caloric expenditure exceeds intake, you have a deficit. The caloric deficit determines the rate of weight loss. If the deficit is 100 calories per day, you will lose a pound every 35 days. If the deficit is 500 calories per day, you'll lose a pound each week. The deficit should never regularly exceed 1,000 calories per day. A daily deficit of 1,000 calories leads to a weight loss of 2 pounds per week. It is neither necessary nor prudent to exceed this rate of weight loss. In fact, if the deficit regularly exceeds 1,000 calories, fatigue, listlessness, and reduced resistance to infection are likely to occur.

Activity

Your weight-control program should include both aerobic and muscular fitness training. The *aerobic fitness* prescription for weight loss or weight control maximizes caloric expenditure (duration) at the expense of exercise intensity. Exercise duration is extended to increase caloric expenditure. Both the duration and frequency of exercise should be increased to achieve the maximal benefit of exercise. Thus, if your fitness prescription suggests 100 to 200 calories of exercise several days per week, you should try to work at the low edge of your training zone (intensity) and increase the caloric expenditure (duration). Also, increase the frequency to daily or twice daily if possible, and add supplemental activities. The addition of moderate exercise to a caloric restriction (diet) program provides advantages in fat utilization, fat loss, and caloric expenditure, even in obese individuals (Kempen, Saris, & Westerterp, 1995).

The *muscular fitness* portion of the weight-control program is aimed at maintaining or increasing lean body weight (muscle) and maintaining the resting metabolic rate (Ryan, Pratley, Elahi, & Goldberg, 1995). Unless you are interested in gaining strength for a particular reason, my recommendation is for muscular endurance training, utilizing at least one set of 15 to 25 repetitions with moderate resistance. Do this for 8 to 10 exercises, two to three times per week, and you will maintain muscle mass and resting metabolic rate, both of which are important to the long-term success of your weight-control program.

Supplemental Activities

There are many ways to increase caloric expenditure aside from your daily exercise session. Walk to work, during work, to lunch, during coffee break, after dinner. Take an exercise break during the day. Climb stairs, jump rope, do calisthenics. Do anything that increases caloric expenditure. If you expend 200 calories in your training session and then expend another 100 walking or climbing stairs, you have accelerated your exercise weight loss by 50%. When you become more fit and are capable of burning 500 calories daily through exercise, you will be able to lose 1 pound per week (3,500 calories) through exercise alone.

Change Lifestyle

The best way to achieve permanent weight loss is to make a change in lifestyle. The change could be to return to old ways of doing things. Avoid unnecessary labor-saving devices (remote control, power mower, snow thrower). Seek out and employ energy-using devices such as the snow shovel, the bicycle, or your own two feet. The best advice is to never use a machine when you can do the job yourself. You will be doing yourself a favor, saving energy (electricity, gas, oil, coal), and reducing pollution, all at the same time.

Perhaps the best idea is to find an active hobby or sport and make it an essential part of your life. Try woodworking, racquetball, or dancing. Get a canoe or cross-country skis, start a garden. Dig out the tennis racquet and give it a try. Go ice-skating in the winter or roller-skating any time of year. You'll enrich your life and lower your weight at the same time. Of course, you'll look better too!

Food Choices (Diet)

Dieting is reducing caloric intake, which is usually accomplished by reducing high-calorie fat in the diet, and little else.

If you're searching for one of those fad diets that regularly come and go, don't look here. *Dieting* is reducing caloric intake, which is usually accomplished by reducing high-calorie fat in the diet, and little else. As I pointed out in chapter 11, each gram of fat contains 9.3 calories, versus only 4.1 for carbohydrate and 4.3 for protein. Almost 40% of the calories in the average diet come from fat. If you've been eating 2,000 calories daily, 800 probably come from fat. The reduced-fat diet is explained later in this chapter. But first let me say what I *don't* mean by dieting.

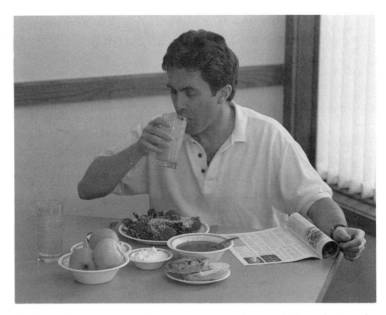

Begin today to reduce the percentage of your daily calories obtained from fat.

When you restrict calories, the daily caloric deficit shouldn't exceed 1,000 calories regularly. Of course, it is entirely possible to restrict caloric intake far below energy needs. However, if you do that for more than a few days you are on a starvation diet. You won't receive the essential nutrients, your energy level will sag, and you will compromise your immune system and lower resistance to infection. Furthermore, the body will interpret the starvation diet as a signal to reduce caloric expenditure; your resting energy expenditure will decline, you'll begin to lose lean tissue, and you will be on your way to increased weight-loss problems.

Diets to Avoid

Almost every popular magazine includes an article on dieting. Many offer a "revolutionary" new diet plan with such promises as "eat all you want," "calories don't count," "quick weight loss," and "superenergy." You've heard of the water diet, the drinking man's diet, high-protein, liquid-protein, low-carbohydrate, and other so-called diets. Unfortunately, most of these plans reach more readers than do the critical editorials and negative reports in medical journals.

FASTING

Fasting is the ultimate form of caloric restriction. It is guaranteed to bring about a dramatic weight loss, as much as a pound a day . . . for a while. An occasional day of fasting will do no harm unless you are under stress or in training for competition. However, the risks of fasting are many, especially if it is continued for an extended period. If you are grossly overweight and eager to fast, check into a clinic and proceed. Otherwise, extended periods of fasting should be avoided.

Be suspicious of any plan that promises rapid results (more than 2 pounds of weight loss per week). Certainly you can lose more weight by fasting or by dehydration. Water is heavy, weighing about 2 pounds per quart. I could try to fool you into losing weight by sweating. You could easily lose 2 pounds in an hour; athletes lose 6 pounds or more in a hard workout. What is so bad about that? Your body needs the water and replaces it as soon as possible, so little weight or fat loss occurs. Question any plan that calls for a low intake of carbohydrate or protein, encourages a high intake of protein or fat, or recommends dehydration as a means of weight loss.

Low-Carbohydrate Diet

One fad diet plan advocates the near exclusion of carbohydrate. The author states that the average overweight man should lose about 7 pounds in the first week of the diet! The diet seems to work because of water loss, not the fat you really want to eliminate. The diet allows a liberal intake of fat and all the protein you want—reason enough to doubt the plan. Low-carbohydrate diets are questionable for another reason: When blood sugar levels are low, the fatty acid molecules from adipose tissue are shipped to the liver, where they are converted to ketone bodies to provide energy for the manufacture of glucose. Excess ketone bodies spill over into the blood and are carried to the tissues, where they are oxidized. During starvation or a low-carbohydrate diet, the production of ketone bodies can exceed the body's ability to remove them metabolically. When this happens, the excess appears in the urine and in the expired air. The condition is called *ketosis*, and the main danger is the lowering of the blood pH (acidosis).

Simple sugars should be avoided, but complex carbohydrates (potatoes, whole-grain products, corn, rice, beans) provide energy and nutrition. They are excellent sources of vitamins and minerals, and many are high in fiber as well. In cultures where the diet consists largely of energy derived from complex carbohydrates, such as the Tarahumara Indians of Mexico, atherosclerosis and heart disease are so low as to be virtually nonexistent!

Low-Protein Diet

Any diet that restricts protein intake below the recommended dietary allowance is idiotic. During adolescence, such a plan could stunt normal development. It is certain to cause muscle loss at any age. And muscle loss makes future caloric expenditure more difficult, leading to increased fat and body weight.

High-Protein Diet

You don't need excessive protein; any excess is stored as fat. Since dietary protein often is associated with fat, as in meat, you are likely to take in more fat and calories on a high-protein diet. Don't be misled into eating more protein than you actually need.

Reduced-Fat Diets

Reducing fat in the diet makes sense, up to a point. Fat is high in calories, and it is related to heart disease, stroke, diabetes, and some cancers, so there are good reasons for reducing the proportion of fat in your diet. However, some fat is required for good nutrition, especially during early childhood. Essential fatty acids must be included in the diet. Moreover, fat-soluble vitamins are not absorbed unless fat is present. Fats improve the flavor of food and make it more filling. I would never suggest complete removal of fat from the diet. I do suggest that you begin now to lower the percentage of your daily calories obtained from fat well below the 40% common in this country to the 25% recommended in the performance diet (see chapter 11). I also suggest that you begin to reduce your intake of saturated fats by replacing butter with vegetable-oil margarine, whole milk with skim milk, and fatty meat with lean (including fish and poultry). How far should you go to reduce the fat content of your diet?

Very Low-Fat Diet

The program recommended by Nathan Pritikin called for the following daily energy intake (percentage of calories):

- 80% from carbohydrate (mostly complex)
- 10% from fat
- 10% from protein

While the research community awaits further proof of the need for this dietary regime, researchers at the California-based Longevity Research Institute have reported dramatic results among patients with heart and circulatory disorders and diabetes. The diet is a surefire way to reduce triglycerides and cholesterol. And when it is joined with an exercise program, as it is at the Institute, it may slow or even arrest the progress of atherosclerosis (Pritikin, 1979). More recently, Dr. Dean Ornish has supported the low-fat diet (10% of calories from fat), with claims that it may reverse atherosclerosis (1993).

The low-fat diet has several advantages in addition to its effect on blood lipids and heart disease. Complex carbohydrates are high in fiber. Low-fiber diets are related to cancer of the colon. The high-carbohydrate diet is an excellent energy diet. When combined with a sensible exercise program it will not lead to the accumulation of fat. In fact, since carbohydrate has only 4 calories per gram, you can eat quite a bit without gaining weight. Finally, since fat seems to inhibit the action of insulin, and since this diet reduces the level of fat in the blood, the low-fat diet could reduce the severity of adult-onset diabetes or the reliance on insulin.

But is there enough protein in the low-fat diet? There may not be enough for vigorous living. Let's assume that your weight is 70 kilograms and your daily caloric intake averages 2,000 calories. If 10% of that energy comes from protein, you will take in 200 calories from protein. Protein averages 4.3 calories per gram, so 200 calories divided by 4.3 equals 47 grams of protein. This falls below the recommended daily allowance for protein published by the National Research Council (0.8 grams of protein per kilogram of body weight multiplied by 70 kilograms equals 56 grams). For this reason I do not recommend this protein intake. Instead I recommend a diet that provides 15% of calories from good-quality protein, including meat, dairy, and plant sources.

How much fat does the very low-fat diet allow? If daily intake is 2,000 calories, the 10% fat allowed equals 200 calories; divide 200 by 9.3 calories per gram of fat, and you get 22 grams of fat, a very small amount. In our culture, this is a difficult diet. The author of the plan found it necessary to retrain the palates of his subjects because the drastic reduction of fat makes food seem bland (Pritikin, 1979). And when one attempts to apply the diet in a restaurant, there is frustration on every page of the menu.

Diet Recommendations

You do not have to change your eating habits overnight, and you don't have to reduce fat intake to 10%, unless your risk of CAD is high. Otherwise, an intake of 25% is both reasonable and attainable. Begin today to reduce the fat content of your diet. If the 10% fat diet becomes necessary, the food industry will respond with alternatives (lean meats, low-calorie dressings, fake fat). In the meantime, try to make some of the substitutions I've mentioned. Begin to experiment with complex carbohydrates. Use beans and corn in a Mexican dinner, rice and soy for an Oriental experience. Use potatoes (with fat-free sour cream), bake whole-grain breads. The proper combination of these low-fat foods provides for energy, protein needs, and other nutrients. Avoid empty calories such as table sugar. Substitute a carrot, celery, or fruit for your usual snacks. You can easily reduce fat intake to 25% as we await the final word concerning the relationship of dietary fat to health and disease.

Does lowering the fat in the diet work? Several years ago, when I cut back on dietary fat in an effort to reduce my cholesterol level, I lost a pound a week for 6 weeks—even though I wasn't trying to lose weight! I substituted fruit for snacks, ate a lot, and still lost weight (yes, my cholesterol came down as well). So, switch to the performance diet and watch performance and health improve.

The dietary program I recommend emphasizes the maintenance of a normal diet, including the energy proportions of the performance diet: 60% carbohydrate, 25% fat, and 15% protein; and adequate levels of vitamins, minerals, and water.

Assess Food Choices

Take a good look at your caloric intake list. If patterns of behavior are not readily apparent, you should continue to count your calories for several days. In addition to what you eat, consider when, where, and why you eat (see figure 14.1). Do you have a doughnut at coffee break just because it's there? Do you have a candy bar at lunch? Do you have a drink now and then? You may be able to eliminate several hundred calories daily by eliminating unnecessary or ritual eating behaviors. Years ago I developed the habit of eating crackers with peanut butter and jelly as a reward for an evening's work. When I realized how quickly the fat calories added up and what was happening to my weight, I vowed to break the ritual. Sure, I still get the urge, and sometimes I am unable to resist. But for the present (an addict is never cured), I reward myself with a nutritious but low-calorie treat such as an apple or orange. In this way, I've reduced both caloric and fat intake.

Modify Meals

Now that you've eliminated the extras, look at the size and content of your meals. You may think that dieting means avoiding meals, often breakfast. That is the worst thing you can do, for several reasons. People work better when they eat breakfast. When you avoid meals, you become weak and hungry. People who are susceptible to low blood sugar may even notice poor performance in sports skills or work. Eventually, you sit down to a meal and overeat. Also, when you eat fewer than three meals a day, the triglyceride and cholesterol levels are higher than when you eat more frequently. By eating more frequent meals, you avoid the feelings of hunger and fatigue often associated with diet, and you reduce blood lipid levels.

Daily Eating Log

Date _____   Weight _____

Time	Place (If at home, exactly where were you?)	What did you eat or drink and how much?	What were you doing before you ate?	What did you do while you ate?	Who were you with when you ate?	What did you do after you ate?

Figure 14.1   Daily eating log.

The easiest way to reduce mealtime calories is to reduce the size and number of helpings you consume. Use a smaller plate, and fill it only once. Refuse second helpings, except for salad or vegetables. And, of course, eliminate high-calorie desserts, toppings, dressings, gravies, and sauces (see table 14.1 for a six-meal plan). Eat all you want of fruits, low-fat cereals, whole-grain breads (without butter), vegetables, and water.

TABLE 14.1   Low-Calorie Six-Meal Plan (1,300 cal)

Meal	Menu
Breakfast	Egg or cheese Slice whole-grain bread Coffee or tea
Mid-morning	Fresh or dried fruit Milk (low-fat)
Lunch	Meat, fish, or peanut butter sandwich Milk, fruit, or vegetable juice
Mid-afternoon	Soup and salad
Dinner	Meat, fish, poultry, or cheese Potato, rice, beans, corn, or whole-grain cereal product Vegetables, including leafy green Coffee or tea
Bedtime	Fruit and low-fat yogurt

Substitute

Substitute low-calorie snacks for high (e.g., pretzels for potato chips or peanuts); substitute low-fat foods for high (skim milk, low-fat meats, no-fat salad dressing, low-fat cheese, etc.).

The final step in this simple plan is to make substitutions. Substitute low-calorie snacks for high (e.g., pretzels for potato chips or peanuts); substitute low-fat foods for high (skim milk, low-fat meats, no-fat salad dressing, low-fat cheese, etc.). Try to stay below 50 grams of fat daily. (If labels don't tell how much fat is in the food, the list of ingredients will help.) And remember to avoid cottonseed, palm, and coconut oils, which are found in many snack foods, in coffee creamers, and in many other processed products. In food preparation, use olive oil and canola oil whenever possible; both are high in monounsaturated fat, preferable to any oil that is hydrogenated. Using this approach, you easily can achieve a daily caloric deficit of 500 calories. Since you are eating at least three meals a day, you won't feel weak and hungry. And when you combine the benefits of diet with those of exercise and fitness, you will be delighted with the results.

Read Labels

To lower the amount of fat in your diet and improve your fat balance, begin by reading the labels and lists of ingredients on everything you eat (see figure 14.2). Ingredients are listed in order of concentration, from highest to lowest. When fat comes early in the list, you are looking at a high-fat food. You probably already know that ice cream and potato chips are loaded with fat, but so are peanuts and many other snacks. If your goal is 25% of calories from fat, and your daily intake is 2,000 calories, you can eat 500 calories of fat, or about 54

Nutrition Facts

Serving Size 1/2 cup (114g)
Servings Per Container 4

Amount Per Serving

Calories 260   Calories from Fat 120

	% Daily Value*
Total Fat 13g	**20%**
Saturated Fat 5g	**25%**
Cholesterol 30mg	**10%**
Sodium 660mg	**28%**
Total Carbohydrate 31g	**11%**
Dietary Fiber 0g	**0%**
Sugars 5g	
Protein 5g	

Vitamin A 4%	Vitamin C 2%
Calcium 15%	Iron 4%

*Percent Daily Values are based on a 2000 calorie diet. Your daily values may be higher or lower depending on your calorie needs.

	Calories:	2000	2500
Total Fat	Less than	65g	80g
Sat. Fat	Less than	20g	25g
Cholesterol	Less than	300mg	300mg
Sodium	Less than	2400mg	2400mg
Total Carbohydrate		300g	375g
Dietary Fiber		25g	30g

Calories per gram:
Fat 9 • Carbohydrate 4 • Protein 4

Figure 14.2   The new nutrition label.

grams (500 divided by 9.3 calories per gram equals 54). If you want to snack, choose pretzels with less than 1 gram of fat per serving instead of chips with 11 grams. Limit saturated fat to one-third of daily fat intake. Read labels and take control of your health.

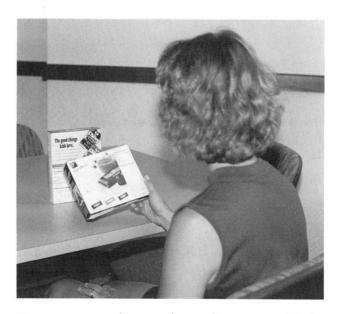

To improve your diet, start by reading nutrition labels.

Behavioral Approach

If you follow the instructions in the previous sections and achieve a negative energy balance (caloric deficit), you will lose weight. With a deficit of 1,000 calories daily, you will lose 2 pounds per week. However, if you are a difficult case and need additional help, this section is for you. Even if you have your weight completely under control, you may learn a lot about yourself and your eating behavior by completing the forms that follow. Behavior therapy (once called behavior modification) is the third and last major weapon in the battle of the bulge. The essentials of the behavioral approach include:

1. Identify the behavior you wish to modify, in this case eating behavior. Keep a food diary that indicates the kind and amount of food you eat—when, where, why, and with whom, what you do while eating, your mood, and your degree of hunger (see figures 14.1 and 14.3).
2. Analyze your customary eating behavior, and plan new eating behaviors. The new behaviors should include dietary adjustments and activity. To reduce cues or reinforcement for old eating behaviors, try the following:

   - Eat in one room only (dining room or kitchen).
   - Wrap your utensils in a napkin; wait several minutes before you begin.
   - Pause between bites; set your utensils down between bites. Don't prepare another bite until you've swallowed the last.
   - Wait 30 minutes before having dessert, or have a low-calorie beverage instead (tea, decaffeinated coffee).
   - Concentrate on what you are eating; take time, and enjoy each bite. Save one item to eat later on.
   - Purchase a new place setting, and eat only from that setting. Use a smaller plate.
   - After the meal, remove all dishes to the kitchen, then brush your teeth—the meal is over.

   When you feel hungry, try to decide if it is real (stomach hunger) or merely boredom for something to do (mouth hunger). Avoid eating in front of the TV set or while reading. If you must snack, be sure the snack is nutritious and/or low in fat, salt, and calories.
3. Plan new reinforcements or rewards to encourage the new eating behavior. Develop a schedule of reinforcement (see figure 14.4), a plan of frequent rewards for good behavior. Since the new eating behavior will soon show up on the scale or the tape measure, you can use small units of weight loss and small reductions in girth as indicators of adherence to the new behavior. Almost any sort of reward is effective (except high fat, high calorie foods)! A tangible, universally accepted reward such as money seems to work for most people. Weigh yourself daily, in the morning after your toilet but before breakfast, and provide a monetary reward for each unit of weight lost. A similar plan to reward reduced girth (waist, thigh) provides added incentive. Spend the reward immediately if you wish, or save it for something you really want but might otherwise refuse to buy. If the plan seems silly, remember this: You will spend far more than the cost of reinforcement on food and medical bills if you do not lose the weight.

Behavior therapy (once called behavior modification) is the third and last major weapon in the battle of the bulge.

Cognitive Supplement to Daily Eating Log

Date _____

Time	What were your thoughts or feelings before you ate?	While you ate?	After you ate?

Figure 14.3   Cognitive supplement to be used in conjunction with daily eating log.

Weight Loss Reinforcement Schedule

Date	Weight	Reward	Girth	Reward	Total[a]

Note. For example, $1 per lb; $1 per 1/2 in. of waist girth.
[a]Start new total when you spend the reward.

Figure 14.4   Weight-loss reinforcement schedule.

The same general principles apply to those who are having trouble starting or staying with an activity program. Review existing behavior, plan the new behavior, and reward yourself each time you jog, play tennis, or walk instead of ride. You may choose a monetary reward or, occasionally, a low-calorie drink or snack. See chapter 19 for suggestions on how you can use behavior therapy to reinforce activity.

Gaining Weight

This section is intended to help underweight individuals achieve sensible non-fat weight gain. It is not meant to help you bulk up for sports such as football. When normal-weight individuals bulk up, they assume a health risk that cannot be ignored. Coaches who encourage such procedures should be held responsible for conducting weight-loss programs when the sport season or career is over.

As with weight loss, the weight-gain program includes exercise, diet, and behavior therapy.

- **Exercise:** Includes a strength-training program to build lean body weight, and a *reduction* in calorie-burning activities (aerobic exercise, sports) to allow a positive caloric balance.
- **Diet:** Includes an overall increase in calories, with 750 extra calories on strength-training days and 250 extra on nontraining days. The extra calories should be largely from low-fat, protein-rich foods (lean meats, low-fat dairy products, nuts). A low-fat protein supplement can be used to provide an extra 20 grams (86 calories) of protein daily.
- **Behavior therapy:** Develop a reinforcement schedule to reward gains in lean body weight. Determine a desirable weight, and make steady progress toward that goal.

This program should lead to a gain of about 1 pound of weight each week. If you attempt to gain weight too fast, much of the gain will be fat. So, determine current eating behaviors, and plan needed modifications (more meals, nutritious snacks, etc.). Start strength training, and watch the scale go up. And remember, return to aerobic exercise and weight control when you achieve the desired body weight.

Health Clubs and Diet Centers

Do health clubs and diet centers figure in your weight control program? While both have experienced considerable growth in recent years, you should be cautious in your approach to their services. It may surprise you to learn that neither clubs nor centers are governed by state or local laws. No professional competence or qualifications are required. Hairdressers need a state license, but anyone can open and operate a health club or diet center. Following are some suggestions to help you become a discriminating consumer.

The American College of Sports Medicine (ACSM) certifies health and fitness instructors and program directors who meet educational and experience standards and successfully complete a rigorous test.

Health Clubs

To help differentiate a good club from a bad one—an effective program and qualified staff from a fly-by-night organization—you should do the following. Visit the club for a tour and introductory session. Is the facility clean and well equipped? Does the equipment meet your needs? Are patrons satisfied, and do they encourage you to join? Ask about the qualifications and credentials of the staff: Do they have degrees in the field from reputable institutions? Do they have experience? Are they certified? Are they all trained emergency responders? The American College of Sports Medicine (ACSM) certifies health and fitness instructors and program directors who meet educational and experience standards and successfully complete a rigorous test. ACSM also publishes a brochure to help you evaluate a health club. Write to ACSM at P.O. Box 1440, Indianapolis, IN 46206-1440, to request the brochure or other services.

When you decide to join a club, be wary of long-term contracts. Be wary also of discounts and other high-pressure come-ons; they may be signs of a failing business or high member turnover. Sign up for a few months so you can be absolutely certain that the club meets your needs. Then become active in a member advisory group that works with management to maintain and upgrade staff qualifications, facilities, and equipment.

Diet Centers

While diet centers provide dieting advice and encouragement, few boast the services of a registered dietitian. Most centers sell expensive vitamins, diet foods, and other products to their clients. Many clients do lose weight, and often at a rapid rate, indicating significant water and protein loss. Some centers advise against exercise, since clients following their program are often too listless to participate.

If you or a friend are considering the services of a diet center, follow the advice I provided regarding health clubs. Visit, ask questions, and by all means, ask about qualifications. Is a registered dietitian on the staff? Is a reputable local physician associated with the center? Most important, ask about the long-term success rate of the program. Then ask to contact some of the diet center's clients. Ask yourself if the diet center provides any service you cannot provide for yourself. The existence of so many centers suggests that the simple facts of energy balance and weight control have reached too few, that individuals lack the information, opportunity, or will to take control of their eating and activity behaviors.

Weight-Control Fallacies

While the fitness and health field is loaded with quacks and fallacies, neither area has more than weight control. Let's review some fallacies and replace them with facts.

Lose Inches, Not Pounds

This is the "come-on" of the figure salon, where they try to appeal to those who don't want to exercise to achieve real fat loss. Of course, it is possible to improve one's appearance with exercises that tone muscles and improve posture. The fallacy is that while you are shaping the body you are ignoring the engine, rusty hoses, and other important parts (i.e., the heart and blood vessels) and missing out on the health benefits associated with body weight and fat loss. Typically, the inches are not lost at all; a slightly tighter pull on the measuring tape gives the impression of progress. Fitness and health, like beauty, are more than skin deep.

DUNLOP'S DISEASE

My friend Ted once tried sit-ups to get rid of "Dunlop's disease," in which his tummy "done lopped" over his belt. He worked up to 400 sit-ups daily with no success. I showed him a study conducted by Dr. Frank Katch and colleagues at the University of Massachusetts. They collected fat biopsies from several fat deposits before and after a 4-week training program consisting entirely of sit-ups. Post-training analysis of fat cells revealed that the fat came from all the fat storage areas measured, not just abdominal fat (McArdle, Katch, & Katch, 1994). What about Ted? He became an ultramarathoner, training for and running 100-mile races, and the tummy roll ceased to be a problem, at least while he was in training. The moral of this story is burn off sufficient calories, and the spots and inches will take care of themselves.

Spot Reduction

There is very limited evidence that fat can be removed from specific areas (spots) by localized exercises. One study showed a mere 1 millimeter of spot reduction after 6 weeks of exercise. Avid tennis players have about the same skinfold on both arms, even though one arm is larger and more active.

Exercise Devices

You've seen the advertisements for passive exercise: electrical stimulation, vibrating machines, sauna shorts, and body wraps, devices that promise weight or fat loss without effort on your part. Sorry, but they don't work. Passive devices don't burn enough calories, electrical stimulation is not equivalent to voluntary exercise, vibrating devices do not break up fat and wash it away in the circulation, and tight pants or wraps do not remove fat with heat and massage. Spend the same amount of time in moderate exercise, and you will get results, including the health benefits you miss during passive exercise.

The advertising usually claims that with a few minutes of "almost effortless" activity you will get a firm, healthy, athletic body. They use attractive models, celebrities, or professional athletes to tout the product, and there is usually a big discount if you act immediately. If you are uncertain, ask your physician or local health club professional (certified by a reputable organization such as the American College of Sports Medicine or the National Strength and Conditioning Association) for advice. My advice: Try the product before you buy. Don't sign a long-term contract for any type of exercise program or device. And remember, a brisk walk burns more calories than most passive devices, and it's a lot more fun.

Drugs and Surgery

Laxatives and diuretics remove only water (dehydration). Amphetamines are sometimes prescribed to suppress the appetite, a dangerous approach to life-long weight control. Reputable physicians prescribe anorectic agents (appetite suppressants) as part of a total program with diet, exercise, and behavior therapy. But they need to avoid increasing doses and the risk of dependency. Current research on the genetic component of obesity may lead to future therapies, but that will never remove the need to balance caloric intake and expenditure.

Lipectomy and liposuction are surgical techniques used to remove unwanted fat. While lipectomy certainly removes fat and reduces weight, some studies suggest that the fat may be regenerated, especially if caloric intake continues to exceed expenditure. Liposuction, which involves vacuuming of fat cells from abdominal, thigh, and other deposits, is generally safe; however, no surgery is without risk. And there is no proof that surgical removal of superficial fat will change heart disease or other risk factors. Other forms of surgery are reserved for cases of morbid obesity, defined as more than 100 pounds overweight. One operation involves bypass of a portion of the small intestine, while a less complicated approach uses staples to fashion a smaller stomach. However, surgery is an expensive and sometimes dangerous approach to the problem.

Eating Disorders

The most tragic fallacy is the adoption of dangerous eating behaviors in an effort to achieve an unattainable ideal: a slim, trim figure. When being thin becomes an obsession, when self-worth becomes associated with slimness, the stage is set for eating disorders. *Bulimia* is a disorder characterized by a binge/purge cycle. Mild cases purge (vomit) occasionally to avoid weight gain, while more serious cases combine binge/purge with laxatives or diuretics, risking serious metabolic and psychological problems.

Anorexia nervosa is a serious psychological problem characterized by a distorted body image and a refusal to eat. Sometimes the behavior is associated with drugs or with obsessive exercise. If not treated, the individual may experience serious medical complications, including death as starvation compromises the heart and other organs. Eating disorders are more common among young women who seek to please others, who try to be perfect. Fortunately, psychological therapy and medical treatments are available to help victims who seek help.

To avoid contributing to the development of eating disorders, don't nag teenagers about weight problems. Minimize the emphasis on body weight, girth, and fat values, and focus on how they feel and function. Schedule family activities followed by family meals. Be aware of eating behaviors, and seek help early if disorders arise.

SMOKING?

It is sad to see young women smoking cigarettes, but it is tragic to hear that they continue the habit to avoid weight gain. While it is true that smokers gain some weight when they quit, the amount is not so excessive that it can't be eliminated with diet and exercise. Moreover, the health consequences of smoking far outweigh the effect of any weight gain. Develop an addiction to exercise to replace the addiction to nicotine.

Summary

This chapter has presented ways to use activity, dieting, and behavioral therapy in your lifelong effort to achieve energy balance and weight control. Most young folks are more active than older people and have more metabolically active tissue, so weight control isn't a problem. With age and responsibilities come less activity and a decline in metabolically active tissue, including muscle. Eventually, weight gain in the winter fails to melt off in the spring, or even the summer, and energy balance becomes a major issue. I've reached the stage of life at which I must exercise more or eat less if I want to maintain my body weight, cholesterol, pant size, and self-respect. Since I already engage in a considerable amount of exercise, and have already reduced the fat in my diet, I am faced with the unhappy prospect of life with fewer calories. But don't feel sorry for me: I've come this far enjoying an enormous appetite and a great love of food, and it is time that I learn some self-control. Guess I'll have to review the section on behavior therapy.

Performance in Work and Sport

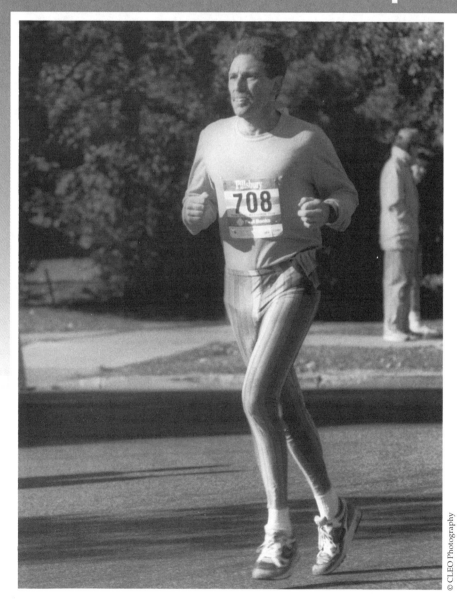

Most of us spend about 8 hours in sleep and 8 hours at work on a typical day. The rest is largely dedicated to preparation for one or the other, or for so-called leisure-time pursuits, including activity and sport. Improve fitness to enhance work capacity or performance in sport, and the sleep will take care of itself.

Beyond health, even beyond fitness, there is the desire to perform at a high level, to achieve one's potential. To do this one must set goals, then design and carry out a systematic plan to achieve them. The final step is to achieve what you trained for, sometimes in a public performance or event. We usually think of performing in sports, races, or other competitions, but some people train for cross-country bicycle trips, mountain climbs, or other private personal goals. And a few train to improve their work capacity, to be industrial athletes capable of impressive performances in the workplace.

This part of the book will help you improve your performance in work or sport. I'll show you how to use simple psychological skills to help you perform better, to play your best game more often. And I'll discuss how to prepare for and perform in a variety of terrestrial environments, including heat, cold, and altitude.

CHAPTER 15

Performance at Work

"In order that people may be happy in their work, these three things are needed: They must be fit for it. They must not do too much of it. And they must have a sense of success in it."

John Ruskin

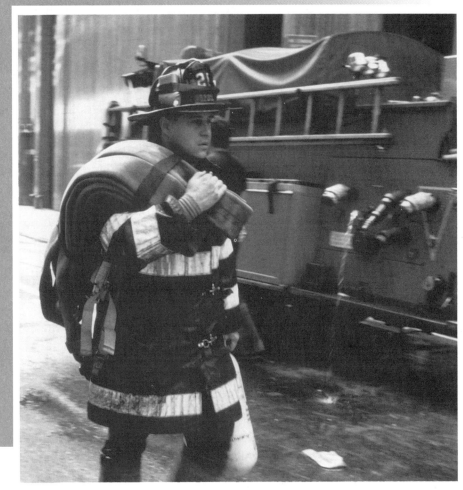

© Richard B. Levine

Until relatively recently in history, the primary source of power for the production of useful work was the contractions of muscles, both human and animal. Of course, people devised ways to augment muscle power with the ingenious use of wind and water, but it was not until the 18th century that mechanization began to reduce the need for muscular work. Machines were designed to supplement or replace human effort. Robots, computers, and other devices have replaced the need for human muscle power. Today, when men and women go to work, few are required to engage in arduous muscular effort.

Much of the credit for the reduction in physical labor must go to the inventors and engineers whose attempts at mechanization and, more recently, automation and robotics have made work relatively effortless. Some credit also is due to specialists in the scientific study of work, ergonomics. Work physiologists, psychologists, and engineers combine to study men and women in their working environment, with the goal of adapting the job to the ability of the average worker. At the same time, labor-saving devices have eliminated the need for muscular work at home, and the automobile makes the task of getting to and from work physically effortless.

The consequences of these trends are obvious: The average worker is incapable of delivering a full day's effort in a physically demanding job, and degenerative diseases associated with inactivity, such as heart disease—the nation's number one killer—are epidemic. If job requirements are continually lowered to meet the ability of the average worker, the trend will continue. Perhaps it is time for a change; perhaps we could benefit by working up to job requirements, not down. Perhaps it is time to adapt the worker to the job rather than just adapting the job to the worker.

THIS CHAPTER WILL HELP YOU

- understand the relationship between fitness and work capacity, and see why fitness is good for business;

- improve work performance and job satisfaction and appreciate the importance of physical maintenance to performance and satisfaction; and

- better integrate your job and your lifestyle.

Fitness and Work

Fit workers are more productive than their sedentary colleagues, are absent fewer days, and are far less likely to incur job-related disabilities or retire early due to heart or other degenerative diseases.

Certain jobs still require strength and endurance at least some of the time. Workers in heavy industry, construction, agriculture, forestry, public safety, and the military are often required to engage in strenuous effort. Without proper conditioning, the stress of arduous work can be unpleasant or worse, so concern for the health and safety of these employees has prompted screening procedures to make sure the worker is capable of meeting job demands. Many companies have instituted employee fitness programs to help workers meet and maintain required levels of work capacity.

Studies show that unfit workers can become a safety hazard to themselves, as well as to co-workers. Fit workers are more productive than their sedentary colleagues, are absent fewer days, and are far less likely to incur job-related disabilities or retire early due to heart or other degenerative diseases. Moreover, physically fit workers have a more positive attitude about work and life in general. For safety, health, production, and morale, fitness is good business.

Work Capacity

Work capacity is defined as the ability to accomplish production goals without undue fatigue and without becoming a hazard to yourself or co-workers. It is the product of a number of factors, including natural endowment, skill, nutrition, aerobic and muscular fitness, intelligence, experience, acclimatization, and lean body weight.

Aerobic or muscular fitness, acclimatization to heat or altitude, even skill and experience, do not ensure work output. A worker may rate high in all of these categories but fail to produce adequately due to lack of motivation. On the other hand, even the most highly motivated workers will fail if they lack strength or endurance, ignore the need to acclimatize to a hot working environment, or lack the physical skills required for the job.

AEROBIC THRESHOLD AND WORK CAPACITY

While aerobic fitness tells a lot about work capacity, a measure called the aerobic threshold is a better predictor of long-term performance. The aerobic threshold indicates the early rise in blood lactate during a progressive exercise test. Those who can do more work before the lactic acid level rises will be able to sustain a higher level of production in prolonged arduous work. It isn't necessary to conduct a laboratory test to determine long-term work capacity. Simply select a job-related work sample and measure performance, the amount of work accomplished by the candidates in 30 to 45 minutes.

Aerobic Fitness and Work Capacity

The body requires energy to perform work, energy that is released in the metabolism of fat and carbohydrate. This process takes oxygen; the tougher the job, the more energy and oxygen are needed. When oxygen and energy needs are light, such as for office duties, work performance isn't strongly related to aerobic fitness, but when oxygen and energy needs are high (more than 7.5 calories per minute), production relates directly to the ability to produce energy aerobically (see table 15.1).

TABLE 15.1   Occupational Work Classifications

Classification	Energy expenditure (cal/min)	Lifting (lb)	Carrying (lb)
Very light work	Under 2.5	Up to 10	Small objects
Light work	2.6-4.9	Up to 20	Up to 10
Medium work	5.0-7.5	Up to 50	Up to 25
Heavy work	Above 7.5	Up to 100	Up to 50
Very heavy work	Above 7.6	Over 100	Over 50

Data from *Dictionary of Occupational Titles* (p. 48) by the U.S. Department of Labor, 1968, Washington, DC: U.S. Government Printing Office.

When heavy work is required, individuals with a low level of aerobic fitness are able to work at only 25% of capacity for 8 hours. Those of average fitness can sustain about 33%, while those with above-average fitness can maintain 40% of their capacity for 8 hours. Only highly conditioned and motivated individuals can sustain levels as high as 50% of their aerobic fitness level for 8 hours. Figure 15.1 illustrates that individuals with comparatively higher fitness levels have the capacity to outperform less fit individuals. In some jobs the fit worker is able to produce 4 to 6 times more than the unfit (Sharkey et al., 1977). Which one would you hire?

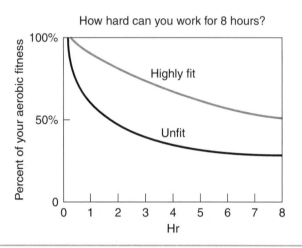

Figure 15.1   Fitness and work capacity.

Muscular Fitness and Work Capacity

Dynamic muscular strength is clearly related to work capacity when very heavy loads must be lifted or when using heavy tools. However, for *repeated* lifting—as in work with hand tools—strength, muscular endurance, and aerobic fitness combine to set the limits of work capacity (figure 15.2).

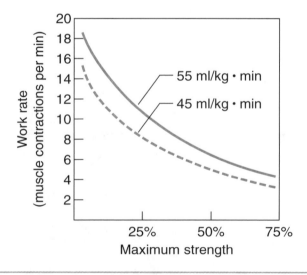

Figure 15.2   Interrelationships of strength, aerobic fitness, and work rate.

Combinations of work rate and percentage of maximum strength that fall to the right of the line that represents your fitness level in figure 15.2 cannot be sustained for a full working day. Highly fit workers (55 milliliters of oxygen per kilogram of body weight per minute (ml/kg · min) can produce more by working at a higher rate. Stronger individuals can lift more with each contraction. The ideal combination includes levels of aerobic fitness and strength adequate to the task.

Most work tasks require more endurance than strength; in fact, many individuals mistakenly use the term strength when they really mean endurance. If an individual has the strength to accomplish a task, physical conditioning should focus on muscular endurance and aerobic fitness. Only those with inadequate strength need engage in strength training. Of course, skill is also needed to work safely and efficiently. Fitness cannot make up for deficiencies in skill. Skill leads to efficiency, and efficiency allows the worker to conserve energy and avoid fatigue.

Body Weight and Work Capacity

Excess fat certainly limits work capacity; when considerable muscular strength is needed on the job, the individual with a high lean body weight (LBW) is more likely to excel (LBW equals body weight minus fat weight). The LBW indicates how much muscle is available. Body weight alone doesn't tell enough about an individual's body composition. The percent body fat can also be misleading: 20% fat sounds high, unless it's on top of 200 pounds of lean weight (muscle). In a study of wildland firefighters, we (Sharkey, Jukkala, Putnam, & Tietz, 1978) found work capacity to be highly related to LBW. LBW has relevance when women engage in heavy work. Since women typically have a greater percentage of body fat than men, men and women of the same weight will not have the same LBW. The female applicant will have to have less fat or weigh more than the average man to have a similar level of LBW.

HOW MUCH STRENGTH?

How much strength is necessary? Generally speaking, for prolonged work, the average load in repetitive lifting should not exceed 20% of your maximal strength in that movement. In other words, strength should be at least five times greater than the load regularly lifted on the job. If the job requires daylong work with a shovel that weighs 10 pounds when loaded, the worker should possess at least 50 pounds of dynamic muscular strength in the arm and shoulder muscles used to perform the task. Once the worker achieves the minimum strength required, further increases in work capacity can be achieved by increasing muscular endurance and aerobic fitness. If the job involves only occasional lifts of very heavy loads (e.g., 100 pounds), the worker can succeed with 100 pounds of strength, plus a margin for safety's sake. The greater the margin, the less is the risk of injury.

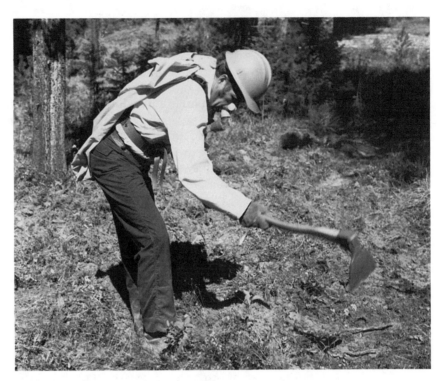

Energy expenditure is determined during a work test.

Fitness Is Good Business

Fit employees are a good investment. Thousands of companies spend billions on fitness and health (wellness) programs for their employees. The expenditure is justified on several grounds.

> Fit workers are less likely to smoke, and smoking costs business and industry billions for health and cleaning expenses, lost and wasted time, and fires.

- **Cost-effectiveness:** Each dollar spent on fitness/wellness in the workplace saves several dollars. Fit workers are less likely to smoke, and smoking costs business and industry billions for health and cleaning expenses, lost and wasted time, and of course, fires.
- **Production:** Fit employees are more productive in any line of work.
- **Safety:** Fit workers are safe workers; they are far less likely to experience debilitating lower back and other injuries, and when injured they miss fewer days.
- **Health:** Fit workers miss fewer days of work; they are far less likely to suffer from degenerative problems such as heart disease. They spend a smaller share of the company's health-care dollar.
- **Morale:** Morale is higher among fit employees and those in the fitness program. Fitness and health programs increase loyalty and reduce turnover.

If your company doesn't already have a fitness/wellness program, talk with management, assemble a group of interested co-workers, and get started. As the program develops consider ways to enhance the activity habit and the climate for fitness.

Flextime

Many employers have adopted an alternative to the rigid 8 to 5 work schedule. Prompted by congestion on highways and parking lots, overcrowding in lunch areas, family responsibilities, and requests for a more accommodating work schedule, employers have tested and confirmed the feasibility of the flexible work schedule. The typical flextime program calls for 8 to 10 hours of work that may begin as early as 6:00 a.m. and end as late as 6:00 p.m. Employees usually are required to be at work during a core period so that company business can be carried out. Flextime can allow individuals to work during their most productive time and to take longer lunch breaks for shopping, exercise, or family. As a result, production goes up, and absenteeism goes down. Flextime allows each worker a freer hand in the creation of his or her own lifestyle.

Four-Day Workweek

Another interesting variation of the traditional work-rest cycle promises even greater individual benefits. The 4-day workweek may provide a simple solution to the overwhelming weekend congestion on roads, beaches, tennis courts, golf courses, and ski lifts, and even in wilderness areas. The 4-day (10 hours per day) workweek has been tried with considerable success in a number of industries. Schedules can be staggered to provide flexible 3-day rest periods. Some possible workweeks are M-T-W-Th, T-W-Th-F, W-Th-F-Sa, even Su-M-T-W. Some people may even prefer to take their "weekend" during the week. When combined with flextime, the 4-day workweek can further humanize the world of work, thereby providing a greater opportunity for a creative adaptation to life.

Home Office

Perhaps the most appealing alternative to the traditional workweek is telecommuting from your home office. Even if this is done only 1 or 2 days each week, it saves money, time, and frayed nerves, and allows a more creative approach for a young or single parent. The time usually spent commuting can be spent at work, freeing other time for family and individual activities, including food preparation and exercise. Money saved on transportation and clothing costs can be used to enhance the quality of life. I belong to an organization that once spent thousands of dollars to bring officers and committee members from around the country to the headquarters office for meetings. Today we accomplish most of our business via teleconference. Soon we'll be able to sit at home and use the computer to meet, share documents, and balance budgets, face to face. While the home office will never replace the need for in-person communication, it does provide another way to free the employee from rigid, outdated workplace requirements.

Occupational Physiology

Physiology, the study of the human body, is becoming increasingly important in the workplace, to determine job demands and aid in the selection of workers; to work-harden, train, and cross-train workers to improve performance and reduce injuries; to rehabilitate injured workers; to confront job discrimination according to age, gender, race, or disability; and to promote health and wellness. This section considers some of the current issues and provides a fair approach to hiring.

Fit to Work

Finding the right person for the job can often be difficult. Employers use high school and college transcripts, written tests, letters of recommendation, background checks, even psychological and drug tests to try to find good employees. When a job demands physical performance, many employers are turning to job-related tests to aid the selection process.

Job-Related Tests

Job-related tests have replaced old-fashioned fitness tests in the workplace. Development of a valid test of work capacity requires a job task analysis to select important work tasks. The candidate (or prototype) test is then administered to successful employees to ensure its usefulness and to determine a minimum passing score. Thereafter, the test can be used to select new employees, to ensure that current employees maintain work capacity, and as an evaluation of readiness to return to work following injury or illness.

Ergonomics

For decades, the goal of ergonomics has been to adapt the job to the worker. Scientists and engineers have attempted to ease the burden on the worker by making adjustments in tools or work processes. When conditions or costs limit these adjustments it makes sense to adapt workers to the job. When the job is demanding, the best approach is to select individuals physically suited for the work, and to maintain their work capacity with an ongoing job-related fitness program. Some companies have begun to view their workers as highly trained *industrial athletes*. They recruit, train, maintain, and cross-train those with the physical capacity to do the work.

Physical Maintenance

Job-related testing accomplishes little if it is used only on recruits. The only way to maintain physical working capacity throughout a worker's career is to

JOB DEMANDS

Dr. Paul Davis has developed a job-related test for municipal (structural) firefighters. The test incorporates actual elements of the job, including carrying hoses up several flights of stairs, a chopping task, pulling a heavy hose, and a victim carry. While some people may argue with the cutoff score used by a particular department, few would say that the test fails to represent the demands of the job. Many departments use this or a similar test to select among the many candidates for the job. Unfortunately, only a few departments demand that their firefighters pass the test annually. Dr. Davis's studies show that the fitness of public service personnel (police, fire) declines at the same rate as that of the sedentary, overweight population at large (Davis and Starck, 1980).

require annual testing and participation in a job-related fitness program. Fire departments are known for the care they give their equipment: They purchase rigorously tested equipment and maintain it with meticulous upkeep. Yet, they will hire employees who barely pass a selection test, and then ignore the need for ongoing physical maintenance. Unfortunately, the need to maintain work capacity has become a pawn in the collective bargaining process.

A well-designed program maintains or builds the aerobic and muscular capabilities required on the job, while meeting the health and wellness needs of the employees. The program also addresses injury prevention with stretching and strengthening exercises, ensures needed heat or altitude acclimatization, and teaches the importance of nutrition and hydration. When job-related fitness is a high priority, work time is provided for it to maintain job performance. This is good business, since fit workers are less likely to sustain disabling injuries and are quicker to return to work after injury. Fitness improves performance in the heat, shortens the time required for acclimatization, and dramatically raises work output. In our studies of wildland firefighters cited earlier, highly fit and motivated workers have outperformed less fit workers by a factor of 3 to 1!

> The only way to maintain physical working capacity throughout a worker's career is to require annual testing and participation in a job-related fitness program.

Equal Opportunity

A major feature of the workplace during the past 25 years has been the effort to provide equal employment opportunities. A series of federal laws has attempted to eliminate discrimination based on age, gender, race, or disability.

Age

The Age Discrimination in Employment Act (ADEA) of 1967 outlawed job discrimination based on age, except when age was a bona fide occupational qualification (BFOQ). The BFOQ requires that the effects of advancing age make it impossible for all or most individuals above a certain age to do a job, and/or it is impossible to assess work capacity with a job-related test. Neither condition of the BFOQ is defensible; age does not make it impossible for all above a certain age to do a job, and job-related tests can be developed to assess work capacity. For a while, Congress exempted fire and law enforcement personnel from the ADEA, assuming that age was a BFOQ. However, a large study commissioned by the Equal Employment Opportunity Commission (EEOC) found that age was poorly correlated with performance, and that job-related tests accurately reflected work capacity (Landy et al., 1992). During the period of exemption from the ADEA, studies of fire and law enforcement personnel indicated the dismal level of physical readiness of these emergency service personnel. Fitness declines rapidly in this relatively inactive population, and body fat levels double during the 20-year career. With this physical decline comes a high rate of heart disease. While heart disease has been called a job-related disability, it clearly is related to lifestyle factors (diet, inactivity). Taxpayers deserve the best qualified and trained public servants available, and age alone does not ensure career-long fitness for duty. The solution is to test recruits and follow up with annual performance evaluations, coupled with a job-related physical maintenance (fitness) and wellness program.

Gender

In the 1970s, with the help of the Civil Rights Act of 1964, women began to seek employment in previously male-dominated jobs, such as fire fighting,

TOO OLD?

Management considered George to be too old to become a "smoke jumper," but not too old to conduct the physical training program for this elite bunch of firefighters. The jumpers are wildland firefighters who parachute into the wilderness to battle wildfires. When the fire is contained, they load up their gear, all 125 pounds of it, and "pack it out" several miles to the nearest trail head. As he approached retirement from his university teaching position, George took advantage of the ADEA and signed up for jumper training. At the tender age of 58 he passed the arduous physical tests, jump training, and field tests such as the 3-mile pack-out with 110 pounds, and he became a smoke jumper. Age alone says little about performance or the size of a person's heart.

law enforcement, and construction. In many cases the transition took place with little fanfare, but in some it has been a struggle. Men still question women's ability to carry out jobs that require considerable upper-body strength. Job-related tests used to select employees have been labeled as discriminatory when they disqualify a large proportion of women. For example, in a test of more than 6,000 recruits for the Chicago Fire Department, no women scored in the top 2,000. Since there were fewer than 200 openings, the test appeared to discriminate against women. The Federal

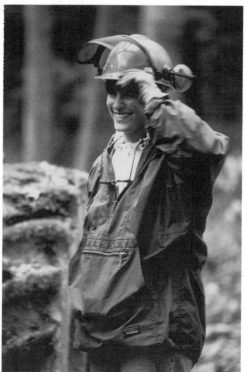

© Terry Wild Studio

Women have worked to achieve success in formerly male-dominated occupations.

Uniform Guidelines for Employee Selection Procedures (1976) state that a selection test has adverse impact when a class of employees scores less than 80% (four-fifths) of the rate of the highest class. Therefore, when women pass at a rate that is less than 80% of the men's pass rate, the employer is required to demonstrate the validity of the test and why it is necessary. When job tasks require upper-body strength it is virtually impossible to avoid adverse impact, since women average 50% of men's upper-body strength.

Unfortunately, many valid tests have been discontinued for fear of adverse impact and the lawsuits brought by state and federal human rights and equal opportunity commissions. In my view, this is a disservice to women. Performance in sport proves that women are capable of training to meet physical challenges. Women's world records in running are just 10% below those of men in distances ranging from 100 meters to the marathon (42 kilometers or 26 miles, 385 yards). My experience with the women of the U.S. Nordic Ski Team and with wildland firefighters has convinced me that many women have what it takes to succeed in physically difficult occupations. Women athletes train to build muscle strength and endurance, and women can train to compete in formerly male-only jobs.

Until women are given the chance to work up to defensible job standards, we'll never know how good they can be. Establish valid job-related tests, advertise the standards, and provide preemployment training programs. If few women qualify, don't panic and lower the standards. Hold firm, and watch as women come forth to accept the challenge.

> Until women are given the chance to work up to defensible job standards, we'll never know how good they can be.

TARA'S STORY

Tara was a graduate student in exercise science and my research assistant when she decided to become a smoke jumper. At that time, only a few women had made it through training to become jumpers. Tara was an endurance athlete who weighed barely enough to qualify for training, so she designed and carried out a weight-training program to gain strength and lean body weight. After several months of serious training she successfully completed the entrance test and training, including the pack-out—a 3-mile hike with a load equal to her lean body weight (110 pounds). This determined lady would not be satisfied with watered-down qualifications. She wanted to be accepted on her merits as a qualified worker, not a token woman or an affirmative-action hire.

Racial/Ethnic Groups

Studies in work physiology do not suggest racial or ethnic differences in work capacity. With some doubting the validity of race as a useful classification, and others downplaying the existence of meaningful racial differences, there is little justification for a lengthy discussion. What is clear is that job-related work capacity tests do not unfairly impact racial or ethnic groups. Indeed, valid work capacity tests can be considered color-blind.

People With Disabilities

The Americans with Disabilities Act (ADA) of 1991 was enacted to ensure employment opportunities and reasonable accommodations for persons with disabilities. The Act also mandates improved access for those with disabilities. The ADA endorses the use of valid preemployment tests as an objective way to determine a person's ability to do the job. It allows postemployment medical examinations so long as the results remain confidential. And it encourages employers to make reasonable accommodations for persons with disabilities.

Summary

Performance in physically demanding work is related to fitness; the harder the work, the higher the relationship to measures of aerobic and muscular fitness. Therefore, when selecting employees for hard work it makes good sense to utilize a job-related work-capacity test in order to hire those most suited for the work. But selection isn't enough: An ongoing job-related fitness or physical maintenance program is necessary to be certain employees maintain the capacity to do the job. The ideal plan involves a job-related selection test, a well-designed fitness program to maintain work capacity, an employee health/wellness program for health, and annual retesting with the work capacity test. When these are combined with ergonomics, safety, and injury prevention, you have a comprehensive approach to employee health, safety, and performance.

Let me add a final note to extol an additional workplace benefit for those who pursue the active life. Studies in the United States and Canada indicate a positive relationship between leisure-time physical activity and personal income; as the level of activity increases so does the level of income. Now, it is true that a correlation does not imply cause and effect, so it doesn't mean that you'll make more money if you become more active. Frequently a relationship can be explained by the fact that behaviors are interrelated, that two are related to a third variable. Indeed, there is a well-known relationship between education level and income: Income rises with education. And there is a positive relationship between education and level of activity, and that helps to explain why activity is related to income (Stephens, Jacobs, & White, 1985).

It is no secret that vigorous, enthusiastic individuals are more likely to be hired. Afterward, raises and promotions should be based primarily on performance. Since activity and fitness improve health, performance, morale, and safety, it seems reasonable that vigorous and enthusiastic workers will be retained, rewarded, and promoted to more responsible positions. In this era of corporate downsizing and layoffs, it is prudent to do all you can to acquire, retain, and enhance opportunities for the attainment of challenging and personally rewarding employment. Don't ignore the role of activity and fitness in the workplace.

CHAPTER 16

Performance in Sport

"Don't play sports to get in shape; get in shape to play sports!"

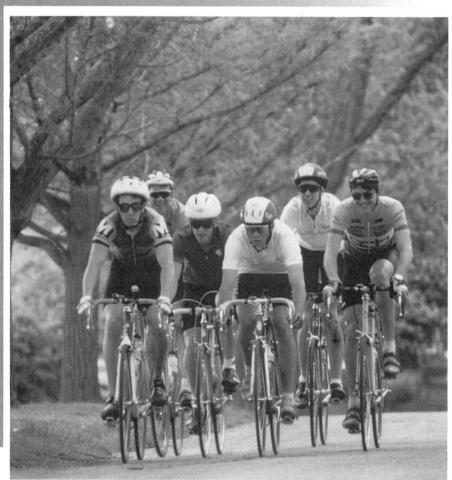

In this chapter, I tell you how to prepare for athletic competition safely and effectively so that you can enjoy the intense pleasure and excitement of sport and competition, without the risk of fatigue, overtraining, injury, or illness. Opportunities for adult (masters, senior, veteran) competition include road races, orienteering, track and field, swimming, alpine and cross-country skiing, tennis, racquetball, handball, golf, softball, volleyball, bowling, judo, karate, and many others. Adults participate according to age group, and it is not unusual to find active athletes of 60, 70, and even 80 years of age. A few, such as the late Larry Lewis, an indefatigable runner, continue to participate in races beyond their 100th birthday. If you like to train and enjoy the thrill of competition, of getting high on your own hormones, this section is for you. But remember, you must train before you compete.

THIS CHAPTER WILL HELP YOU

■ utilize the principles of training,

■ improve performance in your favorite sport,

■ utilize diet to enhance performance, and

■ develop psychological skills to help you play your best game more often.

Principles of Training

This section (adapted from Sharkey, 1986) introduces 12 important physiological principles that you must follow in order to make steady progress in your training and to avoid illness and injury.

Principle 1: Readiness

The value of training depends on the physiological and psychological readiness of the individual. Because readiness comes with maturation, physically immature (prepubertal) individuals lack the physiological preparedness to respond completely to training. Readiness also implies the need for adequate nutrition and rest in order to benefit from training. Psychological readiness refers to the commitment to delay gratification and make the sacrifices involved in sustained training.

Principle 2: Adaptation

Training induces subtle changes as the body adapts to the added demands. Dr. Ned Fredrick, a friend and noted sport scientist, calls training for sport a gentle pastime in which we coax subtle changes from the body. The day-to-day changes are so small as to be unmeasurable; weeks and even months of patient progress are required to achieve measurable adaptations. Try to rush the process and you risk illness, injury, or both.

Typical adaptations include

- increased enzyme proteins or contractile proteins;
- improved respiration, heart function, circulation, and blood volume;

- improved muscular endurance, strength, or power; and
- tougher bones, ligaments, tendons, and connective tissue.

The principle of adaptation tells us that training can't be rushed. The best you can do is to follow a sensible program and be satisfied with the results. Trying to do it all in one season is likely to do more harm than good.

Principle 3: Individual Response

Individuals respond differently to the same training for some of the following reasons.

Heredity

Physique, muscle fiber characteristics, heart and lung size, and other factors may be inherited. But although we inherit certain characteristics, environmental factors such as diet and training also influence the eventual expression of the characteristic. So, although factors associated with aerobic fitness and endurance have been estimated to be approximately 25% genetically determined, the remainder is subject to change.

Maturity

Bodies that are more mature can handle more training. Less mature athletes don't respond as well to training, and they need more energy for growth and development (see Principle 1: Readiness).

Nutrition

Training involves changes in tissues and organs, changes that require protein and other nutrients. Without proper nutrition, the best training program will fail. Remember to eat adequate protein when you lose weight during training.

Rest and Sleep

Although young athletes may require 8 hours or more of sleep per day, adults often get by with less. However, when training gets tough, it is wise to get more sleep or to take short naps. Inadequate rest minimizes the gains associated with training.

Level of Fitness

Improvement due to training is most dramatic when the level of fitness is low. Later, when fitness is high, long hours of effort are needed to achieve small improvements. Less fit individuals fatigue easily and are more prone to illness or injury.

Environmental Influences

Factors in the physical and psychological environment influence the response to training. Psychological factors might include emotional stress at work, home, or school, while physical factors include heat, cold, altitude, and air pollution. Learn to recognize your own ability to tolerate environmental stressors, and slow down when conditions are severe.

Illness or Injury

Of course, illness or injury will influence your response to training. The problem is to spot potential problems before they become serious. Many problems are first noticed during hard effort, and coaches or exercise partners may be the ones to point them out. Try to listen to your body's signals, and if you are injured or ill be certain you have recovered before returning to practice.

Motivation

Individuals work harder and gain more when they are motivated and when they see the relationship of hard work to their personal goals. Your training will be easier if you are involved for personal reasons.

Principle 4: Overload

The legendary tale of Milo, a warrior in ancient Greece, illustrates the overload principle. Milo started lifting a young calf, and as the calf grew, so did Milo's strength. Eventually he was able to lift the full-grown animal. Training must place a demand on the body system if desired adaptations are to take place. To begin, training must exceed the typical daily demand. As you adapt to increased loading, you should add more load. The rate of improvement is related to three factors, which you can remember with the help of the acronym **FIT**:

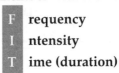

F requency

I ntensity

T ime (duration)

The overload principle is used in all kinds of training. We gradually add more weight to the barbell to achieve increases in strength. Endurance athletes increase training time and intensity to improve race performances. The overload stimulates changes in the muscles and other systems, changes designed to help the body cope with future demands. These changes involve the nervous system, which learns to recruit muscle fibers more effectively; the circulation, which becomes better able to send more blood to the working muscles; and the muscles themselves, where the overload stimulates the production of new protein to help meet future exercise demands.

Principle 5: Progression

To achieve adaptations using the overload principle, training must follow the principle of progression. When the training load is increased too quickly, the body cannot adapt and instead breaks down. Progression must be observed in terms of increases in FIT.

- **Frequency**—sessions per day, week, month, or year
- **Intensity**—training load per day, week, month, or year
- **Time**—duration of training in hours per day, week, month, or year

But progression does not imply inexorable increases, without time for recovery. The body requires periods of rest in which adaptations take place. *Make haste slowly!*

The principle of progression has other implications: training should also progress from the general to the specific, the part to the whole, and quantity to quality.

Principle 6: Specificity

Exercise is specific. When you jog you recruit certain muscle fibers, energy pathways, and energy sources. If you jog every day, you are training, and the adaptations will take place in the muscle fibers used during the exercise. The adaptations to endurance training are different from adaptations to strength training. Endurance training elicits improvements in oxidative enzymes and the muscle's ability to burn fat and carbohydrate in the presence of oxygen. Strength training leads to increases in the contractile proteins that exert force, actin and myosin, but only in the muscles exercised.

This means that the type of training you undertake must relate to the desired results. Specific training brings specific results. You won't get much stronger with endurance training, and you won't improve endurance much with strength training. Cycling is not the best preparation for running, or vice versa. Performance improves most when the training is specific to the activity.

Of course, every rule or principle can be taken to the extreme. Specificity does not mean you should avoid training opposite or adjacent muscles. In fact, you should train other muscles to avoid muscle imbalances that could predispose the body to injury. And you can train adjacent muscles to help you adapt to changes in conditions and to provide a backup when the primary muscle fibers become fatigued. So, some cycling may be good for a runner; it will provide muscle balance, train adjacent fibers, and provide some relief from the pounding of running.

Principle 7: Variation

The training program must be varied to avoid boredom and to maintain your interest. The principle of variation embraces two basic concepts: work/rest and hard/easy.

Adaptation comes when work is followed by rest, when the hard is followed by the easy. Failure to include variation leads to boredom, staleness, and poor performance. Successive sessions of hard work, if not followed by adequate time for rest and recovery, are certain to hinder progress in training.

Achieve variation by changing your training routine and drills. When possible, conduct workouts in different places or under different conditions. Follow a long workout with a short one, an intense session with a relaxed one, or high speed with easy distance. When workouts become dull, do something different. Use variety (cross-training) to diminish monotony and to lighten the physical and psychological burdens of heavy training.

Principle 8: Warm-Up/Cool-Down

A warm-up should always precede strenuous activity to

- increase body temperature;
- increase respiration and heart rate; and
- guard against muscle, tendon, and ligament strains.

The warm-up should consist of stretching, calisthenics, and gradually increasing exercise intensity. Stretching may be more effective after the warm-up.

The cool-down is just as important as the warm-up. Abrupt cessation of vigorous activity leads to pooling of the blood, sluggish circulation, and slow removal of waste products. It may also contribute to cramping, soreness, or more serious problems. High levels of the hormone norepinephrine are present immediately after vigorous exercise, making the heart more subject to irregular beats. The cool-down helps remove excess norepinephrine and lower the body temperature. Light activity and stretching continue the pumping action of muscles on veins, helping the circulation in the removal of metabolic wastes.

Principle 9: Long-Term Training

Changes resulting from the gradual overload of body systems lead to impressive improvements in performance. But it takes years of effort to approach high-level performance capability. Long-term training allows for growth and development, gradual progress, acquisition of skills, learning of strategies, and a fuller understanding of the sport. So, don't rush the process; too much training too soon may lead to mental and physical burnout and early retirement from the sport. Excellence comes to those who persist with a well-planned, long-term training program.

Principle 10: Reversibility

Most of the adaptations achieved from months of hard training are reversible. In general, it takes longer to gain endurance than it does to lose it. With complete bed rest, fitness can decline at a rate of almost 10% per week! Strength declines more slowly, but lack of use will eventually cause atrophy of even the best-trained muscles. To avoid this problem, maintain a year-round program, with periods of hard work followed by periods of relative rest and variety.

Principle 11: Moderation

The principle of moderation applies to all aspects of life; too much of anything can be bad for your health. Temper dedication with judgment and moderation. Train too hard, too long, or too fast, and the body begins to deteriorate. Practice moderation in all things.

SENIOR SUCCESS

Dr. Thomas K. Cureton was a pioneer in exercise physiology and the study of fitness, spending his illustrious career at the University of Illinois during the 1950s and '60s. On weekdays, this indefatigable teacher and researcher taught classes, conducted research studies, and wrote books and articles about fitness. On weekends he took to the road to preach the gospel of fitness and health to the lay public. His YMCA workshops were legendary for the enormous energy exhibited by this traveling prophet of fitness. He was so busy he had little time for himself. Sometime after his retirement he returned to the pool, site of youthful success in competitive swimming. Before long he was setting national and then world records in his age group. I'll never forget his contributions and his delight at finding athletic success in his eighties. It's never too late to start, or start over.

Principle 12: Potential

Every individual has a potential maximal level of performance. Most of us never come close to that potential performance. The highest potential performances are still to be achieved. Regular participation in physical activity will help you achieve your potential and improve the quality of daily living.

Training Fallacies

Before I close this section on principles, let me add some popular fallacies or misconceptions concerning training. These often-quoted "principles" are untrue and have no basis in medical or scientific research.

Fallacy 1: No Pain, No Gain

Although serious training is often difficult and sometimes unpleasant, it shouldn't hurt. In fact, well-prepared athletes can perform difficult events in a state of euphoria, free of pain and oblivious to discomfort. Marathon winners sometimes seem to finish full of vitality, whereas others appear near collapse. Pain is not a natural consequence of exercise or training; it is a sign of a problem that shouldn't be ignored. During exercise the body produces natural opiates, called endorphins, that can mask discomfort during exercise. If you experience real pain during training, you should back off. If the pain persists, have the problem evaluated.

Discomfort, on the other hand, can accompany difficult aspects of training such as heavy lifting, intense interval training, or long-distance effort. Discomfort is a natural consequence of the lactic acid that accompanies the anaerobic effort of lifting or intervals, or of the muscle fatigue, microscopic muscle damage (microtrauma), and soreness that come with long-distance training. I would accept this statement: No discomfort, no excellence. Overload sometimes requires working at the upper limit of strength, intensity, or endurance, and that can be temporarily uncomfortable. If exercise results in pain, it is probably excessive. The next two fallacies are also associated with the "no pain, no gain" misconception.

Fallacy 2: You Must Break Down Muscle to Improve

Microtrauma sometimes occurs in muscle during vigorous training and competition, but it isn't a necessary or even a desirable outcome of training. Runners have shown significant microtrauma at the end of a marathon with long downhill stretches that require eccentric muscular contractions (contractions of a lengthening muscle). Eccentric contractions are a major cause of muscle soreness, which is associated with muscle trauma, reduced force output, and a prolonged (4 to 6 weeks) period of recovery. Excessive trauma doesn't help training; it stops it.

Weight lifters can traumatize muscle with excess weight or repetitions, but that is not a necessary stage in the development of strength. Neither pain nor injury is a normal consequence of training, and you should avoid both.

Fallacy 3: Go for the Burn

This popular statement is often heard among body builders who do numerous repetitions and sets to build, shape, and define muscles. The burn they describe is probably due to the increased acidity associated with elevated levels of lactic acid in the muscle. Although this sensation isn't dangerous, it isn't a necessary part of a strength program designed to improve performance.

Fallacy 4: Lactic Acid Causes Muscle Soreness

This fallacy has been around for years, without any basis in fact. Although lactic acid may be produced in contractions that lead to soreness, the lactic acid isn't the cause of the soreness. Lactic acid is cleared from muscle and blood within an hour of the exercise. Soreness comes 24 hours or more after the effort, long after the lactic acid has been removed or metabolized. Soreness follows unfamiliar exertion or a long layoff and is probably associated with microtrauma to muscle and connective tissue and the swelling that results. After recovery, additional exposure to the activity will yield less soreness.

Fallacy 5: Muscle Turns to Fat (or Vice Versa)

Another common misconception is that when an athlete stops training, muscle can turn to fat. Muscle will no more turn to fat than fat will turn to muscle. Both are highly specialized tissues with specific functions. Muscles are composed of long, spaghetti-like fibers with contractile proteins designed to exert force. Fat cells are round receptacles designed to store fat. Training increases the size of muscle fibers (hypertrophy), and detraining reduces their size (atrophy). Excess caloric consumption causes fat cells to grow in size as they store more fat. The cells shrink when you burn more calories than you eat. But long, thin muscle fibers never change into spherical blobs of fat, or vice versa.

Fallacy 6: I Ran Out of Wind

Athletes often have the sensation of running out of wind when they run too fast for their level of training. The sensation comes from the lungs and reflects another discomfort of exertion. However, it is more likely to be due to an excess of carbon dioxide than a lack of oxygen or air. Carbon dioxide is produced during the oxidative metabolism of carbohydrate, and it is the primary stimulus for respiration. So, when carbon dioxide levels are high, as they are during vigorous effort, they cause distress signals in the lungs. The respiratory system thinks it is more important to rid the body of excess CO_2 than it is to bring in more O_2. Excess CO_2 is a sign that you have exceeded your lactate threshold, that you are working above your level of training. Become familiar with the sensation and what it is telling you; ignore it, and you will soon become exhausted.

The Physiology of Training

The physiology of training, which studies the response of the body to training, has received a great deal of attention in recent years. Working together, coaches, athletes, and sports scientists have contributed to a growing body of knowledge about how the body responds to the demands of systematic training. This section provides an overview of the training along with suggestions to guide the development and conduct of your program.

Energy Training

In order to tailor a training program suited to your needs, you first must know the energy sources required in the activity. Figure 16.1 illustrates the relative contribution of anaerobic and aerobic energy sources in relation to the distance or duration of running events (use the time scale to estimate energy sources for other activities).

Next, it helps to know something about your individual capabilities, both anaerobic and aerobic. If you are eager to prepare for a marathon, for which the energy source is primarily aerobic, you should be as strong as possible in aerobic fitness. If your event is primarily anaerobic, such as a 100-meter swim, you will need anaerobic capabilities, along with the aerobic capacity to support training and enhance recovery. Once you know the energy sources used in the activity and your own capabilities, you can begin to design your training program.

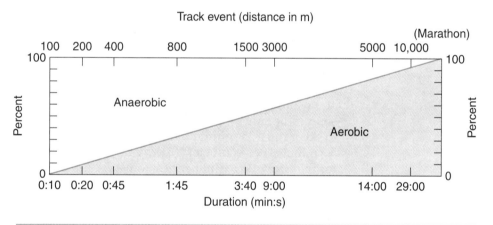

Figure 16.1 Anaerobic and aerobic energy sources in relation to distance and duration of events. Shorter events are primarily anaerobic. For distances greater than 1,500 m (longer than 4 min) training should concentrate on aerobic fitness.

Year-Round Training

While it is possible to make significant improvements in aerobic energy sources in as little as 2 to 3 months, a year-round program is bound to be safer and more effective (see figure 16.2). All training begins with an aerobic buildup, a period of slow distance work that builds stamina and neuromuscular efficiency. Once a sound aerobic foundation has been established, you are ready to train the upper end of your aerobic capability, the anaerobic threshold. This is accomplished by interval training, using long intervals (2 to 5 minutes). Anaerobic training then follows with shorter and faster efforts (30 to 90 seconds). Finally, and only if speed is required in the event, sprints can be added to the program (table 16.1).

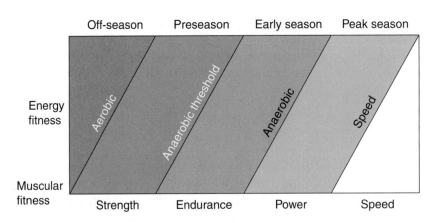

Figure 16.2 Seasonal training goals.

The year-round approach to training provides the strong foundation needed to compete successfully. It minimizes the risk of injury that accompanies anaerobic and speed training. It also leads to a competitive peak that can be sustained for a month or more, and provides for a postseason recovery period prior to a renewed training effort. If you are involved in several activities and cannot devote 12 months to any one, use the same approach but shorten each phase. Always allow at least 1 month each for aerobic and anaerobic threshold buildups. If necessary, use the first few weeks of the competitive season for any speed training, but don't expect your best performances until later in the season (Sharkey, 1986).

Race-Pace Training

To ensure the specificity of training and the development of needed energy sources, be sure to spend part of your time on race-pace training. If your goal is to ski or run a 35-minute 10-kilometer (6.2 miles) course, you'll have to average 3.5 minutes per kilometer. To provide the physiological and psychological base for the effort, do a number of kilometers at that pace (at least 1 in 20, or 5%, at race tempo). If the pace sometimes feels difficult, remember that the excite-

TABLE 16.1   Seasonal Training Goals and Methods

Season	Training goals	Training methods
Off-season	Aerobic fitness of slow twitch fibers	Long, slow distance, medium distance, Fartlek,* hills
Preseason	Raise anaerobic threshold and aerobic fitness of fast oxidative glycolytic (FOG) fibers	Long intervals (2-5 min), Fartlek, pace work, fast distance
Early season	Anaerobic capability and short-term energy and speed	Medium intervals (60-90 s), short intervals (30-60 s), sprints
Peak season	Maintain training gains and achieve peak performances	Reduce training volume, emphasize quality not quantity

*Fartlek—a medium-distance effort that consists of faster sections followed by slower ones for recovery.

ment of the race and the competition provided by others will elicit hormonal support to help ease the burden.

Anaerobic Threshold Training

To run, ski, swim, or cycle fast, you'll need well-trained fast twitch muscle fibers. Faster training (long intervals, pace training) will train fast oxidative glycolytic (FOG) fibers and raise the anaerobic (lactate) threshold, which defines the upper end of sustainable aerobic effort.

HEART RATE MONITORS

Athletes often use heart rate monitors (see figure 16.3) to make sure that they are training at the correct intensity. The best monitors are those that utilize the electrical signal from the heart (ECG). One popular version transmits the signal from the chest to a wrist monitor that displays the rate and stores heart rates for later analysis. If you decide to use a monitor, you will still need to listen to your body, to become familiar with respiratory and other signs of distress. Use the monitor to estimate your anaerobic threshold, then become aware of your breathing at that level of exertion. You'll need to be able to sense your effort when you get in a race.

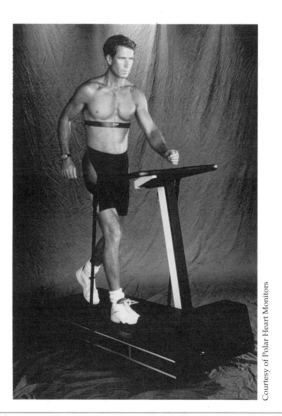

Courtesy of Polar Heart Monitors

Figure 16.3   Athletes use heart rate monitors to gauge the intensity of training.

Anaerobic Training

While aerobic energy sources are developed in long runs, in runs in which fast and slow running are alternated, and in long-interval training, anaerobic training occurs at higher intensities, when you exceed the anaerobic threshold. Since high-intensity effort is fatiguing, it is best to alternate short periods of intense exertion with periods of active rest in the technique called *interval training* (table 16.2). Allow a gradual anaerobic buildup, beginning with longer intervals and rest periods. Increase the pace and shorten the distances as training progresses. Always use active rest (walk or slow jog) to hasten the removal of lactic acid.

The interval training prescription includes the rate and distance of the work interval, the length of the rest period, and the total number of repetitions (e.g., run 6 × 400 meters, each in 75 seconds, with 2 minutes of active rest between run intervals). Rest intervals can be individually tailored by using the recovery heart rate. For example, the heart rate should return to 110 or 120 before attempting the next interval. Since interval runs are accomplished at a faster pace, they require a period of psychological adjustment. Some people never learn to enjoy this form of training; I find it more tolerable when shared with others of similar ability. Incidentally, swimmers often do their intervals in set time periods, such as 4 × 100 meters, each in 80 seconds. Swim fast and the rest is longer; swim slowly and there is little time for rest.

The interval training concept allows a great deal of adaptability to meet individual needs and abilities. It can be relatively mild (e.g., run 4 × 400 meters in 90 seconds) for the neophyte, and it can be made more interesting with a variety of distances (e.g., 200s, 300s, 400s, 600s) and paces. It can also be mind-numbing, like the program used by Buddy Edelen to prepare for the Tokyo Olympic Marathon. Buddy would run 25 × 440 yards to "break the monotony" of long-distance training. Roger Bannister trained until he could run 10 × 440 yards at 60 seconds to prepare for the first 4-minute mile. You, too, can use interval training to prepare for athletic competition. But use it and all intense training in moderation, never doing more than two to three intense workouts a week.

Diet and Performance

This section presents a few basic facts concerning diet and performance. One fact is that athletes use the same sources of energy and nutrients as the rest of us. Granted, they need more calories to fuel hard training, and may need addi-

TABLE 16.2   Interval Training Suggestions

Intervals	Train	Repetitions	Duration	Work/rest ratio*	Max speed (%)	Max heart rate (%)
Long	Anaerobic threshold	4-6	2-5 min	1:1	70-80	85-90
Medium	Glycogen pathway	8-12	60-90 s	1:2	80-90	95
Short	High energy	15-20	30-60 s	1:3	95	100
Sprint	Speed	25+	10-30 s	1:3	100	100

*1:1 means the rest lasts as long as the work interval. 1:3 means the rest is 3 times as long as the work interval.

tional nutrients, but those are usually supplied with an increase in nutritious foods (see chapter 11). Here are some ways to ensure adequate energy for performance.

Carbohydrate Loading

Years before it became popular, researchers had observed that best endurance performances occurred when athletes were on a high-carbohydrate diet, such as the performance diet discussed in chapter 11. That diet provides sufficient energy for continuous events lasting up to 1 hour. Carbo loading goes a step further, to raise muscle glycogen levels for high-intensity performances lasting more than 1 hour. Using a needle to get a sample of muscle tissue (muscle biopsy), researchers studied how performance depends on muscle glycogen levels and how glycogen levels depend on carbohydrate intake.

- **Events lasting 1 to 2 hours:** Use this scheme for events up to 2 hours in length. Four days before the event do a long, hard workout to deplete muscle glycogen stores. This activates an enzyme responsible for packing glycogen into muscle fibers. Next, raise your carbohydrate intake for the next few days by adding extra starches and sugar treats to the diet (fruit sugar, or fructose, doesn't work as well). Be sure to drink lots of water, since carbos are stored with water (hydrated). This scheme will double muscle glycogen stores so long as you reduce (taper) training before the event.

- **Events lasting more than 2 hours:** These events require even more glycogen, so start your depletion efforts 6 days before the event. Do the depletion workout, then another hard workout the next day to further deplete muscle glycogen stores, and keep carbohydrate intake down for those 2 days. Then return to the high-carbohydrate intake, with water and vitamins, and taper training efforts to allow maximum loading. This scheme has raised glycogen levels three to four times, enough to fuel an entire marathon.

Be aware that carbo loading takes place only in the muscles that you deplete with exercise. The glycogen can't be used easily by other muscles, so the effect is specific. Try the short scheme to see how it feels. Some people feel bloated and heavy when they carbo load, but best performances take place when muscle glycogen levels are highest.

- **Gender differences:** Women tend to use more fat and less carbohydrate than men during submaximal endurance events. This difference diminishes as training progresses (Ruby & Robergs, 1994). However, studies show that female endurance athletes do not increase muscle glycogen in response to a carbohydrate loading scheme (Tarnopolsky, Atkinson, Phillips, & MacDougall, 1995). For these reasons, women may decide not to practice carbohydrate loading. Women's preference for fat utilization is hormonally controlled.

Prerace, In-Race, and Postrace Feeding

Generally speaking you should eat the pre-competition meal that works for you. Eat 3 hours or longer before the event to ensure an empty stomach at race time. Emphasize carbohydrates, and avoid difficult-to-digest fats and excess protein. Especially nervous individuals may want to use a liquid meal before competition. I tolerate a peanut butter and honey sandwich before shorter events, and pancakes plus an egg (to slow entry of glucose) for long events, such as a 50-kilometer ski race.

- **Prerace:** Drink 1 to 2 cups of water in the 30 minutes preceding a race, but avoid a high-carbohydrate intake, such as an energy bar, which might raise insulin levels, lower blood glucose, cause hypoglycemia, reduce free fatty acid availability, and increase reliance on muscle glycogen.
- **In-race:** Drink a cup or more of water every 15 to 20 minutes. In longer events, drink water with 4 to 8% (40 to 80 grams per liter) carbohydrate every 15 to 20 minutes to maintain blood glucose levels. Cyclists and skiers are able to tolerate more carbohydrate in drinks or solid food (bananas, energy bars) during competition.
- **Postrace:** Immediately after the event, begin to consume carbohydrate (with some protein) to maximize the replacement of muscle glycogen (Zawadzki, Yaspelkis, & Ivy, 1992). The maximal rate of replacement occurs in the first 2 hours after the event. Select foods with a high glycemic index (see chapter 11, page 210) to maximize replacement of muscle glycogen. Drink lots of juices and water to ensure fluid replacement, but avoid caffeine and alcoholic beverages, which function as diuretics.

Blood Sugar

Low levels of blood sugar (hypoglycemia) certainly can adversely affect behavior and performance.

I have noted how endurance training improves the ability to mobilize and metabolize fat, thereby conserving blood sugar for use by the brain and nervous system. Low levels of blood sugar (hypoglycemia) certainly can adversely affect behavior and performance.

Nerve tissue is dependent on the blood sugar (glucose) as its source of energy. This means that the brain and nervous system require a constant supply of glucose. Blood glucose rises after a meal and then drops until it reaches a normal resting level (about 80 milligrams). Thereafter the liver strives to maintain that level, at least until its supply is depleted. The symptoms of low blood sugar (see table 16.3) indicate its influence on behavior and performance. I recall a day when my tennis game went to pieces. I lost my temper, cursed, threw my racquet, and became enraged. Then I realized that it was mid-afternoon, that I had missed lunch, and that breakfast had been consumed in the early morning. I apologized to my opponent and rushed off to find some nourishment.

TABLE 16.3   Common Symptoms of Hypoglycemia

Nervousness	Anxiety
Irritability	Confusion
Exhaustion	Rapid pulse
Faintness, dizziness	Muscle pains
Tremor, cold sweat	Indecisiveness
Depression	Lack of coordination
Vertigo	Lack of concentration
Drowsiness	Blurred vision
Headaches	

Blood sugar is used by muscles as an energy source; so, long runs, bike rides, or hikes can lead to hypoglycemia. High-energy snacks such as energy bars lead to a big boost of blood sugar, but they also call forth a large secretion of insulin. The insulin speeds the sugar out of the bloodstream, and within a couple of hours one begins to sag again (reactive hypoglycemia). To avoid the problem, simply eat at regular intervals and use snacks and carbohydrate drinks to maintain blood sugar levels.

Muscular Fitness Training

As sport becomes more competitive at every level it becomes necessary to invest more time in muscular fitness training. You should evaluate the muscular demands of your sport as well as your strengths and weak points. Then you can proceed to develop a program to improve the strength, muscular endurance, power, or speed you need to reach your goals.

- **Off-season:** This is the time for strength training. Select important muscle groups in the upper body, trunk, and legs and engage in a program following the prescriptions presented in chapter 10. Don't develop more strength than you need. When your strength is adequate for the sport, move on to the next phase of training.
- **Preseason:** By now you should be moving into power and/or endurance training. As the season approaches, make the exercises more sport-specific, more like the movements of the sport. Power is developed in 15 to 25 repetitions maximum (RM) sets done as fast as possible. Short-term (anaerobic) endurance is improved in sets of 15 to 25 RM also, so this phase of muscular fitness training can achieve two goals.
- **Early season:** From now on the emphasis is on speed and the maintenance of gains in strength, endurance, and power. Practice sport skills at high speed to become more comfortable with speed and to improve neuromuscular coordination. Once-a-week maintenance sessions will retain strength and power gains.

When I took up cross-country ski racing, I found that my upper body lacked the strength, power, and endurance to maintain vigorous poling throughout a race. So, I undertook an off-season strength program to build up the triceps, deltoids, lats, and abdominal muscles used in poling. I did the bench press, dips, and other general exercises for the triceps, along with the more ski-specific modified lat exercise. And I increased the attention usually afforded my abdominal muscles, using weighted sit-ups and the basket hang.

In the preseason I switched to more specific exercises, including the rollerboard for power and short-term endurance, and extended sessions on roller skis for long-term endurance. The early season included some power training with short sprints, using only poles for propulsion.

What did all this effort yield? Well, my technique and race times improved significantly, as did my enjoyment and understanding of the sport (Sharkey, 1984). Evaluate the muscular demands of your sport, and get started on a program. As you proceed to develop particular muscle groups, don't ignore flexibility, and don't forget to maintain balance by training

TABLE 16.4   Developing Your Muscular Fitness Program

1. Determine the muscular fitness requirements of the sport or activity.

2. Identify the major muscle groups and movements involved.

3. Select exercises to develop muscular fitness in upper body, trunk, and leg muscles.

4. Make adjustments for strengths and weaknesses.[a]

5. Establish training goals, set up a schedule, and get started. Remember to keep good records and to test progress every few weeks.

For more on training for sports see Sharkey 1986.

[a]Use fewer sets for strong areas, more for those in need of extra help.

opposite sides of the joint. Excessive attention to one group, such as the quadriceps group on the front of the thigh, could lead to imbalance and a greater risk of injury.

In table 16.4 you'll find a format you can use to develop a program for your sport. Figure 16.4 provides a worksheet for program development, and figure 16.5 illustrates a sample program.

The Psychology of Performance

Sport is a study in cooperation and competition. The quality of the overall experience depends on cooperation. Tennis opponents agree to cooperate by calling lines fairly, keeping track of the score, and observing the written and unwritten rules of the game. Fair, enjoyable competition is impossible without a high degree of cooperation. Top competitors often train together. They share training programs, new ideas, aches, pains, even dreams. Even during competition they cooperate, sharing equipment, encouragement, and the experience itself.

Psychologist Nathaniel Ehrlich (1971) draws a distinction between competitors and performers in athletic competition. *Competitors* evaluate their performances in athletic contests strictly on a relativistic, win-loss basis, with little regard given to the absolute level of performance. *Performers* attach only secondary importance to winning, evaluating performances against an absolute scale, an ideal.

The competitor subscribes to the Vince Lombardi dictum that says, "Winning isn't everything; it's the *only* thing." The performer, on the other hand, would give the nod to "It isn't whether you win or lose; it's how (and how well) you play the game." Ehrlich draws an analogy between competitors and performers and self-esteem and self-actualization, levels of motivation defined by Maslow (see chapter 19). The competitor seeks self-esteem, while the performer works to realize his or her potential. One would hope to find a more mature, self-actualizing approach to competition among adult athletes. Each would be seeking his or her potential, and competition would serve as a means to that end. Performers seek good competition because it helps them achieve their potential. Competitors fear good competition because it threatens their win-loss record, their self-esteem.

The competitor seeks self-esteem, while the performer works to realize his or her potential.

Muscular Fitness Program Planner

Sport _____   Position _____

Season _____   Goals _____

Individual strengths _____

Weak points _____

Body Part	Exercises	Muscle group	Purpose
Arm and shoulder	_____ _____ _____ _____ _____	_____ _____ _____ _____ _____	_____ _____ _____ _____ _____
Trunk			
Legs			
Other:			

Figure 16.4 Muscular fitness program planner.

Muscular Fitness Program Planner

Sport ___Basketball___   Position ___Forward___

Season ___Off-season___   Goals ___Strength and power___

Individual strengths ___Shooting___

Weak points ___Rebounding___

Body Part	Exercises	Muscle group	Purpose
Arm and shoulder	Lat pull-downs (with basketball)	Hands, arms, chest, and lats	Pull-down rebounds
	Bicep curl	Arm flexors	Rebounding
Trunk	Abdominal curl (machine)	Abdominals	Pull-down rebounds
	Back-ups	Lower back	Back strength
Legs	Leaper or power squats	Leg extension and jumping muscles	Sustained power for jumping
	Plyometrics (down jumping)	Leg extension and jumping muscles	Preload and jumping
	Hill (or stair) running	Leg extension and jumping muscles	Sustained power
	Rebounding and fast break drills		Sustained power and endurance in game situations

Note. When sufficient strength is acquired, shift to an endurance, power, or power-endurance program in the preseason (achieve power-endurance with 15-25 reps as fast as possible).

Figure 16.5 Sample muscular fitness program.

Common sense tell us that 100% of the time in a competition, someone loses. If you value your mental health, if you don't want to be frustrated by defeat and lose your self-esteem, become a performer. Competitors realize that someone will soon be able to defeat them. Their many hours of practice and competition ultimately will end in failure. Performers never fail. If their performance is flawed, they know that time and practice will bring them closer to their goal.

Try becoming a performer by focusing on the quality of the experience, not the final outcome. Don't get angry when you lose. Realize that you need good competition. Without it, you would soon lose interest in the sport. Analyze but don't judge your performance. Approach weaknesses positively (I need to get my racquet back earlier), not negatively (my forehand stinks). Set goals in terms of performance instead of wins, medals, or trophies. You may find that the wins and trophies come as performance improves. If not, you can still find satisfaction in the game, and you won't feel regret when it's over.

Playing the Game

Have you noticed that you do well on some days and poorly on others? Did you ever wish you could play your best game all of the time? Sport psychologists Tutko and Tosi (1976) offer suggestions to help you do just that and to improve your ability to deal with the emotional side of your game.

Play your best game more often:

- **Relax:** Contract then relax muscles and say, "let go" as you learn muscle relaxation (Jacobson's *Progressive Relaxation*, 1938). Concentrate on your breathing, and say, "easy" with each exhale (Benson's *Relaxation Response*,

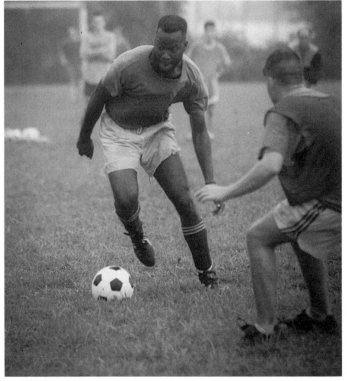

Use relaxation and concentration to help you play your best game more often.

1975). Eventually, the relaxation techniques can be used in competition to help relieve tension.

- **Concentrate:** Focus your attention on an object in the game (e.g., tennis ball) to free the mind of fears and negative judgments and to allow your best performance.
- **Mentally rehearse:** Rehearse mentally before and during practice and before competition to help focus on key elements of the game. Imagine yourself performing well.
- **Rehearse:** Use physical rehearsal to hone skills in days preceding competition, and as skill rehearsal just prior to the event.

You will notice that these sport psychologists neglected to include advice on how to "psych" yourself up for the game. Did they forget it? Of course not. The reason is that most of us fail because we are overly aroused. We are so "psyched up" and concerned, we are tied in knots, unable to execute the skills we worked so hard to perfect. If we think too much and try too hard, we are bound to fail. So Tutko and Tosi provide advice aimed at helping you to free your mind, to relax, to reach the state called *flow*. Then and only then can you produce your best performance. You'll find yourself saying, "I played over my head," "I was out of my mind," "I couldn't miss; everything I hit went in." Don't get me wrong; I'm not suggesting that you enter an event and then forget why you're there. On the contrary, you're there to play well and have fun; you should savor every moment.

MOOD STATES

The Profile of Mood States (POMS) has been used to study the effects of exercise and other therapies on mood, and to determine the effects of overtraining. The POMS test utilizes the responses to 65 words to yield mood scores. Subjects are asked to indicate to what degree they have been experiencing various feelings during the past week, including the day of the test.

Response options are 0—not at all, 1—a little, 2—moderately, 3—quite a bit, and 4—extremely.

Tense	0	1	2	3	4
Hopeless	0	1	2	3	4
Bitter	0	1	2	3	4
Lively	0	1	2	3	4
Worn out	0	1	2	3	4
Bewildered	0	1	2	3	4

Responses are categorized into six mood scores:

Tension/anxiety   Depression/dejection   Anger/hostility
Vigor/activity   Fatigue/inertia   Confusion/bewilderment

The classic iceberg profile depicts an athlete low in all scores except vigor. Overtraining lowers vigor while it raises all the other scales (Morgan et al., 1988).

The theory behind this approach is based on the different roles played by the right and left brains. The left brain is absorbed with details; it is analytical and judgmental, while the right brain is concerned with movements, patterns, and the overall picture. Once skills are learned, they should be performed without the critical review of the left brain. Relaxation and concentration allow us to play our best game more often.

Successful distance runners tend to *associate* during a race. They tune in to their bodies so they will know how fast they dare run. They are consciously aware of pace, position, key opponents, and features along the course. Less successful runners tend to *disassociate*, to lose track of time and place. Form becomes less efficient, and the pace lags.

Learn to handle your emotions, and you'll enjoy the game more. Eliminate the tensions, fears, and frustrations, and you may win more often. Become a performer, and you won't feel you've wasted a day just because you've lost. If you can do all these things and devote sufficient time to practice and training, you will be well on your way to achieving your potential. More important, the enjoyment and success you experience will keep you involved in a lifelong pursuit of excellence.

Performance Potential

I will conclude with some intriguing insights concerning performance limits, insights gleaned from an analysis of the assault on world records in running. Researchers studying the field published a fascinating account of the restraints on performance (Ryder, Carr, & Herget, 1976). Using running records from the previous 50 years, they plotted the rate of improvement and made some surprising conclusions.

On the average, the rate of improvements in distances ranging from 100 meters to 30 kilometers has been a steady but slow 0.75 meters per minute per year. Since record breakers seldom participate in further assaults on the record, they concluded that good runners just don't work as hard after they have set a record. In fact, they contend that running records are still well below human physiological limits, that the restraints on performance largely are physiological and pathological. The major obstacle is not the race but the amount of time devoted to daily training. In recent years, athletes have had to train several hours a day to achieve record-breaking status. Once the record is achieved, the runner is likely to turn attention to other, more mundane matters, such as earning a living, getting married, and having a family.

Thus, *time* is the obstacle, time and the injuries associated with overuse and overtraining. If you feel stymied in your training, if you are stuck on a plateau, invest more time, and progress will resume. Barring injury, you should be able to improve. Following this line of reasoning, progress in world's records will begin to slow when men and women have invested all the training time that is humanly possible. Thereafter, progress will depend on improved equipment and new techniques. For world-class athletes, training has become a full-time job. You and I cannot continue to invest more time in training, so we may define our potential as the level we attain following the maximum possible investment in time and effort.

Even given the limitations imposed by job and family as well as heredity, physique, gender, and age, you can still make dramatic progress toward your potential. Consider the case of petite Michiko Suwa from Japan. She came to the United States at the age of 28, met and married Mike Gorman, and changed her first name to Miki. Five years later she began jogging, and in 1973 at the age of 38 she ran her first marathon. Later that same year she astounded the running world with a woman's world record. Neither physique nor age predicted her potential. Or look at Priscella Welch, a two-pack-a-day smoker who quit smoking, started running, and went on to become a world-class competitor in the marathon. Or consider Sister Marion, a nun who started running in 1979. Within 5 years she qualified for the 1984 Olympic marathon trials at the age of 54!

Overtraining

Training, when overdone, can be a stressor that reduces resistance to infection.

Training, when overdone, can be a stressor that reduces resistance to infection. Yet, athletes at all levels seem prone to overtrain. We grew up believing the adage "no pain, no gain." The risks of overtraining are many, including illness, injury, and lost time.

Symptoms of overtraining include lethargy, fatigue, poor performance, sleep loss, loss of appetite, and illness. Because symptoms arise slowly, overtraining is difficult to diagnose. Contributors to overtraining include boredom, overwork relative to rest, immune suppression due to exhaustion and stress, hormonal imbalance, poor nutrition, and inadequate hydration. Scientists have studied the wake-up heart rate, temperature, body weight, white blood cell count, hormones (cortisol, testosterone), and mood states to identify early stages of overtraining.

The cortisol/testosterone ratio has been correlated with overtraining. Cortisol, a hormone from the adrenal gland, increases when the body is under stress. Testosterone is an anabolic (growth-stimulating) hormone that decreases with overtraining. The ratio is a sensitive but costly indicator of overtraining. If you undertake serious training, you should become familiar with some simple ways to detect overtraining and use them regularly (see table 16.5).

The treatment for overtraining is relative rest. More serious cases demand time off or bed rest, but most respond to reduced training, more time for recovery, attention to nutrition, and a change of pace. Remember that training should be approached as a gentle pastime. Make haste slowly, and you will eventually reach your goals. Overtrain, and you'll lower your resistance to infection.

WHAT TO DO ABOUT AN INFECTION?

What should you do with an upper-respiratory-tract infection? Dr. Randy Eichner recommends the "neck check." If symptoms are above the neck, such as a stuffy nose, sneezing, or a scratchy throat, try a "test drive" at half speed. If you feel better after 10 minutes you can increase the pace and finish the workout. If symptoms are below the neck, with aching muscles or coughing, or if you have a fever, nausea, or diarrhea, take the day off (Eichner, 1995). You can return to training when the fever is gone for at least 24 hours without the aid of aspirin or other anti-fever medications.

TABLE 16.5   Overtraining Indexes

Index	How it's used
Pulse index	Take the pulse rate daily (for 60 s), in the morning before rising. Average the daily rates. When the morning pulse is 5 or more beats above normal you should suspect illness or overtraining.
Weight index	Take the weight daily, in the morning (after toilet but before breakfast). Average daily weights. A rapid or persistent weight loss could indicate impending problems due to poor eating habits, failure to replace fluids, nervousness, or excessive fatigue.
Temperature index	Take the morning temperature daily for a week to establish the "normal." Then use it when the morning pulse is elevated. A fever usually indicates infection. Take a day off.
Fatigue index	Rate your tiredness after you arise.

Rate your tiredness after you arise.

Ready to drop	9
Extremely tired	8
Very tired	7
Slightly tired	6
About average	5
Somewhat fresh	4
Very fresh	3
Extremely fresh	2
Full of life	1

Other useful signs include boredom, weakness, pain in joints, color of urine (dark, concentrated, or cloudy), and skin color (pasty, pale).

Overuse Injuries

As athletes spend more time training, new injuries arise. Young women now experience weight loss, hormonal imbalance, and stress fractures with excessive training. Athletes in many sports develop a wide range of overuse injuries. This has created a demand for athletic trainers, physical therapists, and physicians knowledgable about sports medicine. Progress seldom comes without a cost, or an opportunity.

Cross-Training

The concept of cross-training gained notoriety as the triathlon attracted the attention of multisport athletes. It can be viewed as systematic variety, designed to avoid overuse injuries. It allows addicted athletes to train hard every day, with little risk of overuse or repetitive trauma (e.g., carpal tunnel syndrome) injuries. Some people extol the virtue of training a variety of muscle groups, as in swimming, cycling, and running. Triathletes train for all three disciplines, and they also do sport-specific weight training to enhance performance. Cross-

> **TRIATHLON TRAINING**
>
> I recommend that you train a discipline to a respectable level with at least four training sessions per week, then maintain that level with two to three sessions as you bring up the level of the next discipline. Eventually you'll be doing nine to ten sessions a week, requiring several two-a-day sessions. Serious triathletes may do three or even four training sessions several times a week, with some hard, some easy, some long, and some short. It takes a lot of time and energy to train for the triathlon. So, plan to put other pursuits on hold and to pay special attention to nutrition, hydration, and rest.

Cross-training does not raise performance above the level that can be attained in specific training.

training allows athletes and fitness enthusiasts the option to train more than they could in a single sport, and to achieve balance in their training.

But does cross-training provide special performance benefits? Probably not. Specificity is still the best rule to follow if you want to improve in a sport. Swimming will not improve performance in running or cycling, or vice versa. Cross-training does not raise performance above the level that can be attained in specific training. Activities that use similar muscles may contribute some to performance, but not to the same degree as increases in specific training (Foster, Hector, Welsh, et al., 1995). Of course, cross-training is an absolute necessity if you are preparing for a multiple-discipline event, and it is a great way to remain active and fit as you grow older!

Summary

In this chapter I've included a simple system for the development of a year-round training program. It provides for the systematic development of aerobic and anaerobic energy sources, and for muscular strength, endurance, and power. If you are ready for some **SERIOUS** training, consider the program recommended by Rob Sleamaker (1989). It summarizes this chapter in a single word.

The **SERIOUS** training program includes the following:

S	**peed**
E	**ndurance**
R	**ace or pace**
I	**ntervals**
O	**verdistance**
U	**p or vertical (e.g., hills) if applicable**
S	**trength**

If you are not that serious, forget speed and pace, but don't ignore variety in your training. Alternate hard with easy, short with long, speed with distance—and don't forget to include rest days for recovery. Outline a program, and get started. Keep simple records, and change the program when your goals change. As your interest grows, seek out books or magazines that focus on your activity. In time you will become an expert on training.

CHAPTER 17

The Environment and Performance

"No athlete is crowned but in the sweat of his brow."

St. Jerome

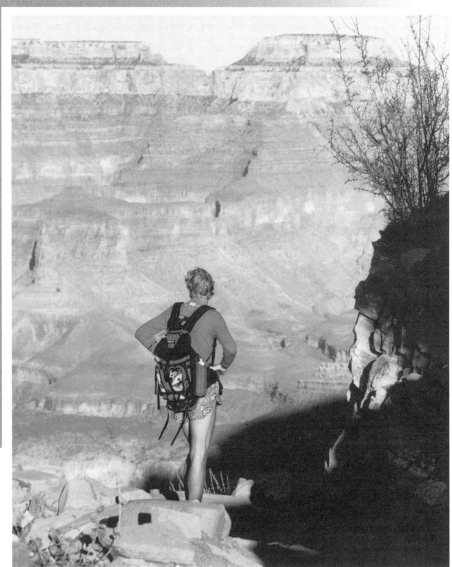

© Richard Echtberger

When I moved to Montana I fully expected to face a cold and sometimes hostile environment, and I looked forward to spending time at higher elevations. What I didn't expect was the potential for high temperatures in the summer months, and I certainly didn't expect the problem of air pollution, not in a state with only 800,000 residents spread out over 150,000 square miles of open space. Over the years I've learned some tricks for coping with and even enjoying environmental extremes.

Environmental factors such as heat and cold, humidity, altitude, and even air pollution can have profound effects on health and performance. Failure to consider these effects can lead to serious problems, even death. On the other hand, it is entirely possible to adjust or acclimate to the environment, enabling you to perform well and comfortably under a wide range of conditions. Let's consider the problems caused by extremes of temperature, humidity, altitude, and air pollution to see how fitness and proper planning can minimize their effects.

THIS CHAPTER WILL HELP YOU

■ anticipate the effects of the environment on performance,

■ take appropriate steps to minimize environmental effects, and

■ understand how fitness enhances your ability to acclimatize and perform in difficult environments.

Temperature Regulation

The body's temperature-regulating mechanism consists of four parts:

- A regulating center located in the hypothalamus, an area at the base of the brain that serves as a thermostat to maintain body temperature at or near 37 degrees Celsius (98.6 degrees Fahrenheit)
- Heat and cold receptors located in the skin to sense changes in environmental temperature conditions
- Regulators such as muscles that increase body heat by shivering
- Vasomotor (nervous system) controls that constrict or dilate arterioles to conserve or lose body heat

The thermostatic regulating center responds to the temperature of the blood flowing by the hypothalamus. If the blood cools, the thermostat sends information to conserve heat loss by constriction of blood vessels in the skin and the extremities. Some heat can also be generated by shivering.

If the blood temperature rises above the desired level (sometimes called a set point), the regulating center can cause dilation of cutaneous (skin) blood vessels and also stimulate the production of sweat. Consequently, blood is brought from the warmer core of the body to the surface, allowing heat loss by conduction (heat transfer via direct contact), convection (heat transfer via movement of a gas or liquid), and radiation, as well as by evaporation of sweat from the surface of the skin. Complete *evaporation* of 1 liter of sweat leads to a heat loss of 540 calories. However, if the sweat *drips* off the body, little heat is lost.

Heat and cold *receptors* in the skin also aid in the maintenance of body temperature. The cold of the ski slopes will cause constriction of blood vessels,

Complete evaporation of 1 liter of sweat leads to a heat loss of 540 calories. However, if the sweat drips off the body, little heat is lost.

especially in the hands and feet. The extremities will stay cold until you elevate the body temperature, warm the blood, and reopen the blood vessels. This can best be done by vigorous exercise. Of course, you can put on more clothing or seek relief in the lodge.

The stifling heat of the tennis court will cause *vasodilation* that diverts a significant amount of blood from the muscles to the surface of the skin. The heart rate increases in an effort to maintain blood flow to the working muscles and the skin. Sweating will eventually reduce blood volume, and unless the water is replaced, your performance will suffer. If you persist in the activity and fail to replace the water loss, you may end up with heat exhaustion or heatstroke. So, you are wise to listen to your body's call for rest, shade, and fluid replacement.

Individual differences in body fat, number of sweat glands, fitness level, and possibly gender may influence your response to heat.

• **Body fat:** Body fat serves as a layer of insulation beneath the surface of the skin. People with more subcutaneous fat may be better insulated from the cold than others, but are they less able to lose excess heat to the environment? Probably not, since the body learns to route blood around the fat for cooling purposes. Excess fat is a handicap in that energy is required just to carry it around.

• **Sweat glands:** Each of us inherits a certain number and pattern of sweat glands. Since evaporative heat loss is the best protection against heat stress, a good supply of active sweat glands is important. Like almost everything else, sweat glands respond to use. If you use them a lot, they become more efficient.

• **Physical fitness:** Fitness seems to enhance the ability to regulate body temperature during work in the heat. It does so by lowering the temperature (set point) at which sweating begins. Thus, fit individuals can work or play with lower heart rates and core temperatures than those of their unfit counterparts. Acclimatization further lowers the point at which sweating begins; therefore, the physically fit and heat-acclimated individual is even better prepared than an unfit or unacclimatized individual for work in the heat (Nadel, 1977). And recent evidence indicates that fitness hastens the process of acclimatization.

• **Gender:** Men produce more sweat than women for a given increase in body temperature, perhaps too much. Women are efficient sweaters; production is more suited to the heat load, so they don't waste water. When men and women are compared on the same task, men seem better able to work in the heat; however, the difference is due to fitness, not gender. When the fitness level is the same or when the workload is equated (e.g., a given percentage of maximal oxygen intake), women seem quite able to work in the heat. In several recent marathons, the women seemed to tolerate the heat as well as or better than many men, probably because they are more efficient sweaters.

Exercising in the Heat

When exercise begins, the temperature-regulating center increases the body's usual set point, and the body temperature is allowed to increase. The rise in temperature depends on the intensity of the exercise. In a moderate environment, the temperature will increase about 1 degree Celsius at 50% of the maximal oxygen intake, and will rise to about 39 degrees Celsius at the maximal level (above 102 degrees Fahrenheit; see table 17.1). This resetting of the core temperature during exercise can be viewed as an adjustment favorable to the enzyme activity within the muscles. It also serves to reduce the problem of heat dissipation. Under moderate environmental conditions, the methods of heat dissipation are not employed until the elevated set point has been reached.

TABLE 17.1   Conversion of Fahrenheit (F) to Celsius (C)

°F	°C
−40	−40
0	−18
32	0
50	10
72	22
85	30
98.6*	37
212	100

*Normal body temperature.

In hot environments, we are able to maintain temporary thermal balance during exercise by virtue of circulatory adjustments and the evaporation of sweat. In a hot, dry environment the body actually gains heat when the air temperature exceeds the temperature of the skin. Under these conditions, the evaporation of sweat allows the maintenance of thermal equilibrium. However, when the humidity also is high and evaporation cannot take place, the body temperature continues to rise, and performance is severely impaired. Blood is diverted from muscles to the skin, blood volume is reduced via sweating, and water and electrolytes are lost in the sweat. Stroke volume declines, heart rate increases, and lactic acid accumulates. Blood may even begin to pool in the large veins, further reducing venous return and cardiac output. This hyperthermia, an alarming rise in body temperature, sets the stage for heat stress and even heatstroke, the potentially fatal collapse of the temperature-regulating mechanism.

Sweating

In a normal day, we lose and must replace about 2.5 liters of water (1 liter equals 1.057 quarts; 1 quart equals 0.946 liters). Of this water loss, about 0.7 liter comes from the lungs and skin (insensible water loss), 1.5 liters from the urine, 0.2 liter from the feces, and about 0.1 liter through perspiration. During heavy exercise in the heat, the water lost through sweating can exceed 2 liters *per hour*. Sweat production may amount to as much as 12 liters per day. Since work capacity becomes impaired as water loss progresses, it is essential that the fluid be replaced. Dehydration in excess of 3 to 5% of body weight leads to a marked decline in work capacity, strength, and endurance. Estimate 1 liter for each 2 pounds of weight loss; therefore, if you weighed 150 pounds and lost 8 pounds, or more than 5%, you would be about 4 liters low on fluid!

> ### THIRST
>
> The thirst mechanism always underestimates fluid loss during work in the heat, and after the work is over. Therefore, it is advisable to take frequent small drinks throughout the work period. If you drink 250 milliliters (about 1 cup) every 15 minutes, you can replace 1 liter per hour. If the sweat rate is higher, it is extremely difficult to keep up with fluid needs. Marathon runners are wise to drink as much as possible (up to 500 milliliters) before the event to offset the tremendous water loss and difficulty of replacement. If during prolonged periods of work in the heat (i.e., several days), weight loss exceeds 2% prior to the next day's effort (e.g., 3 pounds for a 150-pound individual), the individual should be rehydrated before returning to work or exercise.

The thirst mechanism always underestimates fluid loss during work in the heat, and after the work is over.

Sweating rates and evaporative cooling depend on adequate rehydration. Hyperhydration, or excess water intake, allows you to sweat more and work with a lower rectal temperature and heart rate, enabling increased work performance in hot industrial or sporting environments. Recent studies indicate that glycerol contributes to fluid retention during exercise (Montner, Zou, Robergs, et al., 1995). If subsequent studies support this contention, you'll soon see sport drinks containing glycerol.

Electrolytes

Water replacement will not compensate for the loss of electrolytes (sodium, chloride, and potassium) in the sweat. For each liter of sweat lost, approximately 1.5 grams of salt are lost as well. Since the average meal includes 3 to 4 grams of salt, three meals per day will satisfy most salt needs. For long periods of work in the heat (8 hours or more), when considerable water and salt will be lost, workers and athletes are encouraged to salt food liberally (8 hours at 1.5 grams of salt per liter equals 12 grams of salt loss). Salt *tablets* are not recommended for several reasons: They are slow to dissolve and leave the stomach, so they will not provide aid for hours, and while they are dissolving they take needed water from the bloodstream via osmosis. Also, excessive salt intake can cause stomach cramps, weakness, high blood pressure, and other problems.

You have several choices for the replacement of water and salt. Solutions containing the necessary electrolytes as well as some glucose can be obtained commercially (carbohydrate/electrolyte beverages), but remember that you may have to replace several quarts of fluid. That could become expensive. You can save money by using the salt shaker at mealtime, drinking citrus fruit drinks for potassium, and obtaining the balance of fluid needs with water. Or you can prepare your own solution by adding a bit of salt to each quart of half-strength frozen lemonade. Another approach is to replace some of your fluid needs with tomato juice and the rest with water. When long periods of work in the heat make it absolutely necessary to replace electrolytes, use commercially available carbohydrate/electrolyte (C/E) beverages; or add one-fourth teaspoon of salt to each quart of water, and be sure to replace potassium during mealtime with citrus fruits or drinks, bananas, or other potassium-rich foods.

DO YOU NEED A SPORTS DRINK?

Carbohydrate/electrolyte drinks offer several advantages. Their palatability ensures greater fluid intake, they help maintain blood glucose levels and performance during prolonged exertion, and they reduce fluid loss via the urine. Avoid excess glucose (more than 8%) in fluid replacement solutions during running in the heat; the glucose could retard emptying of the stomach and reduce delivery of essential fluid (Costill, Saltin, Soderberg, & Jansson, 1973). In marathon or other long-duration races, runners should drink cool (40-degree Fahrenheit) electrolyte solutions that are relatively low in glucose (less than 40 to 80 grams per liter, or 4 to 8%). Cyclists and cross-country skiers can tolerate higher glucose concentrations during exercise, especially in cool temperatures. Recently developed glucose polymer solutions provide replacement fluid with three times more energy in the form of clumps (polymers) of glucose molecules. Thus, it is possible to provide more energy while replacing essential fluid.

Drink 2 to 3 cups before the event. During the event take a cup or more of fluid every 15 to 20 minutes. After exercise, continue to replace fluids, electrolytes, and energy. You may want to use commercially available carbohydrate/electrolyte drinks to ensure rehydration and to begin replacement of muscle glycogen. Ensure adequate intake of carbohydrates high on the glycemic index (e.g., sugar, honey, white bread) in the first 2 hours after exercise, a critical period for glycogen replacement. Foods with a moderate rating on the glycemic index (e.g., pasta, whole-grain bread, rice) are good choices to continue replacement of muscle glycogen.

Heat Stress

When the body is at rest, metabolic heat production amounts to about 1.2 calories per minute, or 72 calories per hour. Moderate exercise can elevate heat production to 600 calories or more per hour. You can see that exercise, by itself, can create considerable heat. Normally, the heat is lost by convection, radiation, or evaporation of sweat, but when exercise is performed in a hot environment or when the humidity is high, metabolic heat cannot be dissipated, and the body temperature rises.

- **Heat cramps** occur when considerable salt is lost in the sweat. Take lightly salted fluids and use massage to relieve the cramp.
- **Heat exhaustion** occurs when the heat stress exceeds the capacity of the temperature-regulating mechanism. An individual with cold, pale skin, a weak pulse, and dizziness should be given fluids and allowed to rest in a cool environment.
- **Heatstroke** means that the temperature-regulating mechanism has given up. The skin is flushed, hot, and dry; sweating stops; and the body temperature may rise above 106 degrees Fahrenheit. Heatstroke can lead to permanent damage, especially to the temperature-regulating center of the brain, and can even cause death. *Heatstroke is a medical emergency.*

As you may have guessed, heat stress cannot be predicted on the basis of air temperature alone. Relative humidity is an important factor that determines how effective sweating will be. If the sweat cannot evaporate, if it merely drips from the body, little heat is lost, and the water loss only adds to a circulatory problem. Air movement and radiant heat also are important factors to consider in evaluating the effect of a given environment on human comfort and performance. Even the type and color of clothing have an effect on heat loss. Finally, the metabolic heat production due to physical activity must be considered, since it is the major heat source.

The wet bulb globe temperature (WBGT) provides a simple and accurate indication of the effect of environmental factors on active human beings. The index uses dry and wet bulb thermometers to assess air temperature and relative humidity (see table 17.2). The black copper globe thermometer indicates radiant heat as well as air movement. The several temperatures are weighted to indicate their relative contribution to the total heat stress. As indicated in table 17.2, the wet bulb, or relative humidity, is the greatest contributor to heat stress (70% of total).

TABLE 17.2   WBGT Heat Stress Index

	WBGT heat stress index	Example
Wet bulb	= _____ °F × .7 = _____	80 × .7 = 56
Dry bulb	= _____ °F × .1 = _____	90 × .1 = 9
Black globe	= _____ °F × .2 = _____	120 × .2 = 24
WBGT	= _____ °F	WBGT = 89°F

Where: The wet bulb indicates humidity, the dry bulb measures the ambient temperature, and the black copper globe measures radiant heat and air movement.

Standards for Work or Exercise
  Above 80°—utilize discretion
  Above 85°—avoid strenuous activity
  Above 88°—cease physical activity[a]

[a] Trained individuals who have been acclimated to the heat are allowed to continue limited activity.

Reprinted from Sharkey 1974.

The U.S. Marine Corps uses the WBGT to determine when physical training activities should be reduced or canceled, and many high school and college athletic trainers and coaches use it to determine when practice sessions or distance runs should be scheduled. Bear in mind that the WBGT does not allow an estimate of the effect of clothing or energy expenditure. Dark or nonporous clothing can increase radiant heating or reduce evaporation. High levels of energy expenditure can create internal heat problems in rather moderate environments. No simple index tells you everything about heat stress, but for moderate energy expenditures, up to 425 calories per hour, while you are wearing sensible clothing, the WBGT is an excellent indicator of heat stress.

Another approach is to use the heat stress chart (figure 17.1). This chart is based on the shaded air temperature, moderate radiant heat from the sun, a light breeze, and a moderate work rate. Unfit or non-acclimated individuals will suffer at lower levels of heat, humidity, or work.

Heat Stress Chart

When heat and hard work combine to drive the body temperature up, the temperature-regulating mechanism begins to fail and the worker faces serious heat stress disorders. This dangerous—often deadly—combination of circumstances can be avoided by monitoring the environment with simple measurements of temperature and humidity. This chart can help alert individuals to dangerous heat stress conditions.

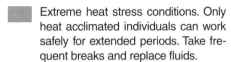 Extreme heat stress conditions. Only heat acclimated individuals can work safely for extended periods. Take frequent breaks and replace fluids.

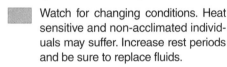 Watch for changing conditions. Heat sensitive and non-acclimated individuals may suffer. Increase rest periods and be sure to replace fluids.

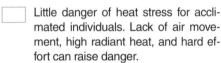 Little danger of heat stress for acclimated individuals. Lack of air movement, high radiant heat, and hard effort can raise danger.

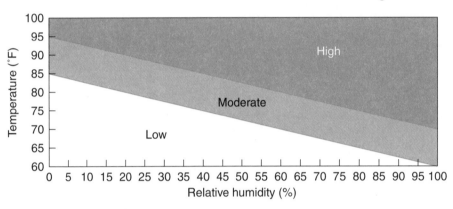

Figure 17.1 Heat stress chart.
Adapted from Sharkey 1979.

Heat Acclimatization

Heat acclimatization occurs after 4 to 8 days of work in a hot environment.

On the first day of vigorous exercise in a hot environment, you may experience a near-maximal heart rate, elevated skin and core temperatures, and severe fatigue. But after just a few days of similar exposure to work in the heat, the same task can be accomplished with a reduced heart rate, made possible by improved blood distribution and increased blood volume. Skin and core temperatures are lower, since sweating begins at a lower temperature (Wenger, 1988). The loss of water in the urine diminishes, and the salt concentration of the sweat gradually is reduced. This increase in circulatory and cooling efficiency is called heat acclimatization, and most of the process occurs after 4 to 8 days of work in a hot environment (increases in sweat rate may take longer).

Highly fit individuals become acclimatized in 4 days, while sedentary subjects take twice as long. The best way to acclimatize is to work in the actual conditions (temperature and humidity) you'll have to endure. However, if you live in a cool climate and don't have a heat chamber in which to achieve acclimatization, high-intensity training can get you halfway there, probably because of the heat generated during vigorous effort. It helps to use a (non-rubberized) sweat suit to increase the temperature close to the skin. Fit individuals start to sweat at a lower body temperature, and they increase sweat production at a faster rate. Acclimatization helps move the set point for sweating even lower.

Less fit individuals should acclimatize using periods of light-to-moderate activity in a hot environment, alternated with rest periods in which fluid is replaced. Electrolytes can be replaced with commercial drinks or the saltshaker at meals, plus potassium-rich citrus fruits or bananas. The vitamin C in the citrus drinks may hasten the acclimatization process.

In summary, the prescription for exercise in a hot, humid environment includes the following advice:

- Wear sensible, porous, light-colored, loose-fitting clothing.
- Acclimatize to the expected environment and workload (i.e., do 50% the first day, 60% the second, and add 10% each day until you do 100% on the 6th day).
- Take 250 to 500 milligrams a day of vitamin C or citrus fruits since Vitamin C may enhance acclimatization.
- Always replace water and electrolytes.
- Find a cool place for rest periods.
- Don't be too proud to quit when you feel the symptoms of heat stress (dizziness, confusion, cramps, nausea, clammy skin).
- Keep a record of body weight during prolonged periods of work or training in the heat. Weigh in before and after exercise to gauge fluid loss. To check for day-to-day rehydration, weigh yourself in the morning, after toilet but before breakfast.
- Maintain aerobic fitness: The enhanced circulatory system and blood volume will help you work better in the heat, acclimate faster, and hold your acclimatization longer.

Exercising in the Cold

Excessive fatigue is the first step toward hypothermia and possible death.

Because of the metabolic heat generated during exercise, cold temperatures do not pose a threat similar to that posed by hot, humid conditions. But severe exposure to low temperatures and high winds can lead to frostbite, freezing, hypothermia, and even death. Constriction of blood vessels (vasoconstriction) increases the insulating capacity of the skin, but it also results in a marked reduction in the temperature of the extremities. It's almost as if the body is willing to lose a few fingers or toes to save the more important parts. Protective vasoconstriction often leads to severe discomfort in the fingers and toes. To relieve the pain, it is necessary to warm the affected area or raise the core temperature to allow reflexive return of blood to the extremities. While shivering may cause some increase in temperature, gross muscular activity is far more effective in restoring heat to the troubled area. Since large muscle activity takes considerable energy, the cold weather enthusiast must maintain a reserve of energy for use in emergencies. Excessive fatigue is the first step toward hypothermia and possible death.

Windchill

The windchill describes the effect of wind speed on heat loss (see figure 17.2). A 10-degree Fahrenheit reading is equivalent to minus 25 degrees Fahrenheit when the wind speed is 20 miles per hour. Runners, skiers, and skaters can create their own windchill. Skiing at 20 miles per hour on a 10-degree Fahrenheit day is equivalent to minus 25 degrees. And if the skier is moving into a wind, the effect is even worse. When possible, run, ski, or skate away from the wind. If you must face into the wind on a cold day, be sure to cover exposed flesh, including earlobes and nose, and be on the lookout for frostbite.

	Actual thermometer reading (°F)											
	50	40	30	20	10	0	−10	−20	−30	−40	−50	−60
Wind speed (mph)	Equivalent temperature (°F)											
Calm	50	40	30	20	10	0	−10	−20	−30	−40	−50	−60
5	48	37	27	16	6	−5	−15	−26	−36	−47	−57	−68
10	40	28	16	4	−9	−21	−33	−46	−58	−70	−83	−95
15	36	22	9	−5	−18	−36	−45	−58	−72	−85	−99	−112
20	32	18	4	−10	−25	−39	−53	−67	−82	−96	−110	−124
25	30	16	0	−15	−29	−44	−59	−74	−88	−104	−118	−133
30	28	13	−2	−18	−33	−48	−63	−79	−94	−109	−125	−140
35	27	11	−4	−20	−35	−49	−67	−82	−98	−113	−129	−145
40	26	10	−6	−21	−37	−53	−69	−85	−100	−116	−132	−148

Little Danger (for properly clothed person)
Increasing Danger
Great Danger
Danger from freezing of exposed flesh

Figure 17.2   Wind chill index.

Note: Wind speeds greater than 40 mph have little additional effect.
Reprinted from Sharkey 1974.

Frostbite

Frostbite is damage to the skin resulting from exposure to extreme cold or wind-chill. As you can see on the windchill index, there is little danger of frostbite at temperatures above 20 degrees Fahrenheit. A temperature or windchill of minus 20 degrees Fahrenheit seems necessary to produce the condition.

At first, frostbite appears as a patch of pale or white skin, due to the constriction of blood vessels in the area. After mild frostbite, the skin appears red and swollen when the blood returns. In severe frostbite, the skin may appear purple or black after it is warmed. Immersion in warm water will hasten the return of blood to the area (hot water may scald the skin). Do not massage the affected part since that could lead to rupture of blood vessels. Protect the groin and other sensitive areas to avoid the excruciating pain that occurs when circulation returns. And if your feet become frostbitten on a winter outing, keep your boots on and walk or ski out before rewarming. Frostbitten feet swell when the boots come off and the feet are warmed. If you're worried about freezing the delicate tissues of the lungs during cold weather exercise, don't be. Cold air may make your breathing uncomfortable because it is so dry, but there is little danger of damage to the tissue. The respiratory system has a remarkable ability to warm and humidify air. Humans tolerate air temperatures well below 0 degrees Fahrenheit without damage. The cold air is warmed to above freezing before it reaches the bronchi. However, when the temperature dips below minus 20, you are advised to modify or curtail your exercise plans. The danger to earlobes, nose, fingers, and toes is great, and at much lower temperatures respiratory tract damage is possible, though unlikely. Very cold air will constrict airways and make vigorous effort difficult.

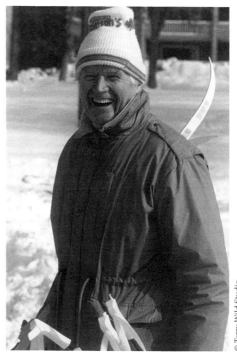

© Terry Wild Studio

Don't allow cold temperatures to limit your activity.

Hypothermia

When your body begins to lose heat faster than it can be produced, you are undergoing exposure. Prolonged exertion leads to progressive muscular fatigue. Shivering and vasoconstriction are attempts to preserve body heat and the temperature of vital organs. Exhaustion of energy stores and neuromuscular impairment lead to the virtual termination of activity. As exposure continues and additional body heat is lost, the cold reaches the brain; you lose judgment and the ability to reason. Your speech becomes slow and slurred, you lose control of your hands, walking becomes clumsy, and you want to lie down and rest. Don't do it! You have hypothermia. Your core temperature is dropping, and without treatment you will lose consciousness and die.

You may be surprised to learn that most hypothermia cases occur in air temperatures above 30 degrees Fahrenheit. Cold water, windchill, and fatigue combine to set the stage for hypothermia. Avoid the problem by staying dry. If you become wet, dry off as soon as possible. Be aware of the windchill and how wind refrigerates wet clothing. During a cold-weather hike or ski tour, take off layers of clothing before you perspire, and put them back on as you begin to cool. Eat and rest often to maintain your energy level. Make camp while you still have energy; don't wait until it's critical.

If someone exhibits the symptoms of hypothermia, transport the victim to a medical facility as quickly as possible. The heart may begin to fibrillate during rewarming, and emergency equipment will be needed. If immediate transport isn't possible, or if the case isn't severe:

- Get the victim out of the wind and rain.
- Remove all wet clothing.
- Provide dry clothing, warm drinks, and a warm, dry sleeping bag for a mildly impaired victim.

Most hypothermia cases occur in air temperatures above 30 degrees Fahrenheit.

- If the victim is only semiconscious, try to keep the person awake, leave him or her stripped, and put the victim in a sleeping bag with another person.
- Build a fire to warm the camp.

Cold Weather Clothing

For extended periods of outdoor exertion when you'll be away from protective shelter and central heating, dress in layers. Layers of clothing provide an insulating barrier of air and can be peeled off as your temperature rises and put back on as it falls. Wool is one of the best fabrics to wear for under and outer garments. It doesn't have the insulating value of dry down, but it is far better than down when wet.

Physiologists rate the insulating value of clothing in "Clo" units, with one Clo unit being equivalent to the dress that will maintain comfort at a room temperature of 70 degrees Fahrenheit (roughly equivalent to cotton shirt and slacks). Table 17.3 and figure 17.3 illustrate how the insulating requirements change during vigorous activity such as cross-country skiing or hiking (heavy work), light work, and rest. That is precisely why it is necessary to dress in layers in cold weather. At a temperature of 0 degrees Fahrenheit, a light shirt will be adequate during vigorous effort, while you may need 2 inches of insulation to maintain comfort at rest, and more for a good night's sleep.

TABLE 17.3   Comfort Data

Effective temperature °F	Thickness of insulation required for comfort (in.)		
	Sleeping	Light work	Heavy work
40	1.5	0.8	.20
20	2.0	1.0	.27
0	2.5	1.3	.35
−20	3.0	1.6	.40
−40	3.5	1.9	.48

These figures are approximate but are a good base for an average healthy person.

Since perspiration is a major problem during exercise in the cold, you would be smart to purchase a set of synthetic (polypropylene) undergarments. This amazing fabric wicks perspiration away from the skin so evaporative cooling won't strip heat from the body. Next comes a wool or fleece layer for warmth. A windproof and rainproof slicker should be all the additional clothing you need during exercise. Invest in a "breathable" slicker if you can afford one, but don't expect any garment to handle the tremendous moisture load created during vigorous skiing or running. A down or pile coat can be carried in your pack for use at lunch or in camp. Modern, light, synthetic fabrics have several advantages over goose down: They are less expensive, are easier to care for, and don't mat and lose insulating qualities when wet.

Of course you'll also need a hat and gloves. I'm a hot exerciser, so I like to wear a polypropylene ear band that allows heat loss from the top of the head. When I stop, I put on a pile or wool hat to retain body heat. The same goes with

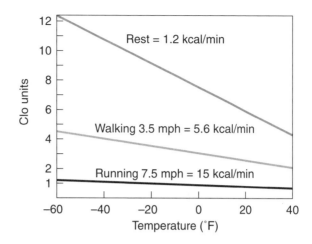

Figure 17.3 Clothing requirements at different energy expenditures in the cold.

gloves: Wear lighter ones during vigorous exercise, but be ready to put on warm mitts for extended breaks. With the right clothing you can enjoy outdoor activity in all but the most severe conditions.

Cold Acclimatization

Are we able to adjust to the cold as we are able to acclimatize to hot environments? If so, what are the physiological mechanisms involved? Specific examples of cold acclimatization do appear in the research literature (Folk, 1974). One mechanism is a metabolic adjustment wherein metabolism is increased as much as 35%. The female divers (Ama) of the Korean Peninsula evidence this adjustment, as well as improved tissue insulation during the winter months when the water temperature falls to 50 degrees Fahrenheit. Australian aborigines are able to sleep in cold conditions via a hypothermic response, a lowering of the core temperature from 98.6 to a more easily maintained 95 degrees. Of course, natural selection and heredity play important roles in the adaptation to cold environments, and a large body mass, short extremities, increased levels of body fat, and a deep routing of venous circulation also help.

It seems that repeated cold exposures can lead to physiological and psychological adjustments that allow one to tolerate and enjoy physical activity in cold environments (Young, 1988). The near-freezing temperatures that seem so bitter in November are perceived as balmy in February. The extra calories I consume in the fall and winter lead to extra weight and an increase in the insulating layer of subcutaneous fat. That's my excuse!

> It seems that repeated cold exposures can lead to physiological and psychological adjustments that allow one to tolerate and enjoy physical activity in cold environments.

Exercising at High Altitude

More than 40 million people live at altitudes above 10,000 feet (3,040 meters; 1 foot equals 0.304 meter), and some live above 17,000 feet. However, no permanent habitations are found above 18,000 feet, indicating that such an elevation may be incompatible with adaptation and long-term survival. Elevations below 5,000 feet have little noticeable effect on otherwise healthy individuals. But as you ascend to higher elevations to ski, hike, climb, or even to live, barometric pressure declines along with available levels of atmospheric and alveolar oxygen (PO_2). When this occurs, the arterial blood is unable to become highly saturated, less oxygen is transported, and the tissues are forced to operate with a reduced supply (see table 17.4). Thus, in spite of the heroic efforts of the oxygen intake and transport systems, altitude always leads to a reduction in aerobic fitness and associated endurance performances.

In this age of rapid transit, it doesn't take long to ascend to a national park or ski resort located above 5,000 feet. When you arrive, your cardiovascular system has to make adjustments. The heart rate is higher, but the stroke volume, the volume of blood pumped with each beat of the heart, may be lower because of a diminished oxygen supply to the heart muscle. More air is brought into the lungs each minute, and this hyperventilation leads to increased carbon dioxide exhalation and the acid-base disturbances associated with mountain sickness. The symptoms—headache, shortness of breath, rapid heartbeat, loss of appetite—appear at 8,000 feet or above. Needless to say, work capacity declines at altitude, as does the motivation to perform hard work.

Does a high level of physical fitness provide some advantage upon arriving at high altitude? On arrival, the conditioned individual maintains his or her sea-level advantage over the unfit, but no more. The trained individual will be able to do less than he or she could at sea level and is just as likely to suffer mountain sickness. At very high elevations, some highly trained endurance athletes have been found to be "nonresponders" whose respiration fails to adjust adequately to the added demands of the altitude (Jackson & Sharkey, 1988).

Acclimatization to Altitude

Profound changes occur soon after one moves to a higher elevation. Pulmonary ventilation is increased, so more air can be moved into the lungs. This increase doesn't take more energy, since the air is less dense at higher elevations. Oxygen transport is gradually enhanced by increases in red blood cells, hemoglobin, and blood volume. Above 15,000 feet the red cells increase from 5 million per cubic millimeter to 6.6 million, while hemoglobin rises from 15 grams per 100 milliliters to above 20. This makes the blood more viscous, but that isn't a problem, since the hypoxia (lower oxygen tension) of altitude serves to vasodilate, or relax, the arterioles. Altitude

TABLE 17.4   Altitude and Oxygen

Altitude (ft)	Barometric pressure (mmHg)	PO_2 in air (mmHg)	PO_2 alveoli (mmHg)	Arterial O_2 saturation (%)	Aerobic fitness (% of sea level)
0	760	159	105	97	100
3,200	680	142	94	96	
6,500	600	125	78	94	90
10,000	523	111	62	90	
14,100	450	94	51	86	75
18,400	380	75	42	80	
23,000	305	64	31	63	50
29,141	230	48	19	30	

exposure also may cause an increase in lung and muscle capillaries; myoglobin, the molecule that serves to store oxygen in muscles, also is increased at higher elevations (Smith & Sharkey, 1984).

It takes about 3 weeks to make a good adjustment to a higher elevation, or about 1 week for each 1,000 feet above 5,000 feet. Once you have acclimated, your oxygen intake and transport systems will be better able to supply oxygen to the working muscles. These adjustments reduce but never eliminate the effect of altitude on aerobic fitness; endurance performances always will be reduced at altitude, regardless of your state of acclimatization. And unfortunately, these hard-earned changes (they occur only when you work at altitude) are reversible; they return to prealtitude values within weeks after you leave the mountains.

Altitude Training

Because of the reduced oxygen intake ability above 5,000 feet, your standard pace will be more anaerobic than usual. You will have several options: Do your usual distance but more slowly, go at your usual pace but for shorter distances, or (my favorite) slow down and enjoy the view. Go sight-seeing, and forget about distance or pace. If you are training to compete at altitude, you should realize that the slower pace may cause your speed to slip a little. Occasional shorter but faster runs should help avoid that problem (athletes sometimes drop to lower elevations for speed work).

For years, coaches and athletes have sought the ultimate training stimulus at moderate altitude (5,000 to 10,000 feet). They believe that reduced availability of oxygen to muscles (hypoxia) is the stimulus that causes changes in aerobic fitness, and that exercise at moderate altitude ensures extreme tissue hypoxia. So, they travel to a training site at 6,000 to 9,000 feet and train for several weeks or months before returning to sea level for a major event such as the Olympic Games. Unfortunately, it may not be worth the effort for all athletes. One study produced a small benefit from altitude training on return to sea level; however, no control group was used in that study. When the study was repeated with a control group, the altitude training was no more effective than equally arduous sea-level training. The subjects were highly trained middle-distance runners, 17 to 23 years old, who trained at sea level, or 7,500 feet, for 3 weeks (Adams, Bernauer, Dill, & Bomar, 1975). It appears that arduous effort at sea level also leads to tissue hypoxia.

Casual observers of the sport scene always will be quick to conclude that a certain athlete's performance is due to his or her residence at high altitude. Several outstanding African athletes have emerged to perpetuate the practice of altitude training. Of course, the athletes do live above 7,000 feet; however, what many people forget is that they were *born* there and lived most of their lives there as well. Their parents were born there and their parents' parents. So, the benefit they seek really is a product of natural selection and long-term residence at a higher elevation, not just a few weeks of altitude training.

The benefits of altitude acclimatization do not seem to help all athletes equally. If they did, if altitude were the only secret to success, all our great distance athletes would reside at higher elevations, and that certainly is not the case. Studies show that about one-third of athletes profit from altitude training. Athletes with low hemoglobin levels may profit from altitude training, but others do no better, and some do worse, perhaps because altitude training is more stressful, or because their already high hemoglobin is raised, making the blood more viscous and difficult to pump at sea level (Smith & Sharkey, 1984).

Air Pollution and Physical Activity

Should you check the local air pollution index before you can safely go outside to exercise? In some cities children's recess and sporting events are canceled when pollution rises. If you fly over any major city in this country, you'll see the pall of pollution that daily diminishes the quality of our lives. While it is true that some forms of pollution are most dangerous for old or weak individuals, young children, and people with respiratory problems, other forms attack physically active, healthy individuals. Exercise increases the volume of air taken into the lungs each minute. Since pollution-related respiratory disorders often are related to the degree of exposure, it seems wise to avoid exercise in polluted atmospheres.

On one warm, humid fall afternoon thousands of cars circled the suburban communities outside New York City. A haze created by the action of sunlight on the hydrocarbon emissions hung heavily in the air. As the players of a suburban New Jersey football team practiced, some began to complain of troubled breathing, chest pains, tightness, nausea, and vomiting. The scene was repeated at other area schools where young, healthy athletes engaged in vigorous physical activity were learning firsthand about the growing problem of air pollution. Adults also were affected as they attempted to mow lawns or work in gardens. The urban East was experiencing the choking pall that forces Los Angeles schoolchildren to cancel games or remain indoors for recess when the photochemical smog is particularly bad.

There are many sources of air pollution, and we are beginning to recognize them as threats to the quality of life and to life itself. Efforts are under way to lower carbon monoxide, dust and soot (respirable particulate), sulfur dioxide, and other pollutants. Some pollutants are relatively harmless by themselves, but in combination with others they are capable of exerting potent biological effects.

The biological effects of air pollution include

- irritation of airways and deadening of ciliary action (by gases and particulate),
- suppresion of the immune system and increased risk of upper respiratory infection,
- loss of diffusing surfaces (e.g., alveolar breakdown in emphysema, pulmonary fibrosis),
- reduction in oxygen-transport capacity (carbon monoxide competes for space on hemoglobin molecule),
- heart disease, and
- lung and other cancers.

In the United States, cigarette smoking is responsible for 400,000 deaths annually.

While many forms of industrial, urban, and automotive pollution are nauseating, troublesome, or even fatal, no single source of pollution is as deadly as the cigarette, which causes all of the biological effects listed above. It can irritate the bronchial tubes; deaden ciliary action and make the smoker more susceptible to infection, chronic bronchitis, and emphysema; reduce oxygen transport; and cause lung cancer and heart disease. In the United States, cigarette smoking is responsible for 400,000 deaths annually.

Carbon Monoxide

Carbon monoxide (CO) is a colorless, odorless gas that results from incomplete combustion. The smoldering cigarette produces high levels of CO, so much that the average smoker is likely to have 5 to 10% of the space on the blood's oxygen-carrying hemoglobin occupied with carbon monoxide (carboxyhemoglobin) (see table 17.5). Carboxyhemoglobin (COHb) occurs when CO unites with hemoglobin, a union that takes precedence over the union of oxygen and hemoglobin. If CO is in the air you breathe, it will find its way into your blood. The level of carboxyhemoglobin depends on its concentration in the air, the duration of exposure, and your air intake, which goes up with vigorous activity. Eventually, blood levels reach an equilibrium with the breathing mixture (about 5% carboxyhemoglobin after 8 hours exposure to 35 parts per million CO; see figure 17.4 and table 17.6). While it takes time to reach equilibrium, it takes almost as long to flush the deadly gas from your system (when exposure stops, COHb levels drop about 50% every 3 hours). Avoid exercising along busy roadways where CO levels are high.

TABLE 17.5   Levels of COHb Produced by Cigarettes

Cigarettes/day	COHb %
10-15	5
15-25	6.3
30-40	9.3

TABLE 17.6   Effects of Carboxyhemoglobin (COHb)

COHb%	Effect
1.0	No apparent effect
1 to 2	Some effect on behavioral performance
2 to 5	Central nervous system effects: Impairment of time interval discrimination, Visual discrimination (sharpness/brightness), Psychomotor function (coordination)
5 to 10	Cardiac and pulmonary function changes
10 to 50	Headaches, fatigue, drowsiness, nausea, dizziness
50 to 60	Intermittent convulsions
70 to 80	Coma, cardiovascular failure, and death

Symptoms may be present at levels below or above those indicated. Nonsmokers may experience headaches and nausea at levels well below 10% COHb.

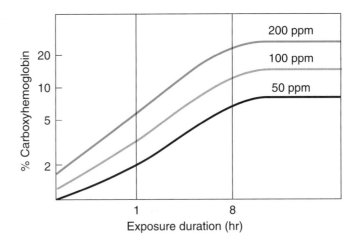

Figure 17.4 Carbon monoxide (ppm) and COHb.
Reprinted from USDA Forest Service. 1991. *Health Hazards of Smoke* 2:2.

The effects of carbon monoxide are additive to those of altitude. If aerobic fitness is down 10% at 6,500 feet, you can lose another 5 to 10% by smoking. While the smoker gets the worst part of the deal, a nearby nonsmoker also is subjected to high levels of CO in so-called secondhand smoke, especially in a crowded or poorly ventilated room or automobile. One study measured levels as high as 166 parts per million inside an automobile with closed windows. It wouldn't be long before the nonsmoker felt symptoms of distress, headache, and nausea. The smoker, on the other hand, has become less sensitive and wouldn't be bothered. Assert your right to an unpolluted atmosphere, and support the public health goal of making the country smoke-free by the year 2000! Tell your friends, "If you must smoke, please do not exhale."

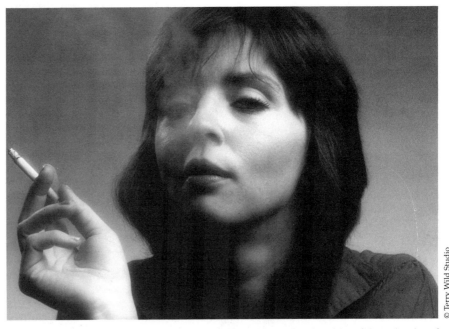

Secondhand smoke kills thousands and impairs the health of hundreds of thousands of young children.

In addition to bronchitis, emphysema, and cancer, the nicotine, carbon monoxide, and other toxic compounds in cigarette smoke combine to dramatically increase the risk of heart disease. Women should never smoke while pregnant, and since secondhand or environmental tobacco smoke causes asthma and other breathing problems for children, parents should never smoke in the house or in the car. Smoking contributes to accidents and illness, and smoking costs business and industry billions of dollars in additional health, cleaning, and other costs.

Respirable Particulate

The soot that clogs the air above major cities contains a range of particles. Large particles become trapped in the upper-respiratory tract. The human respiratory system has a remarkable ability to cleanse itself via the action of the ciliary escalator, which sweeps particles upward so they can be expectorated. When the particulate load is great or sustained, as in smoking or urban pollution, the ciliary mechanism can break down.

Some particles are small enough to find their way deep into the lung. These respirable particles are rendered more dangerous because of carcinogenic compounds that sometimes attach to the particles. A study of six American cities has shown mortality rates to be strongly associated with fine particulate pollution (< 2.5 micrometer). These products of combustion—coming from industry, the automobile, and residential wood burning—penetrate indoors to foul the air we breathe. While air pollution was positively associated with death from lung cancer and cardiopulmonary disease, mortality rates were most strongly associated with cigarette smoking (Dockery, Pope, Xu, et al., 1993).

Many other pollutants are known to irritate respiratory passages, cause bronchitis, allergies, and asthma, contribute to heart and chronic obstructive lung disease, and cause lung and other cancers. Ozone, formaldehyde, asbestos, sulfur dioxide, nitrous oxides, and other by-products from internal combustion engines are a few of the hundreds of compounds considered toxic to humans. Avoid exercise in obviously dangerous areas (along expressways, near industrial pollution) and when air pollution warnings are in effect. That doesn't mean you shouldn't exercise; just find a way to avoid the pollution (exercise indoors, where or when levels are low). We must continue the fight for clean air so our activities need not be regulated in accordance with the air pollution index, and our enjoyment of physical activity need not be compromised by human mistreatment of the environment. Add your voice to the growing fight against all forms of pollution, including the worst of all, the cigarette.

Summary

In this chapter I've outlined the problems encountered in different environments and provided practical advice on how to minimize the problems and maximize performance and enjoyment. Solutions range from improving fitness and acclimatization to dressing properly and maintaining hydration and energy. Fitness, while especially important in the heat, improves performance in all environments. Acclimatization is necessary for heat and altitude, and useful in the cold. Fluid replacement is critical in the heat, but it is also extremely important in the cold and at altitude, where considerable fluid is lost during breathing. Maintenance of energy levels is essential to prolonged performance in any environment. Finally, proper clothing is essential to cope with the demands of the environment.

But what of air pollution? What can be done to minimize its effects? The answers are simple: Minimize exposure, and maintain your immune system with regular exercise, rest, and good nutrition. Include immune-friendly foods in your diet and use antioxidant supplements to counter the free radicals found in pollutants. Minimize exposure by exercising where or when pollution levels are lowest. If you are particularly sensitive to pollutants or allergens, you may want to utilize a dust mask to filter particles, or a mask impregnated with activated charcoal to absorb pollutants.

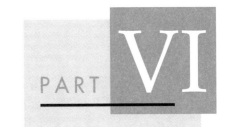

Vitality and Longevity

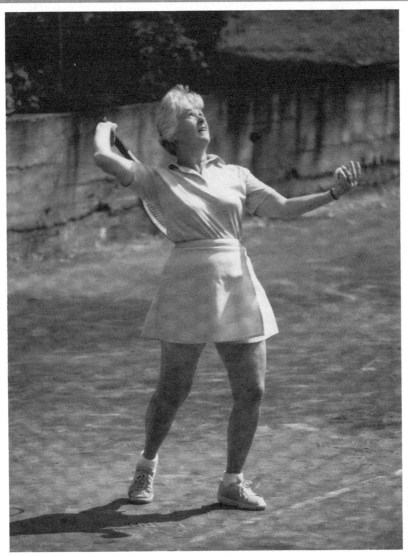

The prevailing scenario of aging is a dreary one, depicting a life of limits and ailments, a vicious cycle with loss of function, frailty, and failure. Fortunately, you do not have to accept this tragic opera as your script. If you are willing to adopt the appropriate lifestyle, you will be able to take command of your role, to write and perform an epic that features a long and satisfying life.

The final chapters of this book are designed to help you develop the daily habits, psychosocial skills, and other behaviors that contribute to a happy, healthy, and vigorous life. Daily habits are an indispensable part of your lifestyle, and the appropriate lifestyle contributes to health and the quality of life. Psychosocial skills are necessary for a full and complete life. Chapter 19 provides ways to utilize psychology to help motivate and maintain your commitment to regular moderate physical activity.

The goal is to be vigorous and fully involved throughout life, to live each stage to the fullest. In return for your efforts you will retain the vitality and mobility needed for a full independent life, and you may even live longer. But the most compelling outcome of the active life is that you'll add life to your years, not just years to your life. Stated simply, you'll extend the prime of life.

CHAPTER 18

Age, Activity, and Vitality

"The daily habits of people have a great deal more to do with what makes them sick and when they die than all the influences of medicine."

Lester Breslow, M.D.

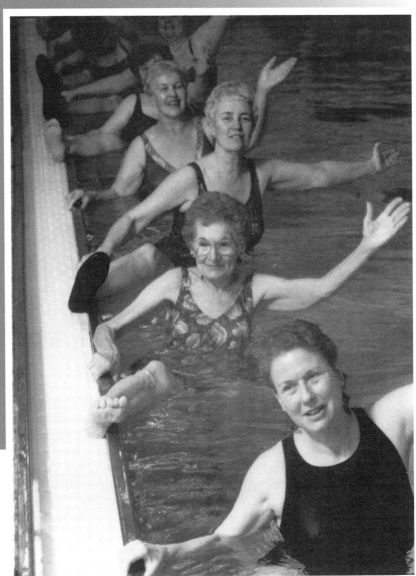

© Terry Wild Studio

Age tells little about your health, your appearance, your fitness, or your ability to perform. While aging inevitably leads to death, it does so at different rates for different people, depending on heredity and on personal decisions about how you choose to age.

Sometime after the peak reproductive years, when the direct evolutionary advantage has passed, virtually all tissues and organs begin to age, and their biological importance begins to wane. Parents remain important at least until the child becomes a young adult, and grandparents may serve to pass on wisdom, or to assist the parents. But when one reaches the 70s there is little survival value for the species in continued life, and indeed life expectancies range from 78 to 79 for women and 73 to 74 for men. But life expectancies, which have risen throughout my lifetime, tell only part of the story.

THIS CHAPTER WILL HELP YOU

- differentiate life expectancy from life span,
- understand how activity and other habits influence longevity,
- see how fitness influences your physiological age, and
- understand how activity and fitness extend the prime of life.

Life Span

People who choose not to age rapidly can reduce morbidity and extend the vigorous years by living an active, healthy life.

Life expectancy has gone up in proportion to declines in infant mortality and infectious diseases. But the attainable life span, the age attainable in a life free of serious accident or illness, has not changed noticeably in the past 200 years. In other words, we are not living longer; we are avoiding premature death. Survival curves point to a theoretically attainable life span of about 85 years, with a standard deviation of 4 years (figure 18.1). Thus, 68% of the population have the potential to live between 81 to 89 years (85 plus or minus 4 years), and 95% of deaths from natural causes would fall between 77 and 93 years (85 plus or minus 2 standard deviations, or 8 years). Rare indeed are the individuals who live more than 3 standard deviations above the mean. The oldest currently living human is a remarkable French woman who just celebrated her 120th birthday.

Postponement of chronic illness has extended the period of adult vigor, so life remains physically, emotionally, and intellectually vigorous until shortly before its close (figure 18.2). Many of the factors believed to be associated with age can be modified, including heart and lung function, bone density, blood pressure, and cholesterol. People who choose not to age rapidly can reduce morbidity and extend the vigorous years by living an active, healthy life (Fries & Crapo, 1981). On the other hand, those who decide to age rapidly are destined to become a burden on family, health care, and community support systems.

Earlier I quoted studies that indicate an increase in longevity for those who lead the active life. Activity adds life to your years as well as years to your life! Unfortunately, some have said, the years you add all come at the end. And it

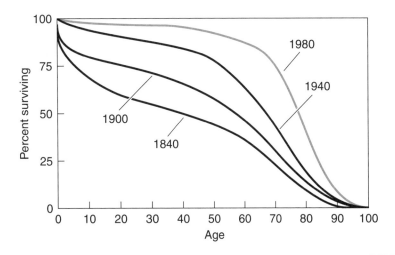

Figure 18.1 Survival curves. With less infant mortality and trauma (accidental death), more people survive to the attainable life expectancy, 85 years. With good health habits, more are able to postpone chronic debilitating illness, to remain vigorous until the last years or months of life.

Adapted from *Vital Statistics of the United States*, 1977 (Vol. 2, Section 5). DHEW Publication PHS 80-1104, National Center for Health Statistics.

has been suggested that the years you add are about equal to the time spent in exercise. Can that be true? One study found at least a 2-year increase in life expectancy associated with activity. If you exercise 1 hour every day for 40 years, you'll spend 14,560 hours engaged in exercise. Divide that number by 24 hours per day, and you get 607 days, or 1.67 years, somewhat less than the 2 years or more you'll earn. Of course you will enjoy the time you spend in exercise, recreation, and sport, and you will extend the years of fun and function, the prime of life.

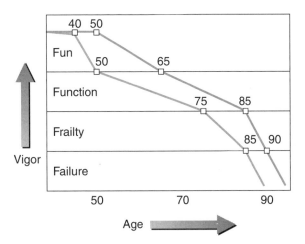

Figure 18.2 Vigor and the active life. Active living extends the periods of fun and function and shortens the time of frailty and failure.

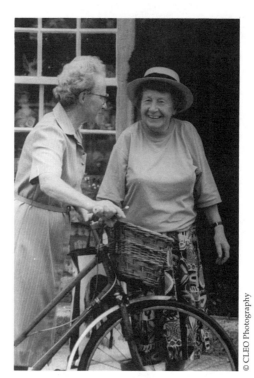

© CLEO Photography

Exercise will extend the prime of life.

Aging

Theories of aging are many, including those dealing with gene defects or chromosomal damage, errors in protein synthesis, and limits to the number of cell divisions (the Hayflick limit). Other factors associated with aging include caloric intake and specific nutrients.

• **Caloric restriction:**   Animal studies have shown that eating fewer calories (up to 40% less) can extend survival time dramatically (28% in one study) when adult animals were put on a low-protein diet. Some researchers have felt that the most important factors determining life span are those that influence body fatness. Animals fed fewer calories also had a lower tumor incidence and less chronic disease (Comfort, 1979). When Alexander Leaf studied healthy old people in three remote parts of the world he found their diets low in calories and fat (1973). Leaf believed that the low-calorie diet, combined with regular activity and a productive and respected role in society, contributed to good health and long life.

• **Free radicals:**   One theory of aging holds that so-called free radicals (reactive molecules with one or more unpaired electrons) prove toxic to vulnerable tissues. In the biologic world, life span is inversely related to metabolic rate. Exercise produces free radicals that could harm the body. But moderate activity enhances antioxidant protection and the immune system. Chronic heavy exertion may produce an excess of free radicals, raise the risk of heart disease, and depress the immune response (Demopolus, Santomier, Seligman, Pietrogro, & Hogan, 1986). The role of free radicals in exercise and aging requires more study. In the meantime, vitamins C and E and beta-carotene are believed to provide some protection against these potentially toxic by-products of oxidative metabolism.

At present, no single theory explains the decline that occurs with age. What is surprising is the realization that the rate of decline or senescence is not fixed but variable, subject to considerable modification. What has emerged is a list of modifiable aspects of aging, markers that are subject to changes brought about by one's personal decisions and behaviors (table 18.1).

A definite pattern emerges from a consideration of the modifiable aspects of aging, a pattern that points to the importance of daily habits as the way to improve your health span, your active life expectancy.

Health Habits

Since 1962, researchers at the Human Population Laboratory of the California Department of Health have studied the relationship of health to various behaviors or habits. Health and longevity are associated with the following:

- Adequate sleep (7 to 8 hours per day)
- A good breakfast
- Regular meals—avoid snacks
- Weight control
- Not smoking cigarettes
- Moderate alcohol consumption
- Regular exercise

TABLE 18.1   Modifiable and Non-Modifiable Aspects of Aging

Aging Marker	Personal Decision/Behavior
Modifiable Aspects	
Cardiac output	Exercise
Glucose tolerance	Exercise, diet, weight control
Osteoporosis	Weight-bearing exercise, diet
Pulmonary function	Exercise, nonsmoking
Blood pressure	Exercise, diet, weight control
Endurance and strength	Exercise
Reaction time	Training, practice
Cholesterol	Diet, weight control, exercise
Arterial wall rigidity	Diet, exercise
Intelligence and memory	Training, practice
Skin aging	Avoid sun
Non-Modifiable Aspects	
Elasticity of skin	Avoid sun, nonsmoking
Graying, thinning of hair	
Kidney reserve	
Cataracts	

From: *Vitality and Aging* by Fries and Crapo. Copyright 1981 by W.H. Freeman and Company. Used with permission.

The study found that men could add 11 years to their lives and women 7 years, just by following six of the rules (Breslow & Enstrom, 1980). Let's examine each practice to see if it fits your current lifestyle. Then you can decide if changes are in order.

Sleep

When men or women sleep 6 hours or less per night they are not as healthy as when they sleep 7 or 8 hours. Those who sleep 9 hours or more are slightly below average in health. Thus, 7 to 8 hours of sleep is most favorable, and as you might expect, too little sleep is more of a problem than too much.

Sleep is characterized by alternating stages. One stage involves rapid eye movements (REM) and changes in heart rate, blood pressure, and muscle tone. This stage may serve as a rest period for the inhibitory nerve cells of the brain. It usually is accompanied by dreams, and if it is interrupted we become anxious and irritable. This REM sleep constitutes about 20% of the night's total, while deeper or quieter periods provide the rest necessary for recovery from fatigue. If you miss some sleep one night, the body will not make any serious attempt to recover the sleep deprivation. However, if a substantial amount of the loss is REM sleep, more REM sleep will occur on subsequent nights (figure 18.3). Going without sleep seems to impair creative capabilities, which suggests that another function of sleep is to restore a cerebral cortex fatigued by consciousness.

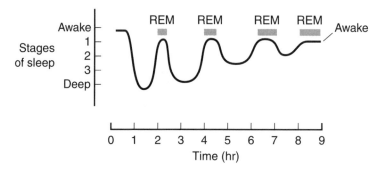

Figure 18.3   The stages of sleep.

Moderate physical activity seems to enhance the ability to fall into deep sleep without altering the time spent in REM sleep. Too little or too much exercise appears to result in sleep disturbance, and significant sleep loss seems to suppress the immune system.

Breakfast

In the California study, individuals who ate breakfast almost every day experienced better health than those who ate breakfast only some of the time (Breslow & Enstrom, 1980). Furthermore, a good breakfast may be a prerequisite to good performance in work and sport. Breakfast often comes 12 hours after the evening meal, so you can see why it is important for energy and cellular metabolism. A few researchers suggest that breakfast should be the largest and most important meal, and everyone agrees that it should include more than a cup of coffee and a donut.

Regular Meals

Erratic eaters have poorer health than those who eat regular meals. Those who seldom or never eat between meals have better health than those who eat between meals regularly. Unfortunately, this study did not include for comparison the health status of those who eat smaller but more numerous meals, but it does indicate the effects of erratic eating behavior and snacking. We can only guess at the content of the between-meal snacks, but chances are that they were junk foods high in simple sugars and saturated fat and low in nutrients.

Weight Control

When weight is more than 20% above or more than 10% below the desirable weight, health status declines. For example, if your desirable weight is listed as 150 pounds, your health status is most favorable when you maintain your weight between 135 (minus 10%) and 180 (plus 20%), a broad margin of error indeed. It would be interesting to compare the effects on health of low body weight (more than 10% below desirable) due to malnutrition, illness, or smoking, and low weight due to habitual vigorous exercise. Personal observations indicate that having a low body weight associated with vigorous exercise and good nutrition is at least as healthy as being at or above the desirable weight.

Smoking

Smoking, especially cigarette smoking, is dangerous to your health. If you don't smoke, don't start. If you do, stop. It could be the best thing you ever did for yourself. And if you can't stop for your own health, think of loved ones, especially children, who are exposed to your habit. Secondhand tobacco smoke is responsible for asthma and respiratory problems for many thousands of children, not to mention lung cancers. Is quitting worth the trouble? Data from numerous studies show that quitting has many benefits, including better oxygen-carrying capacity, lower blood pressure, improved night vision, and increased effectiveness of prescription drugs. And while some diseases, such as emphysema, cannot be reversed, others seem to repair with time. Repair time for smoking-induced illnesses include 10 years for heart disease and 10 to 15 years for cancer. Quit today, and help make the nation smoke-free by the year 2000.

Alcohol

Some studies show that those who drink one or two alcoholic drinks daily have a lower risk of heart disease, perhaps because alcohol is associated with higher levels of HDL cholesterol.

Poor health is associated with heavy alcohol consumption (five or more drinks at one sitting). Those who never drink and those who drink moderately (one to two drinks a day for men, one to three per *week* for women) enjoy the same level of good health. The French Paradox ponders why the French seem to tolerate rich foods without an increase in heart disease risk. The answer may lie in the regular consumption of wine. Some studies show that those who drink one or two alcoholic drinks daily have a lower risk of heart disease, perhaps because alcohol is associated with higher levels of HDL cholesterol (Gaziano, Buring, Breslow, et al., 1993). This should not be construed as a broad endorsement of alcohol consumption. Some level of alcohol consumption, if continued for a sufficient period, may lead to degenerative effects on the liver, even when nutrition is adequate. The best advice is to drink moderately, or don't drink at all. And don't save your drinks for a weekend binge, because the liver can only handle so much at a time.

Regular Activity

Researchers in the California study compared the health benefits of five types of activity: active sports, swimming or long walks, garden work, physical exercises, and hunting and fishing. Only hunting and fishing (seasonal and infrequent) were *not* associated with improved health. For all the others, those who participated most often experienced the best physical health. The best health was associated with active sports, followed by swimming or walking, physical exercise, and gardening. Lowest death rates were recorded for people who were often active in sports, while the highest rates were for those who chose not to engage in any exercise.

In summary, physical health, longevity, and the rate of aging are associated with your daily health habits and your lifestyle. These habits have more to do with your health and longevity than all the influences of medicine. The California study indicated that a man of 55 years who follows all seven health habits has the same health status as a person 25 to 30 years younger who follows fewer than two. Moreover, the researchers found a positive relationship between physical and mental health. You know that an association or relationship between variables does not imply cause and effect, that good physical health doesn't necessarily cause good mental health, but you are probably familiar with psychosomatic illnesses and should realize that the opposite effects are possible. A healthy body is an important aid to good mental health, and you can help maintain physical health by following the recommended health habits.

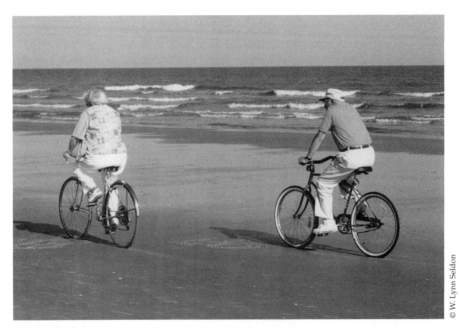

© W. Lynn Seldon

Those who age successfully engage in daily routines that require activity.

Longevity

One key to longevity, to what it takes to live well beyond normal life expectancy, is your lifestyle. Observations of healthy older individuals (aged 75 years and over) provide intriguing insights into the personality traits and living habits associated with long-term survival.

The following characteristics are associated with longevity:

- **Moderation:**   Moderation is a common denominator in all phases of life, including diet, vices, work, and physical activity. Long-term survival in a footrace or the human race depends on pacing.
- **Flexibility:**   Psychological flexibility implies the ability to bend but not break, to accept change, to avoid rigid habits.
- **Challenge:**   Accept challenges. Create them if necessary; don't allow life to become too easy. But when a challenge becomes too great, say so and seek an alternative.
- **Health habits:**   Long-term survival is characterized by a relaxed attitude toward health. Elderly "survivors" are rather unconcerned about their health. They eat a wide variety of foods, do not seek out organic or other fad foods, and are not terribly concerned about avoiding items such as cholesterol. They are moderate in their use of alcohol, and some even smoke now and then.
- **Relationships:**   Seasoned citizens enjoy other people; they maintain an interest in and continuous contact with friends and family. They enjoy their marriages.
- **Outlook:**   Healthy elders maintain a positive outlook. They recognize the effects of advancing age and *plan* to enjoy each phase of life. They realize that long life means growing old, and they are prepared to enjoy them both.
- **Active life:**   Of course, those who age successfully are engaged in daily routines that require activity. They find reasons to be socially and physically active. Involvement in daily chores provides the purpose, rhythm, and activity everyone needs.

The active life can benefit you in a number of ways, including:

- **Health:**   Both physical and mental health are enhanced with regular activity.
- **Mobility:**   Regular aerobic activity, supplemented with resistance exercises, retains or restores mobility and the capacity for a free and independent life.
- **Economy:**   Walk, jog, or ride a bike, and save money. Cross-country skis are cheaper than a snowmobile and better for you.
- **Ecology:**   The active life, with emphasis on human (muscle) powered sport and recreation, helps conserve limited energy supplies. Physically active individuals have less impact on the environment than their sedentary counterparts who use energy-consuming recreational vehicles.
- **Adaptability:**   The active individual retains the ability to adapt to changes in the economy or the environment.
- **Survival:**   Seniors are survivors. Along the way they accumulate wisdom and insights that have value to coming generations. The axiom in nature applies to the human race as well: The *fittest* survive.

Active individuals view each moment as one to be lived. They avoid people who depress them; when they feel moody or depressed they *do* something. They take risks, engage in life, and enjoy it; they don't waste the present with moods, worry, or immobilizing thoughts about the future. Depression, worry, guilt, and anger can lead to (or be caused by) subtle changes in brain chemistry and hormone levels. Physical activity can have a direct effect on the moods and the chemistry of behavior; it can also divert the attention and provide enjoyment and a sense of self-satisfaction that minimizes or eliminates self-defeating behavior.

You are free to think, feel, and act as you choose. You are not bound by circumstances, biorhythms, behavior traits, or deep-seated psychological problems. You can create the life you desire, if you really want to. Don't fall back on excuses like: "I haven't got the time," "I'll start next week (month, year)," or "I'm too busy right now, but when the kids are a little older . . ."

Age and Performance

As I've said, chronological age is a poor predictor of health or performance. Health is a function of health habits, heredity, environment, and previous illness. Performance in work or sport is a function of the physiological age.

Physiological Age

The physiological (biological or functional) age is a composite of health, physiological capacity, and performance measures. The best single measure of physiological age is probably the aerobic fitness score. It tells you about the health and capacity of the respiratory, circulatory, and muscular systems. Moreover, a considerable body of evidence shows an inverse relationship between aerobic fitness and a number of risk factors. Thus, it is possible at age 60 to have the health and performance capabilities of the average 30-year-old. This fact has considerable relevance when it comes to changing our society's view of aging and its consequences, such as age discrimination in hiring. Age does not connote a rapid decline in performance, and when physical performance is important, the physiological age is a more accurate predictor of performance potential than chronological age (Sharkey, 1987).

Other indicators of physiological age include your family history; health habits; and measures such as blood pressure, cholesterol, strength, reaction time, vision, hearing; and other variables.

Chronological age is a poor predictor of health or performance.

Aerobic Fitness and Age

Long-term (longitudinal) studies show that aerobic fitness declines at the rate of 8 to 10% per decade. However, when moderately active individuals are studied, the rate of decline is 4 to 5%, and when trained individuals are investigated the rate of decline is 2% or less (figure 18.4). When body weight and fat gains are avoided, the rate of decline in fitness is minimized. Dr. Paul Davis has shown that a significant portion of the decline in fitness and performance associated with age can be accounted for by increasing body fat (Davis & Starck, 1980).

The beneficial effects of a weight- and fat-control program on fitness, performance, and health are clear. The quality of life depends on the ability to pursue a variety of activities. Negative factors that affect this capacity for activity, such as excess body fat, should receive attention before irreversible physiological deterioration occurs. Excess fat restricts exercise capacity, causing a decline in fitness, which further reduces activity, resulting in additional fat accumulation—a vicious circle indeed. A reduction in body fat allows and promotes a more active life, and minimizes the decrease in fitness and performance previously blamed on increasing age.

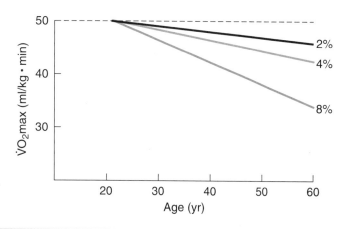

Figure 18.4 Decline in fitness with age.

Strength and Age

Strength declines rather slowly with age until the fifth decade, when the rate of decline increases. Those who use their strength regularly, such as auto mechanics, retain strength even longer. Some weight lifters have achieved personal bests in their 40s. And recent evidence suggests that even very elderly men and women (average age 87 years) can counter muscle weakness and frailty with resistance training. Activities of daily living including gait velocity, stair climbing power, and spontaneous physical activity all improved in the training group. And muscle mass increased, in contrast to a decline for the control group (Fiatarone et al., 1994).

Summary

We're all concerned that we save and invest well enough during our working years to ensure financial security in retirement. But fiscal fitness is only part of the story. In order to ensure a vigorous and independent retirement, you need to invest in physical fitness as well. In personal finance, the sooner you start to invest the better, in order to enjoy the fruits of compound interest. The same is true with fitness: Maximum gains are achieved with an early start. The best time to begin the active life is when you are young; the second best time to start is now.

In many ways, the active life and fitness represent money in the bank, by reducing future medical costs, minimizing the need for long-term care, and eliminating future burdens on family, friends, and society. They represent an investment in vitality and vigor that will pay off many times over in your retirement years. In crass financial terms, several years of extended life imply a greater return on retirement funds, annuities, and social security. But the greatest return is having the vigor and independence to pursue life to the fullest, throughout all your days.

Activity and training maintain fitness and other measures of performance that normally decline with age. Reaction and movement times, which typically slow down with age, are maintained by tennis players and other avid sports participants. The body doesn't wear out; it rusts out. So the adage "Use it or lose it" is worth noting. Humans were not designed for a sedentary life. With good genetics and a careful diet, you may live a long life, but the final years of your life may be spent in a nursing home if you don't do something to slow the rate of aging.

CHAPTER 19

The Psychology of Activity

"It is impossible to
live pleasurably
without living
wisely, well, and
justly, and impos-
sible to live wisely,
well, and justly
without living
pleasurably."

Epicurus

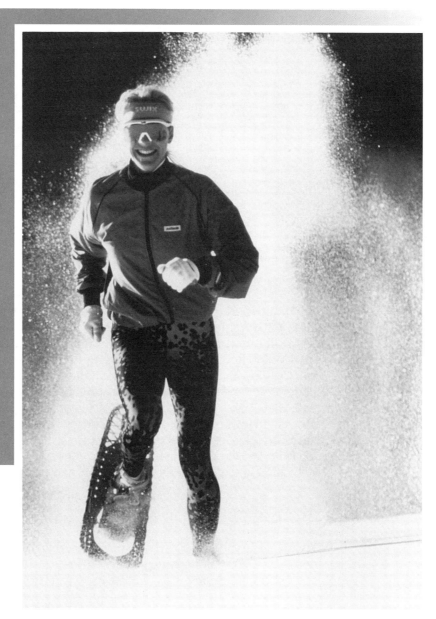

It is safe to say that from a health standpoint, the people likely to benefit the most from regular moderate physical activity seem most resistant to adopting or maintaining the behavior. As a teacher, researcher, and writer I have devoted my career to the proposition that increased knowledge concerning the health benefits of activity and fitness will lead to increased participation. Unfortunately, for the vast majority, this has not been the case. Indeed, feelings related to well-being, enjoyment, and pleasure seem more important in initiating and maintaining activity than concerns about health or factual knowledge. So, I am forced to journey beyond the comfortable landscape of physiology into the realm of psychology in search of answers to questions of motivation and adherence to regular moderate physical activity.

This chapter presents ways to help you begin and maintain a healthy, active life. It deals with motivation, the reasons to become involved in regular activity; and adherence, how to sustain that involvement throughout life. Central to the discussion will be the concepts of enjoyment, pleasure, satisfaction, and having fun. The active life is not a monastic existence, an exercise in asceticism. Rather it is a vital, vigorous, and joyful life, replete with satisfactions, healthy pleasures, and even thrills.

THIS CHAPTER WILL HELP YOU

- understand the importance of enjoyment, pleasure, and satisfaction in activity and other life choices;

- appreciate the role of motivation, goal setting, and feedback in the initiation of and adherence to the active life;

- identify your current involvement in physical activity;

- develop systematic changes in your activity plan; and

- construct a reinforcement schedule to reward new behaviors.

Motivation

What motivates individuals to engage in regular activity? Is it to look or feel good, for weight control, or to improve and maintain health? Far fewer than half of all Americans follow the health recommendation of the Centers for Disease Control and Prevention (CDC) and the American College of Sports Medicine (ACSM), that every U.S. adult should accumulate 30 minutes or more of moderate-intensity physical activity on most, preferably all, days of the week (Pate et al., 1995). Among those who do, fewer than 20% do so in a way that will bring about improvements in fitness. The rest lack the interest or motivation necessary to ensure regular participation. Let's examine the psychology of motivation in hopes of finding ways to motivate ourselves, family members, and friends. Motivation involves the arousal, direction, and persistence of behavior.

Arousal

Physiological motives or drives are triggered by basic biological needs such as food, water, elimination, and sex. Safety and health needs are next in the hierarchy of human motives or needs—to be safe from threat, to be secure. Then come love and belonging—needs involving genuine affection and a place in one's group. Next in the hierarchy are the esteem needs—to be liked and respected and to respect oneself. At the top of the hierarchy is the need for self-actualization, to realize one's potential (Maslow, 1954). Any of these needs may serve to arouse an individual to action (see figure 19.1).

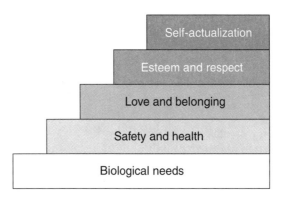

Figure 19.1 Hierarchy of needs.

Directing Behavior

The direction of behavior—that is, where and how one behaves when aroused—is a complex study involving a multitude of learned behaviors and their interaction with ever varying situations. Kenyon (1968) attempted to categorize the reasons why individuals engage in physical activity. They included

- social reasons—to meet or be with people or part of a group;
- pursuit of vertigo (the thrill of speed and change of direction while remaining in control;
- aesthetic reasons—the beauty of movement;
- catharsis—relief from stress and tension;
- ascetic reasons—self-denial, discipline, training; and
- health and fitness.

Many forms of activity may satisfy an individual's needs. One could walk, jog, run, swim, or cycle for health and fitness; or climb, kayak, ski, mountain bike, or windsurf in pursuit of vertigo. The direction chosen will depend on a number of factors, including the level of arousal, previous exercise experiences, opportunity, the physical and social environment, and a bit of chance.

Before I moved to Montana some 30 years ago, I had never seen a pair of skis, let alone a real mountain. Yet, I was motivated to give skiing a try, probably because my friends and co-workers were skiers (social reason). It didn't take long to realize that skiing was for me. Soon I was doing it not to belong or for esteem, but because it was exciting, because it felt good, to test myself, to find my potential. Now I am hopelessly hooked, positively addicted.

It strikes me that Kenyon's list of reasons why people engage in physical activity needs to be updated. A study of runners indicated additional reasons why people participate, including challenge, centering, afterglow, and because it feels good (Johnsgard, 1985). What a surprise—people engage in activity because it feels good and brings them enjoyment.

What reasons have you given for your lack of participation in regular moderate physical activity?

Interested but:

- ☐ Can't afford the time; maybe when I'm not so busy
- ☐ Lack of opportunity
- ☐ Not convenient
- ☐ Too expensive
- ☐ Don't know how to start

Not interested:

- ☐ Low priority at this point in my life
- ☐ Concerned about my health
- ☐ Don't want to be embarrassed
- ☐ Bad childhood experiences
- ☐ Never have enjoyed it

What would you say to motivate a family member or friend who expressed one of these reasons for not participating in regular activity?

The Pleasure Principle

In their book *Healthy Pleasures*, Ornstein and Sobel (1989) describe the pleasure principle and its role in the motivation of behavior. Pleasurable sensations reverberate in the nervous system, releasing endorphins and other opiate-like chemicals. These chemicals find their way to receptors and satisfy physiological needs. The authors reason that the human desire for enjoyment evolved to enhance survival. They cite eating, reproductive behavior, and caring for others as examples of pleasures that are good for health and survival of the species. And they suggest that measurable, pleasurable, benefits of physical activity for mind and body may be as close, easy, and even as fun as a walk in the park. Their advocacy of natural pleasures, of things that feel good, is consistent with the CDC/ACSM activity recommendations and the active life. Exercise doesn't have to hurt to be good; it only has to be regular and moderate to bestow the benefits and healthy pleasures.

That does not mean that all healthy pleasures are easy or immediately gratifying. Pleasure is synonymous with enjoyment and satisfaction. Some of the hardest things I have ever done are the most satisfying, such as running or skiing a marathon, climbing a mountain, or completing a triathlon. The training is always satisfying and sometimes enjoyable. But you must be willing and able to delay gratification if you are to experience the pleasure and relief that come with completion of a difficult task.

You must be willing and able to delay gratification if you are to experience the pleasure and relief that come with completion of a difficult task.

Intrinsic Motivation

Intrinsic or self-directed goals are more effective than impersonal sources in long-term motivation and adherence to exercise. Extrinsic or external sources

TYPE T

Type T (for thrill) is a personality type that describes individuals who are hooked on excitement, risk, and tempting fate. Jack, a physician friend, is the quintessential Type T. Over the years he has raced motocross, climbed mountains, kayaked rivers, and sailed a catamaran. He mastered downhill skis, moved on to Telemark skis, and is now a board skier. His latest passion, windsurfing, takes him to the Columbia River, the mecca for the sport. Type Ts fit Kenyon's category "pursuit of vertigo," defined as the thrill of speed and change in direction while remaining in control. There is pleasure and satisfaction in pushing the limits, in gaining mastery, flirting with danger while remaining in control, if just barely. It has been said that Type Ts get high on their own hormones. Certainly this behavior can become addictive, leading to tougher climbs and more challenging descents. Or it can become somewhat less dangerous, taking the form of in-line roller skating, scrambling up peaks, or even caving. It isn't necessary to follow the thrills to an untimely end. The addiction can be channeled into demanding but safer pursuits, compatible with the needs of family and career.

of motivation may arouse and direct efforts to win a prize, medal, trophy, or scholarship, or to gain social acceptance, but the motivation necessary to persist, to ensure lifelong participation in the active life, must come from within, from the upper reaches of the hierarchy of human needs (self-respect, self-actualization), and from the pleasure principle. Consider the former athletes who lose interest in their sport when the glory fades and the medals tarnish. Then look at your habitually active friends, the hikers, runners, tennis and racquetball players, and skiers. What keeps them going? Do they seek health, a trophy, or a championship? They go out each day because they must, because they are addicted, and because it feels good. They go out to be themselves, and in the process they come closer to their potential.

Persistence

Defined as the ability to go on resolutely or stubbornly in spite of difficulties, persistence is the key to success in physical activity and in life. Calvin Coolidge summed up its importance in the following lines:

> "Nothing in the world can take the place of persistence. Talent will not; nothing is more common than unsuccessful men with talent. Genius will not; unrewarded genius is almost a proverb. Education will not; the world is full of educated derelicts. Persistence and determination alone are omnipotent."

Persistence is needed to meet fitness, performance, weight-control, or other goals, especially on cold, windy, or rainy days. It implies faith in the eventual outcome, the ability to delay gratification, and confidence in your ability to cope with adversity. Without it I could never leave my cozy home and venture forth in cold and snow. Persistence helps to sustain effort over a prolonged period in order to obtain a goal. It is the foundation of adherence.

Adherence to Activity

Adhere means to maintain loyalty, to stick fast, to cling. Why do some people stick with the active life while others drop out? The range for dropouts—those who begin an exercise program and then cease participation—is from 20% to more than 50%. Lack of time is cited most often as the reason for dropping out, as well as for not starting in the first place. Family, career, or other responsibilities make it difficult for many people who say they are just too busy. I think of our recent presidents when I hear this excuse. They found time for physical activity in their schedules. Effective time management is one of the hallmarks of success, as is involvement in the active life. Other reasons for dropping out include: no place to exercise, fatigue, inadequate information, inconvenience, and lack of willpower.

Studies have shown a number of factors associated with dropping out, including a sedentary youth and previous unfavorable exercise experience, which underscores the need for enjoyable activity experiences, for having fun in school physical education and youth sports programs (Willis & Campbell, 1992). Education and income have also been linked positively with adherence. In personality tests, adherers were found to exhibit more self-confidence and emotional stability than dropouts. And cigarette smoking is almost always linked with a higher rate of dropping out (Willis & Campbell, 1992). Adherence is enhanced with family and peer support, and hurt by excessive work demands.

A number of factors that influence continued participation have been identified; some relate to individual participation and others to exercise programs. Some people thrive in an individual program, while others enjoy group participation and supervision. One local company's wellness program provides for both types: individual time-share programs (in which employees match personal exercise time with an equal amount of company time), and fitness club memberships that provide group or individual programs. Convenience, good facilities, likable leadership, and social support are all related to adherence in group programs. Another determinant is how well the program meets the participants' needs. Finally we return again to the pleasure principle. Programs that are enjoyable and foster a sense of achievement and satisfaction are more likely to encourage adherence.

> **Programs that are enjoyable and foster a sense of achievement and satisfaction are more likely to encourage adherence.**

The Climate for Adherence

With maturation comes the satisfaction of lower-order needs and the opportunity to seek self-actualization. The self-actualized individual is free to determine his or her lifestyle and personal goals and to pursue them without anxiety and without the necessity to conform, except superficially, to society's conventions and restraints. Self-actualized individuals seek *to be, not to become.* They enjoy their lives as they seek to realize their capacity. They require neither the attention nor the adulation of the crowd, only a personal sense of satisfaction and achievement.

Sometimes it is difficult, even for the self-actualized individual, to make the necessary sacrifices. It is hard to pursue any goal when those around you are nonsupportive. Fitness studies have shown that the emotional climate created by *significant others* is highly related to a participant's adherence to a program. When wives, husbands, and loved ones offer encouragement and support, the participant is likely to continue. Why would someone deprecate a loved one's efforts in a fitness or sports training program? Spouses may complain about the amount of time involved, the cost, upset schedules and vacations. Of course, it is possible that some complain because, secretly, they envy their spouse's dedication and satisfaction, or because they fear losing their rejuvenated loved one, or because other shared experiences are lost.

To avoid emotional conflicts, discuss your interests and goals with loved ones. Realize how your participation may affect them, and try to minimize the effects. Schedule shared experiences to make up for the time spent in your personal quest for excellence. A supportive emotional climate is certain to prevail when *both* husband and wife are happily involved in active lifestyles. It isn't necessary for both to be involved in the same activity, although there are many such cases. If both seek excellence in tennis, it isn't absolutely necessary that they play mixed doubles. What matters is that each understands how important participation is to the other, and that the emotional climate they create influences enjoyment and adherence.

Improving Adherence

We've considered some of the reasons people drop out and the factors associated with adherence to physical activity. And we've discussed the emotional climate and the importance of pleasure and having fun. Now let's turn our attention to psychological concepts that shed light on ways to enhance adherence. One concept is the therapeutic use of physical activity as a means of coping with moods, stress, anxiety, depression, and other problems. With a daily schedule, the activity becomes preventive, an inoculation against moods that interfere with life satisfaction and adherence.

Internals Versus Externals

The psychological construct called locus of control separates people into *internals*, those who believe they can control outcomes in their lives, and *externals*, who believe their lives are controlled by chance or by others. Internal controllers are more likely to adhere to healthy behaviors than are externals. Which better fits your view of life? Can your locus of control be modified to enhance adherence to healthy behavior, such as regular activity? I believe it can.

Self-Efficacy

The theory of self-efficacy suggests that coping behaviors such as physical activity are influenced by the perception of acquiring mastery in that area. Perception of mastery influences performance, and it is theorized that this perception is altered by positive experience. Thus, an activity may be reinforced by successful experience, leading to continuation of the behavior. It has even been suggested that enhanced self-efficacy in one behavior may generalize to others.

Extol your virtues, and you'll boost self-esteem, adherence, and possibly, performance.

If the perception of mastery reinforces behavior, perhaps we can influence that perception with *affirmative statements*, positive reinforcements of progress and performance. Elite athletes use affirmative statements to build confidence and aid performance. It's part of the positive internal dialogue that leads to success, in sport and in life. If it works for athletes, you can use positive self-talk to reinforce your sense of success, thereby enhancing adherence. Recognize your sacrifices, your progress, and your achievements. Celebrate your epic adventures. At the same time, you must eliminate negative self-talk. Extol your virtues, and you'll boost self-esteem, adherence, and possibly, performance.

INTERNAL DIALOGUE

The first step toward a positive internal dialogue is to eliminate negatives, irrational thinking, and cognitive distortions from your internal dialogue. Stop blaming yourself, focusing on negatives, overgeneralizing, magnifying, and minimizing. Don't undervalue your accomplishments. Change the negative "I look flabby" into the positive "I need to improve muscle tone." Then select positive affirmations to reinforce your behavior. Add simple statements to your internal dialogue, such as "I can do this," "I'm making progress," "I'm looking good," "I'm achieving my goals." Use them regularly, and you'll feel better about yourself and your program.

Goal Setting

A goal is an aim or a purpose, what an individual seeks to accomplish. Goals serve to help focus and regulate behavior; thus, they affect both motivation and adherence. Goal setting has a beneficial influence on the performance of a task. While most folks use goals to a certain extent, few take full advantage of their influence on the motivation for and adherence to physical activity. By utilizing short- and long-term goals, one is able to devise a strategy to achieve the desired result.

Goal setting works best when *process-oriented goals* are utilized. For instance, a process-oriented goal is to gradually work up to 30 miles of running per week, or to complete a 10-kilometer (6.2-mile) race. An *outcome-oriented goal* would be to run the 10-kilometer race in less than 40 minutes, an outcome that might be very difficult to achieve. Outcome-oriented goals have their place, but they need to be reasonable and adaptable. If the day of the 10-kilometer race is hot and humid, you'll need to adjust your goal.

I use goals to prepare for upcoming events and adventures, such as our annual winter ski trip in Yellowstone Park. In the fall I engage in muscular fitness training to build strength and endurance in skiing muscles. As soon as the snow flies I begin training so I'll be able to keep pace with my partners in February. Of course, I thoroughly enjoy every phase of the preparation. And I particularly enjoy the sense of accomplishment at the end of a long, hard trail. Set long-term goals as targets and short-term goals to help attain them. Write down your goals, and keep records as you progress. Back when I considered myself a serious runner I set training targets and would record my daily mileage on the calendar. At the end of the week I'd add up the total to see if I was on target to reach my goal. Use figure 19.2 to identify and record your goals.

Set realistic goals, such as 30 minutes of moderate physical activity, most days of the week. When the goal becomes too easy and loses its motivational effect, set a new, more challenging goal. Challenging goals get better results than easy ones. Use specific goals; don't just plan to "work hard." Finally, keep the list simple; don't set too many goals. As you achieve success you may expand the list. But for now begin with one or two long-term targets and some short-term steps to guide progress toward the targets (Locke & Latham, 1985). When you achieve a significant long-term goal, celebrate!

Goal Setting

Write down your goals in each category.

Dream Goal (long-term)   What is your long-term dream goal? What is potentially possible if you stretch all your limits?

Dream Goal (this year)   What is your dream goal this year? What is potentially possible if you stretch all your limits?

Performance Goals   What are some intermediate goals that you must reach in order to achieve this year's dream goal?

Realistic Goal (this year)   What do you feel is a realistic performance goal that you can achieve this year, based on your present fitness level, your potential for improvement, and your current motivation?

Daily Goal   Set a personal goal for tomorrow's training session. Write down one you would like to accomplish or approach with a special focus or intensity. Try to set a personal goal for every training session.

Figure 19.2   Short- and long-term goals questionnaire.
Adapted from Orlick 1986.

Behavioral Change

This section outlines important steps in the initiation and maintenance of regular physical activity. It begins with the intention to change, perhaps the best indicator of success. We then look at the early stages of behavior change, followed by factors associated with program maintenance or adherence. Behavior therapy is then reviewed as a strategy to aid the initiation and maintenance of the activity program.

Intention to Change

Influences on one's intention to adopt a new behavior include information, role models, authoritative figures (e.g., physician), previous experience, and social pressure. It may take time for an individual to move from disinterest to being ready to change. While no single approach works every time, the following seem to help.

- Inquiries from the fitness program leader concerning the individual's interest in information or changing behavior
- Continued gentle reminders
- Crises or scare tactics such as literature on health risks
- Enjoyable experiences

One of the best indicators of future success is an individual's readiness to change. If people say they are ready they probably are.

Initiating Behavior

Early success is associated with reasonable expectations and goals, gradual change, appropriate reinforcement, social support, and cognitive strategies (relaxation, dissociation). Relax during activity by focusing on your breathing.

Dissociation involves diverting attention from how you feel during exercise by focusing on other topics or conversation with a partner. For some people, the first 20 minutes of activity are the hardest, until pain-killing endorphins kick in. Similarly, the first few weeks of a new program are the toughest. So, it helps to have ways to survive until appreciable changes become evident or until you become addicted. Behavior therapy seems to work for difficult cases.

Behavior Therapy

Once called *behavior modification*, this approach provides a way to identify a desired behavior and to make progress toward its acquisition. The essentials of the approach are threefold:

1. Identify the behavior you wish to modify (e.g., physical activity), and maintain an accurate record of your current behavior. Maintain a weeklong record of all your physical activity (figure 19.3). Include the intensity and duration of your involvement, and complete the cognitive question for fitness training and recreational activities.
2. Analyze the current behavior, and then plan needed modifications. Do you need to burn more calories, increase intensity, or do specific training (e.g., muscular fitness)? Plan appropriate modifications to meet your

Daily Activity Log

Date _____

Time	Place	Exercise	Intensity	Duration	What were your thoughts during exercise?

Note. Include all forms of physical activity, including work, walking, and household chores.

Score	Intensity
5	Sustained heavy breathing and perspiration
4	Intermittent heavy breathing and perspiration—as in tennis
3	Moderately heavy—as in recreational sports and cycling
2	Moderate—as in volleyball, softball
1	Light—as in fishing, walking

Score	Duration
4	Over 30 min
3	20 to 30 min
2	10 to 20 min
1	Under 10 min

Figure 19.3   Daily activity log.

needs and interests. For example, you could increase your activity to meet the new CDC/ACSM guidelines: 30 minutes or more of moderate-intensity physical activity, most days of the week.

Develop a contract with specific goals and a schedule of rewards to reinforce the new behavior.

3. Develop a contract with specific goals and a schedule of rewards to reinforce the new behavior (figure 19.4). Use activity benchmarks (minutes or miles per day or week), weight loss, or other indicators of successful adoption of the new activity. A tangible, universally accepted reward such as money seems to work for most folks. Spend the reward immediately or save it for something you really want but might otherwise not purchase. Don't worry about the expense; the new behavior will save more than the cost of the reward in medical and other costs. In time the new behavior will become a healthy habit, and you will be able to focus on new goals or a new behavior (e.g., time management).

Maintenance

Adherence to a newly adopted behavior can be difficult; 50% of participants drop out of exercise programs within the first year. Certain strategies help to improve the odds of success, according to Taylor and Miller (1993). Activity tends to be continued if

- it meets a need,
- it is fun,
- there is social support, and
- there is evidence of change.

To ensure lifelong participation, the individual must move from extrinsic to intrinsic motivation, must become self-sufficient, independent of the instructor and the setting, and must develop strategies to deal with threats to continued participation. Work, illness, or family crises may interrupt but must never terminate participation in regular moderate activity.

Develop a network of support systems to help you guarantee adherence. Support is available from family and friends, interest groups, professionals, clubs, programs, publications, and organizations:

• **Family:** My wife and I provide support by taking a sincere interest in each other's activity, and we often participate together. Gifts are often selected to encourage or enhance activity, and trips usually revolve around a shared experience, such as hiking, canoeing, or skiing.

• **Friends:** Most of my long-time friends are those who share my interests. The shared interests are the foundation of the relationship. Their presence gets me out and keeps me going. Together we do more than any of us could do alone.

• **Interest groups:** I have access to hiking, skiing, and running clubs, and more. The local canoe racing group welcomes neophytes to join their Wednesday evening sessions. If you can't find a group with your interests, start one.

• **Professionals:** From personal trainers to fitness instructors, a wide array of help is available. Seek experts out for advice and for motivation. Get professional instruction to improve your performance and enjoyment of skiing or other recreational sports.

Activity Reinforcement Schedule

Date	Activity	Distance or time	Reward[a]	Total

Total for month

Note. Daily reward—for meeting activity goal (e.g., 2 mi); weekly reward—for meeting activity goal (e.g., 12 mi); monthly reward—for meeting activity goal (e.g., 50 mi; improved fitness score). Adjust goals as fitness improves.

[a]Rewards: daily—a small monetary award (e.g., $1) or a cool drink; weekly—a larger monetary reward (e.g., $5) or a special favor (e.g., movie); monthly—a substantial monetary reward (e.g., $20) or a very special favor (e.g., concert, dinner out). Rewards can be saved for a special purpose (e.g., new warm-up outfit, tennis racquet).

Figure 19.4 Activity reinforcement schedule.

- **Clubs:** When you join a health and fitness club you gain access to equipment, instruction, and an added bonus, the social support of fellow members. Club-based programs often succeed when home-based programs fail because of social and psychological support.

- **Programs:** Take advantage of your workplace wellness program, and become involved in new activities. The wellness program at the university with which I'm affiliated has provided me with weight lifting, swimming, in-line skating, slide board, and ski clinics, and many classes. Our campus recreation program has welcomed me on winter trips and in canoe and kayak classes.

- **Publications:** Many books are available to help you maintain or expand your interests. Magazines cater to general (*Outside*) or specific interests (*Backpacker*). Videos and computer programs on compact disc provide instruction in everything from golf to mountain biking.

- **Organizations:** The American College of Sports Medicine (ACSM) provides information and publications on fitness, exercise science, and sports medicine. ACSM also publishes position papers on a wide range of topics. Sport organizations such as the United States Tennis Association provide sport-specific pamphlets, instruction, and tournaments.

Sometimes a new piece of equipment will revive interest in an activity. For example, an adjustable ski pole has increased my interest and enjoyment in backcountry travel. The pole aids uphill travel, relieves aging knees on the downhills, and provides balance while crossing logs and streams. Sporting goods stores and equipment catalogs provide ways to make activity more pleasurable. Take advantage of these and other support systems to bolster a lifelong involvement in physical activity.

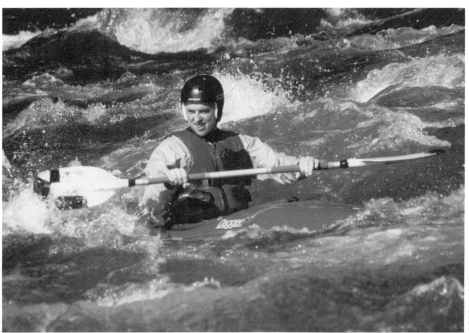

A new sport or piece of equipment will add interest and enjoyment, and bolster participation in the active life.

Relapse

It is not uncommon for participants to relapse, to slip back to inactivity after an initial change for the better. Relapse occurs for many reasons, ranging from emotional and social to physical. Since the event is so common, you should not let it bother you. It is part of the process of change, for athletes as well as newcomers. In dieting, relapse is par for the course. The question is: What can you do to prevent or recover from relapse? Studies in this relatively new area of research suggest some potential for relapse prevention (Brownell, Marlatt, Lichtenstein, and Wilson, 1986). One approach suggests a planned relapse, just to test the reaction when instructor support is available. To date most relapse-prevention programs have been labor-intensive, teaching how to anticipate and cope with relapse with strategies we have already discussed, such as behavior therapy and goal setting. Most have yielded modest results.

My suggestion is to search for intrinsic motivation and to strive for internal control. Free yourself from the need for external validation from fitness instructors. Their responsibility is to lead you to a level of independence where you will no longer rely on them for information or encouragement. Wean yourself from dependence on their motivation and control. Then develop your own approach to relapse prevention. Build the social support and emotional climate you need to keep going. Don't depend on one activity; be ready to adapt in the event of injury or chronic illness. When relapse comes, and it will, return to your goals, to behavior therapy, and to your support systems. People who develop behavioral or cognitive strategies, such as positive self-talk, are more successful at coping with relapse (Willis & Campbell, 1992). Devise your own solution, and you'll be better prepared for the future. But if all else fails don't hesitate to consult a professional.

The Active Personality

Do activity and improved fitness influence the personality, or are some personality types more likely to be active? Personality is a frame of reference used by psychologists in the study of behavior. More than a mask but less than reality, it is a product of heredity and the environment, usually studied with paper-and-pencil tests or in-depth interviews, but it has never really been defined or measured. That should not deter scientists in their search. The day may come when we will be able to define and measure this elusive concept of personality and thus understand, predict, or even improve behavior and health.

Cattell suggests that one's personality indicates what one will do when in a given mood and placed in a given situation. He developed the Cattell 16 Personality Factor Questionnaire, a personality test used widely by researchers (Cattell, Eber, & Tatsuoka, 1970). The test, typical of the paper-and-pencil approach, presumes to score the subject on each of 16 factors, or personality "traits" (see table 19.1). Assuming this approach is valid, let's use it to consider how activity and personality are related.

Using the Cattell questionnaire, studies of the personalities of middle-aged men have shown that highly fit subjects are more unconventional, composed, secure, easygoing, emotionally stable, adventurous, and intelligent than the low-fitness subjects. The most pronounced personality differences were those related to emotional stability and security.

TABLE 19.1   Cattell's 16 Personality Factors

Low score description	Personality factors	High score description
Aloof, cold	A	Warm, sociable
Dull, low capacity	B	Bright, intelligent
Emotional, unstable	C	Mature, calm
Submissive, mild	E	Dominant, aggressive
Glum, silent	F	Enthusiastic, talkative
Casual, undependable	G	Conscientious, persistent
Timid, shy	H	Adventurous, "thick-skinned"
Tough, realistic	I	Sensitive, effeminate
Trustful, adaptable	L	Suspecting, jealous
Conventional, practical	M	Bohemian, unconcerned
Simple, awkward	N	Sophisticated, polished
Confident, unshakable	Q	Insecure, anxious
Conservative, accepting	Q_1	Experimenting, critical
Dependent, imitative	Q_2	Self-sufficient, resourceful
Lax, unsure	Q_3	Controlled, exact
Phlegmatic, composed	Q_4	Tense, excitable

However, the presence of differences between high- and low-fitness groups does not prove that the differences are due to fitness. It could be that in our culture, emotionally stable and secure men are more likely to engage in a fitness program. In fact, when researchers studied the effects of a 4-month fitness program on these subjects, little personality change was noted among the low-fitness subjects, in spite of a conspicuous improvement in fitness. The researchers reasoned that it takes years to become fit or unfit, and that a few months of activity is insufficient to bring about significant personality changes (Ismail & Young, 1977). Studies using more elaborate personality instruments, such as the Minnesota Multiphasic Personality Inventory (MMPI), have produced mixed results. Longitudinal studies are necessary to confirm or reject the hypothesis that personality improves with activity or fitness.

Perception

There was a time when we researchers felt that perceptions were too subjective, too prone to error and variation. When an athlete said he was too tired to go on, we doubted his motivation. But Swedish psychologist Dr. Gunnar Borg changed all that when he developed his ratings of perceived exertion (RPE). Borg (1973) realized that the sensory stimuli generated during physical effort are integrated by the brain into a perception of effort. Stimuli from muscles, respiratory distress, pain, and the sensation of a pounding heart are perceived and evaluated. Subsequent studies have shown that these "subjective" estimates of effort are highly related to workload, heart rate, oxygen consumption, even lactic acid and hormones. In other words, our subjective estimate of work intensity provides a rather accurate estimate of the load itself, as well as the

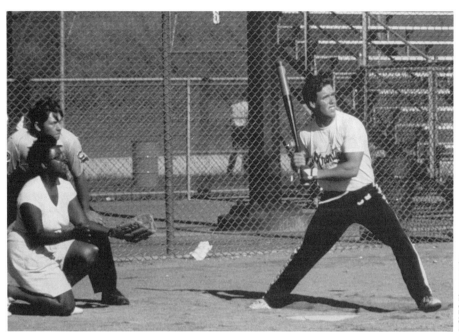

© CLEO Photography

Build the social support and emotional climate you need to keep going.

internal factors affected by the work. Of course, our subjective perception of effort is also closely tied with the pleasure we derive from participation.

Since we are able to accurately judge our effort in an exercise such as cycling or running, and since the heart rate and metabolic cost of the effort are closely related to those ratings, we should be more inclined to listen to our bodies during exercise. If the exercise feels too difficult, it probably is. The use of the heart rate training zone in exercise prescription is an attempt to employ important physiological criteria in the determination of a safe and effective dose of exercise. You may find that running at your training heart rate feels "somewhat hard." Thereafter, you can use that sense of difficulty to guide your exertion. If high temperatures cause your heart rate to rise, your perception of effort will adjust your pace to a more prudent level. Eventually this sense of effort is all you need to gauge exercise intensity.

While we're on the subject of perception, let me spend a moment on the concept of *preferred exertion*. Experienced exercisers seem to require a certain level of exertion to be satisfied. If the exertion is too easy, it diminishes their sense of satisfaction. Training increases the preferred exertion, while inactivity lowers it. People who have been involved in highly competitive sports often have learned to prefer a high level of exertion. Some erroneously believe that exercise has to hurt to be good (it does not), or no pain, no gain (also untrue); therefore, when they resume activity after a layoff, they overdo and end up with soreness or injury.

The preference for exertion is learned. For most Americans, it consists of the minimum, of walking to and from the car. It could be different: If parents and school and community leaders demonstrate and encourage sensible and inexpensive exercise habits, more kids will grow up with a predisposition to regular activity. If parents become involved, the kids will make it a family affair. Elementary, high school, and even college students should be encouraged to participate in healthful activities. Community organizations can sponsor activities for which participation is the major goal. The objective is to raise the level of preferred exertion to that required to achieve the health benefits of regular moderate physical activity.

The preference for exertion is learned.

Summary

This chapter has looked at motivation and adherence in order to help you initiate and maintain involvement in enjoyable, life-long physical activity. We've learned that motivation involves the arousal, direction, and persistence of behavior, and that intrinsic motivation is more persistent than extrinsic. We've also learned that internals, those who believe they are in control of their lives, are more likely to adhere to healthy behaviors than externals, those who believe their lives are controlled by chance or by others. We've seen that success or the perception of mastery reinforces participation and aids adherence. The chapter provides a way to identify current activity patterns, to establish realistic goals for new behaviors, and to utilize reinforcement to help ensure the attainment of those goals.

Throughout this book I have advocated realistic goals, minor adjustments, and gradual change as a proven approach to improvements in activity and other health behaviors. This approach is supported by research and by common sense. Most people won't need a radical change if they just stick with minor adjustments, such as taking daily walks or substituting low-fat foods for high-fat. However, one school of thought suggests that moderate changes are hard to measure and easy to ignore, making a slip back into bad habits more likely. Gradual change may not provide the results and positive feedback required to reinforce the behavior, while big changes in health behaviors are more likely to yield big results. If you think you might prefer this "big-change" approach, set some lofty goals, such as running a marathon or switching to a very low-fat diet. Make a major commitment, and see what happens. Use the approach that works for you.

Active individuals seem to be better able to cope with life's problems. These hardy people share several characteristics: a sense of being in control, a sense of involvement and purpose, and the flexibility to adapt to challenges and opportunities (Kobasa, 1979). Robust good health and resistance to illness don't absolutely require regular moderate activity, not if you are blessed with superb genes. But if you are like most of us, the activity provides a coping mechanism that contributes to health, adaptability, and resistance to stress. And more important, it's fun.

It's been said, "Begin; the rest is easy." Of course, that isn't true—the rest isn't easy. But unless you begin you'll never know how easy or hard the road may be. Life is a journey, not a destination.

CHAPTER 20

Activity and the Quality of Life

"Every age has its pleasures, its style of wit, and its own ways."

Nicolas Boileau-Despreaux

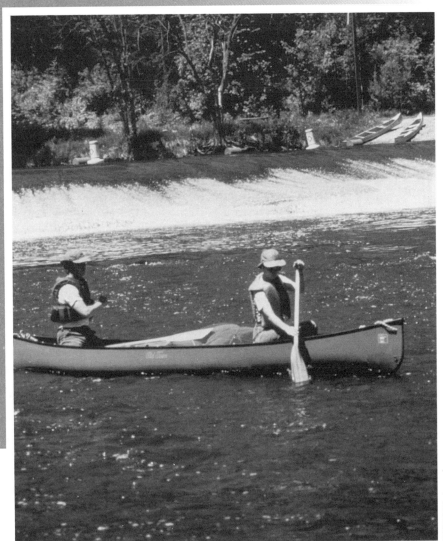

What began with a catalog of health benefits associated with the active life now concludes with a consideration of the contribution of physical activity and fitness to the quality of life. We'll begin with a consideration of quality, and ways to measure it and success in life. Then we'll consider how the definition of success shifts with the seasons of life. We'll conclude with an invitation to action, a challenge to maintain and improve the quality of life in your community.

THIS CHAPTER WILL HELP YOU

- define your definition of quality and success in life,
- understand how the definitions change at different stages of life,
- influence the quality of your experiences,
- understand your responsibility to maintain and improve the quality of life, and
- appreciate the dimensions of the active life.

Quality of Life

Quality of life, quality time—just what is this quality thing all about? The dictionary definition of quality includes: "degree of excellence"; "a distinguishing attribute." Quality is necessarily a subjective, personal response, not an absolute. Quality is easily distinguished from quantity: For example, for competitive runners, quantity of training simply refers to the miles run, while quality refers to the race-pace training that leads to improvement in performance. Similarly, while some people find quality in a difficult mountain climb, others prefer the tranquility of a hike in the forest below.

Objective measurement of this subjective concept has just begun. The health care debate has prompted discussion of quality-of-life issues in reference to treatment decisions, such as surgery, chemotherapy, radiation, or drugs. Will surgery or some other therapy improve the quality of life? Removal of the prostate gland may excise a cancer, but it often comes at a terrible cost (incontinence, impotence). You make quality-of-life decisions daily. Make certain you understand the options and the factors that contribute to your personal defini-

QUALITY TIME

A recent addition to the lexicon of pop-psych, *quality time*, or QT, usually refers to time spent with loved ones. Its value is that it reminds us to do the obvious: Spend time with those we value. But QT means more than just spending time; it means being there in mind as well as body. Put aside work or diversions, turn off the TV, and become fully engaged in the moment. Play games with the kids, walk and talk with your significant other, or simply sit and watch the sunset. Don't wait for an accident, a heart attack, or some other disaster to remind you of the things that really matter.

tion of quality. Do you value family or friends above wealth and fame, excitement over tranquility, sociability above privacy? Try to be certain that your decisions are consistent with the things you value. To do this you'll have to arrive at your own definition of success.

Success

Your definition of success may have a lot to do with how you view the quality of life.

Definitions of success differ among individuals and may change as one ages. Many people set out to be successful in business, or a profession, or to earn wealth and fame. In time the definition may be modified to include family, friends, and financial security. Take the time to list the things you associate with success.

You don't need fame, status, power, or a pile of money to be successful, just a favorable or satisfactory outcome or result. Few of us look back and wish we had spent more time working or acquiring wealth, while many of us wish we had spent more time with family and friends, or in healthy pursuits. Your definition of success may have a lot to do with how you view the quality of life.

The inane bumper sticker, "He who has the most toys wins," describes the credo of the motorized recreationist, owner of powerboat, jet ski, all-terrain vehicle, motorcycle, and snowmobile. While these methods of transportation have a legitimate purpose—access to recreation or work—they have become an end instead of a means. One loud, polluting machine can spoil the tranquility of lake or forest, ruining the quality of experience for human-powered paddlers, hikers, mountain bikers, and cross-country skiers. Worse yet is the realization that this lifestyle is being handed down to the next generation of overweight, underactive kids.

Perception of Quality

Psychologists and sensory physiologists long have known how to measure the quantity of stimulus (e.g., sound, light, exertion). It is far more difficult to assess the quality of an experience, yet it is the quality of an exercise experience that provides pleasure and brings us back for more. Ask someone to rate the quality of an exercise experience, and he or she will respond with a long-winded evaluation of the physical environment, weather, companions, personal sensations, expectations. Many factors are involved in the quality of an exercise experience.

A creek-side run on a tree-shaded path amid the beauty of the mountains is an experience to be savored and long remembered. Cover the same distance on a short, crowded running track or along a busy city street, and the experience becomes an ordeal—unless, of course, you are with company you enjoy, or glad for the chance to get away from the office. You can control the factors that enhance the quality of your exercise experiences. If you abhor noisy, crowded public tennis courts and are bothered by players who either don't know or won't practice the etiquette of the sport, build your own court, join a private club, play before the crowds arrive, or encourage the city recreation department to teach court etiquette. Your exercise experiences will be more enjoyable if you follow these guidelines:

- **Be flexible:** Don't depend on one activity, time, or place for satisfaction.
- **Plan ahead:** Plan your participation, your companions, the time of day, the place. If the afternoon winds diminish the quality of tennis, plan to play in the morning.

- **Set realistic goals:** If you set out to run 10 miles on a hot, humid day and don't finish, you may feel you've failed, but you haven't. You just set an unrealistic goal.
- **Recognize your moods:** We all get depressed, concerned, worried. Sometimes exercise can help you calm down when you're too excited, or pick you up when you're depressed, but a really foul mood can ruin a friendly game.
- **Be prepared:** Keep your equipment in good condition, get adequate rest, eat sensibly, take along extra food or drink if it may be needed, and have tools and extra parts available.
- **Learn to relax:** Sit in a quiet room, and focus on your respiration. Think "easy" with each exhale. Practice daily, and when you become proficient start using the technique in your sport, while driving in traffic, or whenever the need arises.

It is up to you to enhance the quality of your exercise experiences.

It is up to you to enhance the quality of your exercise experiences. If your daily activity is satisfying, it may bubble over and affect other phases of life. If it isn't, you may feel cheated, lose interest in the activity, and quit. In that case, you will be the loser.

The Seasons and Stages of Life

Physical activity should be spontaneous and enjoyable. Excessive planning can inhibit spontaneity and induce the kind of drudgery found in many fitness programs. On the other hand, a well-conceived plan can contribute to the flow of life, helping one season melt into the other. Just this once, give your physical life the same attention you spend on finance, education, travel, or other aspects of life. We'll look first at the seasons of the year, then the stages of life.

Annual Plan

Once a year take the time to outline the activities in which you intend to participate during the coming year. Fill in the sports or recreational activities you enjoy each season. When you come upon a blank season, consider a new activity, a supplement, or preparation for an upcoming season (figure 20.1). This brief mental exercise will also show you how one activity can blend into the next, removing the need for extensive physical preparation. Year-round activity is the ideal way to maintain the desired level of fitness. It minimizes the discomfort associated with the first few days of exercise. It also maintains fitness and optimizes energy balance and weight control. Of course, most of us remain active because we enjoy the experiences.

Stages of Life

Each of us is engaged in a lifelong search for meaning. The seasons of our lives are marked by an ebb and flow of purpose and confidence, periods of satisfaction followed by doubt. Our goals shift as the stages unfold.

- **Young adult:** This stage usually requires severing ties, acquiring an education, finding a mate, establishing a career, and perhaps, starting a family. So it isn't surprising to find definitions of success framed in financial and material terms.

Seasonal Activity Planner

	Winter	Spring	Summer	Fall
Major activities				
Minor activities				
Supplements				

Figure 20.1   Seasonal activity planner.

• **Adult:** By avoiding divorce and major career changes, the 30-something adult may be able to put down roots, even purchase a home. But that goal is often threatened by uncertainties in the workplace or the economy. And this period sometimes brings the midlife crisis, a realization that time to reach goals is running out.

During the decade from 45 to 55 years, what some call *middle age*, we begin to accept ourselves and our lives, and redefine our goals for success and the quality of life. Thereafter we may be refreshed or resigned, facing the best time of life if we let go of old roles and definitions, and find a renewal of purpose (Sheehy, 1976).

• **Senior:** Sometimes called the golden years, the senior stage may be the best of all, finally providing the time and resources to fulfill goals. Limited resources won't diminish satisfaction if the goals are qualitative rather than quantitative.

• **Elder:** Sometime after the age of 80 folks say they begin to slow down, but not stop. Many artists and musicians continue to create and perform. In spite of crippling rheumatoid arthritis, my independent mother continued to play the piano in musical programs until shortly before her death at the age of 84. Gardening and swimming helped maintain the physical vitality she needed to pursue her passion for music.

Too busy to do all the things you want to do? Some activities, such as football, should be attempted only by the young, whereas others, such as tennis or golf, are perfectly suited for adults, seniors, or even elders. Activities such as fishing or sailing can be enjoyed at any stage of life. So, relax; there is time for everything you want to do. Give some thought to activities you want to take up in the future, when you'll have time to enjoy them.

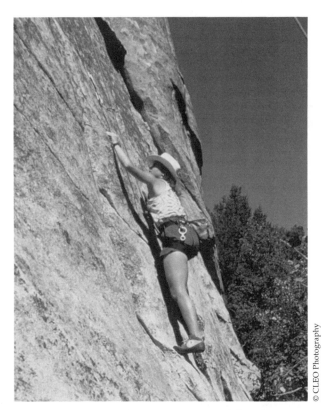

© CLEO Photography

Remain open to peak experiences and flow.

As you advance in years you will find new challenges and new adventures, and although you may temporarily put aside favorite activities, you'll never forget well-learned skills. Competition becomes more difficult as you approach the top of an age group, but when you enter a new age classification, it's like being a kid again. Eventually you'll seek less competition and more cooperation; you'll discover the quiet world of sailing, the solitude of wilderness, or good companions in golf and tennis. For everything there is a season, so keep active, and you'll find the time to enjoy the seasons and stages of life.

Dimensions of the Active Life

This book began with a physiological analysis of the active life and its benefits. Eventually it dealt with less measurable but no less meaningful aspects of psychology and their relationship to fitness and health. As we approach the end of the book I want you to know about another dimension of exercise and fitness, a dimension that provides meaning far beyond the measurable. I refer to the transcendent, peak, or even mystical experiences frequently reported by those who regularly engage in exercise and sport.

These moments of perfection are characterized by total involvement, control, concentration, and ease of movement, and a sense of *flow*, described as a smooth sequence of movement without conscious effort. These rare moments can occur in training or competition, in individual or team sports, and at all levels of ability. They are more likely to occur when you are relaxed and nonjudgmental than when you are critical or dissatisfied. When they come they impart meaning and satisfaction that transcends the physiological benefits of physical activity and fitness.

So, as you pursue the pleasures and values of the active life, remain open to peak experiences and flow. Don't become preoccupied with time, distance, or pulse rates. Set aside a time during each exercise session during which you just let it happen. Ignore form so you can enjoy sensations, forget time so you can experience the timelessness of flow. Once you do you will come back day after day to repeat the experience. And activity will take on new meaning in your life.

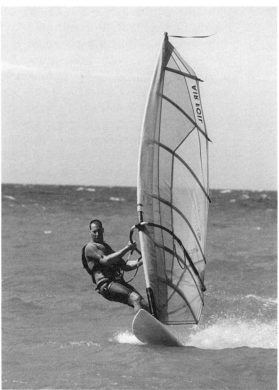

The stages of life provide many challenges and opportunities.

Responsibility

If you're still with me this late in the book you've probably accepted the importance of the active life and the positive health habits it fosters. No doubt you are engaged in regular moderate activity and practicing healthy habits, most of the time. You are taking responsibility for your behaviors and your health. If so you are ready for a new responsibility.

It is not enough that you work to improve your health and the quality of life; you must strive to do the same for family, friends, and the community. As you become convinced of the contribution and potential of the active life, you will appreciate your responsibility to extend the message and the opportunity to others. We need to redirect a society caught in a cycle of inactivity and overindulgence, of energy-wasting, polluting, motorized recreation, of declining health and vitality. This effort is important if we are to reduce disease and disability, and gain control of spiraling health care and worker's compensation costs. We need to restore a sense of personal responsibility for our health and our actions. Also essential is the need to preserve the physical, emotional, and social environments we want for our children and our children's children.

Act Locally

It is not enough that you work to improve your health and the quality of life; you must strive to do the same for family, friends, and the community.

What can you do to reverse the trend toward inactivity? Begin with little acts of kindness to family and friends. Find the time to acquaint others with the pleasures of the active life. Invite a friend for a walk. Plan a hike with the family. Give gifts that encourage activity, then find ways to make certain that they are used. While my grandson wanted another video game for Christmas, I presented him with cross-country skis, boots, and poles. Then one sunny winter day I took him skiing, masking the effort with drinks and snacks. Fortunately, we didn't have to go very far to find good ski trails.

If you believe, as I do, that the quality of life is closely tied to the environment, then you may accept my challenge and work to preserve and improve the features you enjoy. I'm currently serving as a member of our local Air Pollution Advisory Committee. Our mountain valley traps pollutants during the air inversions common to winter months. Wood-burning stoves, automobiles, and industrial pollution contribute to a problem that threatens to grow with the population. With health department efforts and citizen cooperation, the community has seen substantial improvements in air quality. Wood stove emissions have been controlled, and new regulations prohibit installation of polluting stoves. These efforts have helped to clear the air for this and future generations.

What Can You Do?

Be a volunteer in local causes and clean-up efforts. Join the PTA and work for improved activity programs and facilities for the kids and the community. Help start a worksite wellness program, or work to improve the one you have. Write letters to policy makers and agencies to encourage better use of the environ-

HAPPY TRAILS

Gordon, an avid cross-country skier, came to our community as a graduate student and stayed on to pursue a career and raise his family. He used his term as president of our Nordic Ski Club to expand our local ski trails. Due to his efforts, as well as those of club volunteers, and the cooperation of local agencies and ski stores, we now have a fine network of trails located minutes from town. Other trailblazers helped create a local wilderness area, with trails for hikers, runners, skiers, mountain bikers, and horses. And we have been blessed with river walks, hillside trails, and other pathways to the active life, all because individuals made the effort.

ment, limits on motorized recreation, and preservation of open space. Vote for bond issues that are designed to preserve open spaces or improve the environment. Contribute to the work of organizations that share your goals. With some thought and attention, you'll find dozens of ways to promote activity, enhance the environment, and improve the quality of life.

As you pursue your cause, be patient, be positive, and be persistent. Employ persuasion, avoid confrontation, and seek mutually beneficial solutions. Keep a sense of humor, and you'll be more likely to get results and enjoy the experience. Good luck—I look forward to hearing of your successes.

Health Impact Analysis

Public policy influences health behavior. People are more likely to quit smoking when it is banned in the workplace, in public buildings, on airline flights. On the other hand, people are more likely to participate in sedentary, energy-consuming, polluting activities (snowmobile, motorboat, all-terrain vehicle) when they are allowed or even encouraged in local, state, and national parks. Sometimes the contrasts are perplexing, as when Yellowstone National Park grooms trails for snowmobile use but bans mountain bikes and arrests runners who use park trails for a race. The contrast is even more perplexing when you realize that Glacier National Park bans the snowmobile, and Crater Lake National Park encourages running with an annual marathon. Based on the acknowledged contribution of physical activity to health, Congress and the Public Health Service should endeavor to make participation in physical activity and other healthy behaviors a high priority in decision-making for all government agencies.

Local, state, and national laws and policies should be designed to encourage healthy behavior. Just as land use policies require environmental impact analyses prior to approval, we should require health impact analyses prior to the approval of any and all laws and policies. Wouldn't this tend to hurt the economy? On the contrary, healthy behaviors are usually good for the economy and the environment. Nonmotorized physical activity conserves fuel and is nonpolluting, easy on the environment, and far less expensive for participants. If manufacturing jobs are lost, for example, with the elimination of motorized golf carts on public courses, others would be created in the construction of quality, light-weight golf bags. Encourage your local, state, and national legislators and bureaucrats to consider the impact of laws and regulations on health and the quality of life.

Encourage your local, state, and national legislators and bureaucrats to consider the impact of laws and regulations on health and the quality of life.

Summary

The stages of life provide many challenges and opportunities. We need an arsenal of activities and coping strategies to help us through the lows as we regain confidence and establish new goals. While faith, family, and friends provide the major sources of support, the active life serves by providing vitality, discipline, challenge, and time for reflection. It is my hope that this book helps you to improve your health and the quality of life, and to experience and appreciate all the dimensions of the active life.

Glossary

acclimatization—Adaptation to an environmental condition such as heat or altitude

actin—Muscle protein that works with the protein myosin to produce movement

adenosine triphosphate (ATP)—High-energy compound formed from oxidation of fat and carbohydrate, used as energy supply for muscle and other body functions; the energy currency

adipose tissue—Tissue in which fat is stored

aerobic—In the presence of oxygen; aerobic metabolism utilizes oxygen

aerobic fitness—Maximum ability to take in, transport, and utilize oxygen

agility—Ability to change direction quickly while maintaining control of the body

alveoli—Tiny air sacs in the lungs where oxygen and carbon dioxide exchange takes place

amino acids—Chief components of proteins; different arrangements of the 22 amino acids form the various proteins (muscles, enzymes, hormones, etc.)

anaerobic—In the absence of oxygen; nonoxidation metabolism

anaerobic threshold—More properly called the lactate threshold, the point at which lactic acid produced in muscles begins to accumulate in the blood; defines the upper limit that can be sustained aerobically

angina pectoris—Chest pain (also called necktie pain) associated with narrowed coronary arteries and lack of oxygen to heart muscle during exertion

anorexia nervosa—An eating disorder characterized by excessive dieting and subsequent loss of appetite

arrhythmia—Irregular rhythm or beat of the heart

asymptomatic—Without symptoms

atherosclerosis—Narrowing of coronary arteries by cholesterol buildup within the walls

atrophy—Loss of size of muscle

balance—Ability to maintain equilibrium while in motion

behavior therapy—A system of record keeping and motivation designed to help change a behavior (e.g., overeating)

blood pressure—Force exerted against the walls of arteries

body composition—The relative amount of fat and lean tissue

bronchiole—Small branch of airway; sometimes undergoes spasm, making breathing difficult, as in exercise-induced asthma

buffer—Substance in blood that soaks up hydrogen ions to minimize changes in acid-base balance (pH)

bulimia—An eating disorder characterized by alternate bouts of gorging and purging

calorie—Amount of heat required to raise 1 kilogram of water 1 degree Celsius; same as kilocalorie

capillaries—Smallest blood vessels (between arterioles and venules) where oxygen, foods, and hormones are delivered to tissues and carbon dioxide and wastes are picked up

carbohydrate—Simple (e.g., sugar) and complex (e.g., potatoes, rice, beans, corn, and grains) foodstuff that we use for energy; stored in liver and muscle as glycogen, while excess is stored as fat

cardiac—Pertaining to the heart

cardiac output—Volume of blood pumped by the heart each minute; product of heart rate and stroke volume

cardiorespiratory endurance—Synonymous with aerobic fitness or maximal oxygen intake

cardiovascular system—Heart and blood vessels

central nervous system (CNS)—The brain and spinal cord

cholesterol—Fatty substance found in nerves and other tissues; excessive amounts in blood have been associated with increased risk of heart disease

Clo units—The insulating value of clothing

concentric—Contraction that involves shortening of the contracted muscle

contraction—Development of tension by muscle: concentric muscle shortens and eccentric muscle lengthens under tension; static contractions are contractions without change in length

cool-down—Postperformance exercise used to dissipate heat, maintain blood flow, and aid recovery of muscles

coronary arteries—Blood vessels that originate from the aorta and branch out to supply oxygen and fuels to the heart muscle

coronary-prone—Having several risk factors related to early development of heart disease

creatine phosphate (CP)—Energy-rich compound that backs up ATP in providing energy for muscles

defibrillator—Device that applies a strong electric shock to stop irregular heart action and restore normal heart rhythm

dehydration—Loss of essential body fluids

delayed onset muscle soreness (DOMS)—Muscle soreness that peaks 24 to 48 hours after unfamiliar exercise or vigorous eccentric contractions

deoxyribonucleic acid (DNA)—The source of the genetic code housed in the nucleus of the cell

diastolic pressure—Lowest pressure exerted by blood in an artery; occurs during the resting phase (diastole) of the heart cycle

duration—Distance or length of time (or calories burned, in the case of the exercise prescription)

eccentric—Contraction that involves lengthening of a contracted muscle

electrocardiogram (ECG)—A graphic recording of the electrical activity of the heart

electrolyte—Solution of ions (sodium, potassium) that conducts electric current

endurance—The ability to persist or to resist fatigue

energy balance—Balance of caloric intake and expenditure

enzyme—An organic catalyst that accelerates the rate of chemical reactions

epinephrine (adrenaline)—Hormone from the adrenal medulla and nerve endings of the sympathetic nervous system; secreted during times of stress and to help mobilize energy

ergometer—A device, such as a bicycle, used to measure work capacity

evaporation—Elimination of body heat when sweat vaporizes on the surface of the skin; evaporation of 1 liter of sweat yields a heat loss of 580 calories

Fartlek—Swedish term meaning speed play; a form of training in which participants vary speed according to mood as they run through the countryside

fast-twitch muscle fibers—Muscle fibers that contract quickly but are susceptible to fatigue

fat—Important energy source; stored for future use when excess calories are ingested

fatigue—Diminished work capacity, usually short of true physiological limits; real limits in short, intense exercise are factors within muscle (muscle pH, calcium); in long duration effort, limits are glycogen depletion or central nervous system fatigue due to low blood sugar

fitness—A combination of aerobic capacity and muscular strength and endurance that enhances health and the quality of life

flexibility—Range of motion through which the limbs or body parts are able to move

frequency—Number of times per day or week (in the case of the exercise prescription)

glucose—Energy source transported in blood; essential energy source for brain and nervous tissue

glycogen—Storage form of glucose; found in liver and muscles

heart attack—Death of heart muscle tissue that results when atherosclerosis blocks oxygen delivery to heart muscle; also called myocardial infarction

heart rate—Frequency of contraction, often inferred from pulse rate (expansion of artery resulting from beat of heart)

heart rate range—The difference between the resting and maximal heart rates

heat stress—Temperature-humidity combination that leads to heat disorders such as heat cramps, heat exhaustion, or heatstroke

hemoglobin—Iron-containing compound in red blood cells that forms a loose association with oxygen

high-density lipoprotein (HDL) cholesterol—A carrier molecule that takes cholesterol from the tissue to the liver for removal; inversely related to heart disease risk

hypoglycemia—Low blood sugar (glucose)

hypothermia—Life-threatening heat loss brought on by rapid cooling, energy depletion, and exhaustion

inhibition—Opposite of excitation in the nervous system

insulin—Pancreatic hormone responsible for getting blood sugar into cells

intensity—The relative rate, speed, or level of exertion

interval training—Training method that alternates short bouts of intense effort with periods of active rest

ischemia—Lack of blood to a specific area such as heart muscle

isokinetic—Contraction against resistance that is varied to maintain high tension throughout range of motion

isometric—Contraction against an immovable object (static contraction)

isotonic—Contraction against a constant resistance

lactic acid—A by-product of glycogen metabolism that also transports energy from muscle to muscle and from muscle to the liver; high levels in muscle poison the contractile apparatus and inhibit enzyme activity

lean body weight—Body weight minus fat weight

lipid—Fat

lipoprotein—A fat-protein complex that serves as a carrier in the blood (e.g., high-density lipoprotein cholesterol)

low-density lipoprotein (LDL) cholesterol—The cholesterol fraction that accumulates in the lining of the coronary arteries and causes ischemia

maximal oxygen intake (consumption)—Aerobic fitness; best single measure of fitness with implications for health; synonymous with cardiorespiratory endurance

metabolic equivalent (MET)—Unit of measure; 1 MET is resting metabolism

metabolism—Energy production and utilization processes, often mediated by enzymatic pathways

mitochondria—Tiny organelles within cells; site of all oxidative energy production

motoneuron—Nerve that transmits impulses to muscle fibers

motor area—Portion of cerebral cortex that controls movement

motor unit—Motor nerve and the muscle fibers it innervates

muscle fiber types—Fast twitch fibers are fast contracting but fast to fatigue; slow twitch fibers contract somewhat more slowly but are fatigue-resistant

muscular fitness—The strength, muscular endurance, and flexibility needed to carry out daily tasks and avoid injury

myocardium—Heart muscle

myofibril—Contractile threads of muscle composed of the proteins actin and myosin

myogenic—Training that influences the muscles

myosin—Muscle protein that works with actin to produce movement

neurogenic—Training that influences the nervous system

neuron—Nerve cell that conducts an impulse; basic unit of the nervous system

nutrition—Provision of adequate energy (calories) as well as needed amounts of fat, carbohydrate, protein, vitamins, minerals, and water

obesity—Excessive body fat (more than 20% of total body weight for men, more than 30% for women)

osteoporosis—Weakening of bones via the loss of bone minerals

overload—A greater load than normally experienced; used to coax a training effect from the body

overtraining—Excess training that leads to staleness, illness, or injury

oxygen debt—Postexercise oxygen intake that exceeds resting requirements; used to replace the oxygen deficit incurred during exercise

oxygen deficit—Lack of oxygen in early moments of exercise

oxygen intake—Oxygen used to provide energy via oxidative pathways

perceived exertion—Subjective estimate of exercise difficulty

peripheral nervous system—Parts of the nervous system not including the brain and spinal cord

pH—Acidity or alkalinity of a solution; below 7 is acid, and above 7 is alkaline

physiological age—Also called functional age; as contrasted to chronological age, defines an individual's ability to perform physically

plaque—A growth of cellular debris and low-density lipoprotein cholesterol that impedes blood flow in the coronary artery

plyometrics—A form of power training that uses vigorous contractions with resistance

power—The rate of doing work

progressive resistance—Training program in which the resistance is increased as the muscles gain strength

protein—Organic compound formed from amino acids; forms muscle tissue, hormones, and enzymes

psychoneuroimmunology—A new field of study that explores links among the brain and nervous system and the immune system, or among thoughts and emotions and sickness and health

pulse—The wave that travels down the artery after each contraction of the heart (see heart rate)

rapid eye movement (REM)—A stage of sleep associated with dreams

relaxation response—Proven method to achieve relaxation

repetition maximum (RM)—The maximum number of times you can lift a given weight (1 RM is the most you can lift one time)

respiration—Intake of oxygen (from the atmosphere into the lungs and then to the blood and to the tissues) and exhalation of carbon dioxide (from tissues to the blood, to the lungs, and to the atmosphere)

ribonucleic acid (RNA)—A cellular compound that carries messages from the nucleus (DNA) to the rest of the cell (messenger RNA) or transfers amino acids to the ribosome for protein synthesis (transfer RNA)

ribosome—A cellular organelle that synthesizes protein from amino acids

risk factors—Factors associated with a higher risk for a certain disease (e.g., coronary risk factors)

sarcomere—The contractile unit of the muscle

somatotype—Body type; ectomorph is linear or thin, mesomorph is muscular, and endomorph is fat

slow-twitch muscle fibers—Muscle fibers that contract more slowly than fast-twitch fibers but are more resistant to fatigue

specificity—A principle of training that states that the type of training undertaken must relate to the desired results (i.e., you get what you train for)

speed of movement—The sum of reaction time (time from stimulus to start of movement) and movement time (time to complete the movement)

strength—Ability of muscle to exert force

stroke volume—Volume of blood pumped from the ventricle during each contraction of the heart synapse—Junction between neurons

systolic pressure—Highest pressure in arteries that results from contraction (systole) of the heart

tendon—Tough connective tissue that connects muscle to bone

testosterone—Male hormone

threshold—The minimal level required to elicit a response

tonus—Muscle firmness in absence of a voluntary contraction

training stimulus—The type of exercise that elicits the desired adaptation to training

training zone—The heart rate zone within which training is likely to produce the desired effect

triglyceride—A fat consisting of three fatty acids and glycerol

Valsalva maneuver—Increased pressure in abdominal and thoracic cavities caused by breath holding and extreme effort

variable (or accommodating) resistance—A machine or system that matches resistance to the capability of the muscle group

velocity—Rate of movement or speed

ventilation—The amount of air inhaled per minute; the product of tidal volume and frequency

ventricle—Chamber of the heart that pumps blood to the lungs (right ventricle) or to the rest of the body (left ventricle)

warm-up—A preperformance activity used to increase muscle temperature and to rehearse skills

weight training—Progressive resistance exercise using weight for resistance

wellness—A conscious and deliberate approach to an advanced state of physical, psychological, and spiritual health

windchill—Cooling effect of temperature and wind

work capacity—The ability to achieve work goals without undue fatigue and without becoming a hazard to oneself or co-workers

References

Adams, W.C., Bernauer, E.M., Dill, D.B., & Bomar, J.B., Jr. (1975). Effect of equivalent sea level and altitude training on $\dot{V}O_2$max and running performance. *Journal of Applied Physiology, 39*, 262-268.

Ainsworth, B., Haskell, W., Leon, A., Jacobs, D., Jr., Montoye, H., Sallis, J., and Paffenbarger, R. (1993). Compendium of physical activities: Classification of energy costs of human physical activities. *Medicine and Science in Sports and Exercise, 25*, 71-80.

American College of Sports Medicine. (1995). *ACSM Guidelines for Exercise Testing and Prescription* (5th ed.). Baltimore: Williams & Wilkins.

Anderson, T., & Kearney, J. (1982). Effects of three resistance training programs on muscular strength and absolute and relative endurance. *Research Quarterly for Exercise Science and Sport, 53*, 1-7.

Ardell, D. (1984). *The history and future of wellness.* Pleasant Hills, CA: Diablo Press.

Armstrong, R. (1984). Mechanisms of exercise-induced delayed-onset muscular soreness: A brief review. *Medicine and Science in Sports and Exercise, 16*, 529-538.

Åstrand, P.O., & Rodahl, K. (1970). *Textbook of work physiology: Physiological bases of exercise* (2nd ed.). New York: McGraw-Hill.

Baker, D., Wilson, G., & Carlyon, B. (1994). Generality versus specificity: A comparison of dynamic and isometric measures of strength and speed-strength. *European Journal of Applied Physiology and Occupational Physiology, 68*, 350-355.

Balke, B. (1963). *A simple field test for the assessment of physical fitness.* Report no. 63-6. Oklahoma City: Civil Aeronautic Research Institute, Federal Aviation Agency.

Balke, B. (1968). Variation in altitude and its effects on exercise performance. In H.B. Falls (ed.), *Exercise physiology.* New York: Academic Press.

Barham, J. (1960). *A comparison of the effectiveness of isometric and isotonic exercise when performed at different frequencies per week.* Unpublished doctoral dissertation, Louisiana State University, Baton Rouge.

Barnard, R.J., Gardner, G.W., Diaco, N., & Kattus, A.A. (1972). *Ischemic response to sudden strenuous exercise.* Paper presented at the annual meeting of the American College of Sports Medicine, Philadelphia.

Benson, H. (1975). *The relaxation response.* New York: Harper & Row.

Blackburn, H., & Jacobs, D. (1993). Physical activity and the risk of coronary heart disease. In J. Boustet (ed.), *Proceedings of the fifth world congress on cardiac rehabilitation* (403-418). Hampshire, UK: Intercept.

Blair, S. (1993). Physical activity, physical fitness, and health. *Research Quarterly for Exercise Science and Sport, 64*, 365-376.

Blair, S., & Kohl, H. (1988). Physical activity or physical fitness: Which is more important for health? *Medicine and Science in Sports and Exercise, 20*, S8.

Blair, S., Kohl, H., Barlow, C., Paffenbarger, R., Gibbons, L., & Macera, C. (1995). Changes in physical fitness and all-cause mortality: A prospective study of healthy and unhealthy men. *Journal of the American Medical Association, 273,* 1093-1098.

Blair, S., Kohl, H., Paffenbarger, R., et al. (1989). Physical fitness and all-cause mortality: A prospective study of healthy men and women. *Journal of the American Medical Association, 262,* 2395-2401.

Blomqvist, C.G., & Saltin, B. (1983). Cardiovascular adaptations to physical training. *Annual Review of Physiology, 45,* 169-185.

Boileau, R., McKeown, B., & Riner, W. (1984). Cardiovascular and metabolic contributions to the maximal aerobic power of the arms and legs. *International Journal of Sports Cardiology, 4,* 67-75.

Borensztajn, J. (1975). Effect of exercise on lipoprotein lipase activity in rat heart and skeletal muscle. *American Journal of Physiology, 229,* 394-400.

Borg, G. (1973). Perceived exertion: A note on history and methods. *Medicine and Science in Sports and Exercise, 5,* 90-93.

Bouchard, C., Holimann, W., Venrath, H., Herkenrath, G., & Schlussel, H. (1966). *Minimal amount of physical training for the prevention of cardiovascular disease.* Paper presented at the 16th World Conference for Sports Medicine, Hanover, Germany.

Bray, G. (1983). The energetics of obesity. *Medicine and Science in Sports and Exercise, 15,* 32-40.

Breslow, L., & Enstrom, J. (1980). Persistence of health habits and their relationship to mortality. *Preventive Medicine, 9,* 469-483.

Broeder, C., Burrhus, K., Svanevik, L., & Wilmore, J. (1992). The effects of aerobic fitness on resting metabolic rate. *American Journal of Clinical Nutrition, 55,* 795-801.

Brooks, G. (1988, May). *Lactate as a metabolic intermediate.* Symposium presented at the annual meeting of the American College of Sports Medicine, Dallas.

Brown, M., & Goldstein, J. (1984). How LDL receptors influence cholesterol and atherosclerosis. *Scientific American, 233,* 58-67.

Brownell, K. (1995). Exercise and obesity treatment: Psychological aspects. *International Journal of Obesity, 19,* S122-S125.

Brownell, K., Greenwood, M., Stellar, E., & Shrager, E. (1986). The effects of repeated cycles of weight loss and regain in rats. *Physiology and Behavior, 38,* 459-464.

Brownell, K., Marlatt, G., Lichtenstein, E., & Wilson, G. (1986). Understanding and preventing relapse. *American Psychologist, 41,* 765-782.

Brownell, K., & Rodin, J. (1994). Medical, metabolic, and psychological effects of weight cycling. *Archives of Internal Medicine, 154,* 1325-1330.

Bruce, R.A., & Kluge, W. (1971). Defibrillatory treatment of exertional cardiac arrest in coronary disease. *Journal of the American Medical Association, 216,* 653-658.

Brynteson, P., & Sinning, W. (1973). The effects of training frequencies on the retention of cardiovascular fitness. *Medicine and Science in Sports and Exercise, 5,* 29-33.

Butterfield, G. (1987). Whole-body protein utilization in humans. *Medicine and Science in Sports and Exercise, 19,* S157-S165.

Campbell, W., Crim, M., Young, V., & Evans, W. (1994). Increased energy requirements and changes in body composition with resistance training in older adults. *American Journal of Clinical Nutrition, 60,* 167-175.

Carey, T., Garrett, J., Jackman, A., et al. (1995). The outcomes and cost of care for acute low-back pain among patients seen by primary-care practitioners, chiropractors, and orthopaedic surgeons. *New England Journal of Medicine, 333,* 913-917.

Caspersen, C. & Merritt, R. (1995). Physical activity trends among 26 states, 1986-1990. *Medicine and Science in Sports and Exercise*, 27, 713-720.

Cattell, R.B., Eber, H.W., & Tatsuoka, M.M. (1970). *Handbook for the sixteen personality factor questionnaire*. Champaign, IL: Institute for Personality and Ability Testing.

Christensen, E.H., & Hansen, O. (1939). Arbeitsfähigkeit und shrnährung [Working capacity and diet]. *Scandinavian Archives of Physiology*, 81, 160-172.

Comfort, A. (1979). *The biology of senescence*. New York: Elsevier.

Consolazio, C.F., Johnson, R.E., & Pecora, L.J. (1963). *Physiological measurements of metabolic functions in man*. New York: McGraw-Hill.

Cooper, K.H. (1970). *The new aerobics*. New York: Bantam.

Cooper, K.H., Purdy, J.G., White, S.R., Pollock, M.L., & Linnerud, A.C. (1975). Age-fitness adjusted maximal heart rates. In D. Brunner & E. Jokl (eds.), *The role of exercise in internal medicine* (Medicine and Sport, vol. 10). Basel, Switzerland: Karger.

Costill, D., Saltin, B., Soderberg, M., & Jansson, L. (1973). *Factors limiting the ability to replace fluids during prolonged exercise*. Paper presented at the annual meeting of the American College of Sports Medicine, Seattle.

Coyle, E. (1995). Substrate utilization during exercise in active people. *American Journal of Clinical Nutrition*, 61, 968-979S.

Coyle, E., Hemmert, M., & Coggan, A. (1986). Effects of detraining on cardiovascular responses to exercise: Role of blood volume. *Journal of Applied Physiology*, 60, 95-99.

Cureton, T. K. (1969). *The physiological effects of exercise programs upon adults*. Springfield, IL: Thomas.

Davis, P., & Starck, A. (1980). Age and performance in a police population. *Law Enforcement Bulletin*. Washington, DC: Federal Bureau of Investigation, 15-21.

DeLorme, T., & Watkins, A. (1951). *Progressive resistance exercise*. New York: Appleton-Century Crofts.

Demopolus, H., Santomier, J., Seligman, M., Pietrogro, D., & Hogan, P. (1986). Free radical pathology: Rationale and toxicology of antioxidants and other supplements in sports medicine and exercise science. In F. Katch (ed.), *Sport, health, and nutrition: 1984 proceedings of the Olympic Scientific Congress* (139-189). Champaign, IL: Human Kinetics.

deVries, H.A. (1986). *Physiology of exercise* (4th ed.). Dubuque, IA: Brown.

deVries, H.A., & Adams, G.M. (1972). Electromyographic comparison of single doses of exercise and meprobromate as to effects on muscular relaxation. *American Journal of Physical Medicine*, 51, 130-141.

deVries, H. & Housh, T. (1994). *Physiology of exercise*. Madison: Brown & Benchmark.

Dintiman, G., & Ward, R. (1988). *Sportspeed*. Champaign, IL: Human Kinetics.

Dockery, D., Pope, C., Xu, X., Spengler, J., Ware, J., Fay, M., Ferris, B., & Speizer, F. (1993). An association between air pollution and mortality in six U.S. cities. *New England Journal of Medicine*, 329, 1753-1759.

Docktor, R., & Sharkey, B.J. (1971). Note on some physiological and subjective reactions to exercise and training. *Perceptual and Motor Skills*, 32, 233-234.

Ehrlich, N. (1971). Acquisition rates of competitors and performers: A note on the theory of athletic performance. *Perceptual and Motor Skills*, 33, 1066.

Eichner, R. (1995). Contagious infections in competitive sports. *Sports Science Exchange*, 8, #3, 1-4.

Enos, W.F., Beyer, J.C., & Holmes, R.H. (1955). Pathogenesis of coronary disease in American soldiers killed in Korea. *Journal of the American Medical Association*, 158, 912-917.

Ernst, E. (1993). Regular exercise reduces fibrinogen levels: A review of longitudinal studies. *British Journal of Sports Medicine*, 27, 175-176.

Equal Employment Opportunity Commission, Departments of Labor and Justice. (1978). Uniform guidelines on employee selection procedures. *Federal Register*, vol. 43, 38290-38315.

Equal Employment Opportunity Commission (1991). Equal employment opportunity for individuals with disabilities: Final rule. *Federal Register*, 56, 29, CFR Parts 1602 and 1627.

Fiatarone, M., O'Neill, E., Doyle Ryan, N., Clements, K., Solares, G., Nelson, M., Roberts, S., Kehayias, J., Lipsitz, L., & Evans, W. (1994). Exercise training and nutritional supplementation for physical frailty in very elderly people. *New England Journal of Medicine*, 330, 1769-1775.

Fleck, S. (1992). Cardiovascular response to strength training. In P. Komi (ed.), *Strength and power in sport*. Oxford: Blackwell Scientific Publications.

Fleck, S., & Kraemer , W. (1987). *Designing resistance training programs*. Champaign, IL: Human Kinetics.

Folk, G.E. (1974). *Environmental physiology*. Philadelphia: Lea & Febiger.

Food and Nutrition Board. (1989). *Recommended daily allowances* (7th ed.). Washington, DC: National Academy of Sciences.

Foster, C., Hector, L., Welsh, R., et al. (1995). Effects of specific versus cross-training on running performance. *European Journal of Applied Physiology and Occupational Physiology*, 70, 367-372.

Fosterpowell, K., & Miller, J. (1995). International tables of glycemic index. *American Journal of Clinical Nutrition*, 62, S871-S890.

Frederick, E.C. (1973). *The running body*. Mountain View, CA: World Publications.

Friedman, M., & Rosenman, R. (1973). Instantaneous and sudden death. *Journal of the American Medical Association*, 22, 1319-1328.

Fries, J., & Crapo, L. (1981). *Vitality and aging*. San Francisco: W.H. Freeman.

Frisch, R., Wyshak, N., Albright, T., et al. (1985). Lower prevalence of breast cancer and cancers of the reproductive system among former college athletes compared to non-athletes. *British Journal of Cancer*, 52, 885-891.

Froelicher, V.F. (1984). *Exercise testing and training*. Chicago: Year Book Medical.

Gaziano, J., Buring, J., Breslow, J., Goldhaber, S., Rosner, B., Vandenburgh, M., Willett, W., & Hennekens, C. (1993). Moderate alcohol intake, increased levels of high-density lipoprotein and its subfractions, and decreased risk of myocardial infarction. *New England Journal of Medicine*, 329, 1829-1834.

Glasser, W. (1976). *Positive addiction*. New York: Harper & Row.

Gordon, E.E. (1967). Anatomical and biochemical adaptations of muscle to different exercises. *Journal of the American Medical Association*, 201, 755-758.

Greenleaf, J.E., Greenleaf, C.J., VanDerveer, D., & Dorchak, K.J. (1976). *Adaptation to prolonged bedrest in man: A compendium of research*. Washington, DC: National Aeronautics and Space Administration.

Gruber, J. (1986). Physical activity and self-esteem development in children: A meta-analysis. American Academy of Physical Education Papers, 19, 30-48.

Gwinup, G. (1970). *Energetics*. New York: Bantam.

Hettinger, T., & Müller, E.A. (1953). Muscle strength and training. *Arbeitsphysiologie*, 15, 111-126.

Hickson, R. (1980). Interference of strength development by simultaneously training for strength and endurance. *Journal of Applied Physiology*, 45, 255-263.

Hill, S.R., Goetz, F.C., & Fox, H.M. (1956). Studies on adrenocortical and psychological responses to stress in man. *Archives of Internal Medicine*, 97, 269-298.

Holloszy, J.O. (1967). Biochemical adaptations in muscle: Effects of exercise on mitochondrial oxygen uptake and respiratory enzyme activity in skeletal muscle. *Journal of Biological Chemistry*, 242, 2278-2282.

Holloszy, J.O., Dalsky, G., Nemeth, P., Hurley, B., Martin, W., & Hagberg, J. (1986). Utilization of fat as a substrate during exercise: Effect of training. In B. Saltin (ed.), *Biochemistry of Exercise IV* (pp. 183-190). Champaign, IL: Human Kinetics.

Ikai, M. (1970). *Training of muscle strength and power in athletes.* Paper presented at F.I.M.S. Congress, Oxford, England.

Ikai, M., & Steinhaus, A.H. (1961). Some factors modifying the expression of human strength. *Journal of Applied Physiology*, 16, 157-163.

Ismail, A.H., & Young, R.J. (1977). Effects of chronic exercise on the personality of adults. In P. Milvy (ed.), *The marathon.* New York: New York Academy of Sciences.

Issekutz, B., & Miller, H. (1962). Plasma free fatty acids during exercise and the effect of lactic acid. *Proceedings of the Society of Experimental Biology and Medicine*, 110, 237-239.

Jackson, C., & Dickinson, A. (1988). Adaptations of skeletal muscle to strength or endurance training. In W. Grana, J. Lombardo, B. Sharkey, & J. Stone (eds.), *Advances in sports medicine and fitness* (45-59). Chicago: Year Book Medical.

Jackson, C., & Sharkey, B. (1988). Altitude training and human performance. *Sports Medicine*, 6, 279-284.

Jackson, J., Sharkey, B.J., & Johnston, L.P. (1968). Cardiorespiratory adaptations to training at specified frequencies. *Research Quarterly*, 39, 295-300.

Jacobson, E. (1938). *Progressive relaxation.* Chicago: University of Chicago Press.

Jenkins, D., Taylor, R., & Wolever, T. (1982). The diabetic diet, dietary carbohydrate and differences in digestibility. *Diabetologia*, 23, 477-485.

Jensen, M., Brant-Zawadzki, M., Obuchowski, N., Modic, M., Malkasian, D., & Ross, J. (1994). Magnetic resonance imaging of the lumbar spine in people without back pain. *New England Journal of Medicine*, 331, 69-73.

Johnsgard, K. (1985). The motivation of the long distance runner. *Journal of Sports Medicine*, 25, 135-143.

Kanehisa, H., & Miyashita, M. (1983). Specificity of velocity in strength training. *European Journal of Applied Physiology*, 52, 104-110.

Kanter, M. (1995). Free radicals and exercise: Effects of nutritional antioxidant supplements. In J. Holloszy (ed.), *Exercise and sports science reviews.* Baltimore: Williams and Wilkins.

Kasari, D. (1976). *The effects of exercise and fitness on serum lipids in college women.* Unpublished master's thesis, University of Montana.

Kempen, K., Saris, W., & Westerterp, K. (1995). Energy balance during an 8-week restricted diet with and without exercise in obese women. *American Journal of Clinical Nutrition*, 62, 722-729.

Kenrick, M.M., Ball, M.F., & Canary, J.J. (1972). *Exercise and fat loss in obese patients.* Paper presented at the annual meeting of the American Academy of Physical Medicine and Rehabilitation, San Juan, Puerto Rico.

Kenyon, G. (1968). Six scales for assessing attitudes toward physical activity. *Research Quarterly*, 37, 566-574.

Keul, J. (1971). Myocardial metabolism in athletes. In B. Pemow & B. Saltin (eds.), *Muscle metabolism during exercise.* New York: Plenum.

Kline, G., Pocari, J., Hintermeister, R., Freedson, P., Ward, A., McCarron, R., Ross, J., and Rippe, J. (1987). Estimation of $\dot{V}O_2$max from a one-mile track walk, gender, age, and body weight. *Medicine and Science in Sports and Exercise*, 19, 253-259.

Klissouras, V. (1976). Heritability of adaptive variation. *Journal of Applied Physiology*, 31, 338-344.

Kobasa, S. (1979). Stressful life events, personality and health: An inquiry into hardiness. *Journal of Personality and Social Psychology*, 37, 1-11.

Komi, P. (1992). Stretch-shortening cycle. In P. Komi (ed.), *Strength and power in sport*. Oxford: Blackwell Scientific Publications.

Komi, P., & Buskirk, E.R. (1972). Effect of eccentric and concentric muscle conditioning on tension and electrical activity of human muscle. *Ergonomics*, 15, 417-422.

Kramsch, D., Aspen, A., Abramowitz, B., Kreimendahl, T., & Hood, W. (1981). Reduction of coronary atherosclerosis by moderate conditioning exercise in monkeys on an atherogenic diet. *New England Journal of Medicine*, 305, 1483-1489.

Kraus, H., & Raab, W. (1961). *Hypokinetic disease*. Springfield, IL: Thomas.

Lakka, T., Venalainen, J., Rauramaa, R., Salonen, R., Tuomilehto, J., & Salonen, J. (1994). Relation of leisure-time physical activity and cardiorespiratory fitness to the risk of acute myocardial infarction in men. *New England Journal of Medicine*, 330, 1549-1554.

Landy, F., et al. (1992). Alternatives to chronological age in determining standards of suitability for public safety jobs. Vol. 1, Technical Report, Pennsylvania State University.

Leaf, A. (1973). Getting old. *Scientific American*, 229, 45-55.

Lee, I-Min, Hsieh, C., & Paffenbarger, R. (1995). Exercise intensity and longevity in men: The Harvard alumni health study. *Journal of the American Medical Association*, 273, 1179-1184.

Leibel, R., Rosenbaum, M., & Hirsch, J. (1995). Changes in energy expenditure resulting from altered body weight. *New England Journal of Medicine*, 332, 621-628.

Lemon, P. (1995). Do athletes need more protein and amino acids? *International Journal of Sports and Nutrition*, 5, S39-S61.

Leon, A., Connett, J., Jacobs, D., & Rauramaa, R. (1987). Leisure-time physical activity levels and risk of coronary heart disease and death: The multiple risk factor intervention trial. *Journal of the American Medical Association*, 258, 2388-2395.

Leonard, J., Hofer, J., & Pritikin, N. (1974). *Live longer now*. Mountain View, CA: World Sports Library.

Lieber, C.S. (1976). The metabolism of alcohol. *Scientific American*, 234, 25-33.

Locke, E., & Latham, G. (1985). The application of goal setting to sports. *Journal of Sports Psychology*, 7, 205-222.

Lopez, S.A., Vial, R., Balart, L., & Arroyave, G. (1974). Effects of exercise and physical fitness on serum lipids and lipoproteins. *Atherosclerosis*, 20, 1-9.

Lubell, A. (1988). Blacks and exercise. *The Physician and Sportsmedicine*, 16, 162-176.

Mackinnon, L. (1992). *Exercise and immunology*. Champaign, IL: Human Kinetics.

Malina, R., & Bouchard, C. (1991). *Growth, maturation, and physical activity*. Champaign, IL: Human Kinetics.

Malmivaara, A, Hakkinen, U., Aro, T., Heinrichs, M., Koskenniemi, L., Kuosma, E., Lappi, S., Paloheimo, R., Servo, C., Vaaranen, V., & Hernberg, S. (1995). The treatment of acute low back pain: Bed rest, exercises, or ordinary activity? *New England Journal of Medicine*, 332, 351-355.

Manson, J., Willett, W., Stampfer, M., Colditz, G., Hunter, D., Hankinson, S., Hennekens, C., & Speizer, F. (1995). Body weight and mortality among women. *New England Journal of Medicine*, 333, 677-685.

Markoff, R., Ryan, P., & Young, T. (1982). Endorphins and mood changes in long-distance running. *Medicine and Science in Sports and Exercise*, 14 (l), 11-15.

Maslow, A.H. (1954). *Motivation and personality*. New York: Harper.

Massey, B.H., Nelson, R.C., Sharkey, B.J., & Comden, T. (1965). Effects of high-frequency electrical stimulation on the size and strength of skeletal muscle. *Journal of Sports Medicine*, 5, 136-144.

Mayer, J., & Bullen, B.A. (1974). Nutrition, weight control and exercise. In W.R. Johnson & E.R. Buskirk (eds.), *Science and medicine of exercise and sport*. New York: Harper & Row.

McArdle, W., Katch, F., & Katch, V. (1994). Essentials of exercise physiology. Philadelphia, Lea & Febiger.

Mitchell, J.H., Reardon, W., McCloskey, D.I., & Wildnethal, K. (1977). Possible roles of muscle receptors in the cardiovascular response to exercise. In P. Milvy (ed.), *The marathon* (232-252). New York: New York Academy of Sciences.

Móle, P.A., Baldwin, K.M., Terjung, R.L., & Holloszy, J.O. (1973). Enzymatic pathways of pyruvate metabolism in skeletal muscle: Adaptations to exercise. *American Journal of Physiology*, 224, 50-54.

Móle, P.A., Oscai, L.B., & Holloszy, J.O. (1971). Adaptation of muscle to exercise: Increase in levels of palmityl CoA synthetase, carnitine palmityl-transferase, and palmityl CoA dehydrogenase, and in the capacity to oxidize fatty acids. *Journal of Clinical Investigation*, 50, 2323-2329.

Móle, P.A., Stern, J., Schultz, C., Bernauer, E., & Holcomb, B. (1989). Exercise reverses depressed metabolic rate produced by severe caloric restriction. *Medicine and Science in Sports and Exercise*, 21, 29-33.

Molz, A., Heyduck, B., Lill, H., Spanuth, E., & Rocker, L. (1993). The effect of different exercise intensities on the fibrinolytic system. *European Journal of Applied Physiology and Occupational Physiology*, 67, 298-304.

Montner, P., Zou, Y., Robergs, R., Murata, G., Stark, D., Quinn, C., & Greene, J. (1995). Mechanism of glycerol-induced fluid retention and heartrate reduction during exercise. *Medicine and Science in Sports and Exercise*, 27, S19.

Morgan, W. P. (1979). Negative addiction in runners. *The Physician and Sportsmedicine*, 7, 57-70.

Morgan, W.P., & Goldston, S. (1987). *Exercise and mental health*. New York: Hemisphere.

Morgan, W., O'Conner, P., Ellickson, A., & Bradley, P. (1988). Personality structure, mood states and performance in elite male distance runners. *International Journal of Sport Psychology*, 19, 247-263.

Morris, J., & Crawford, M. (1958). Coronary heart disease and physical activity of work. *Journal of the British Medical Association*, 2, 1485-1496.

Morris, J.N., & Raffle, P. (1954). Coronary heart disease in transport workers. *British Journal of Industrial Medicine*, 11, 260-272.

Morrissey, M., Harman, E., & Johnson, M. (1995). Resistance training modes: Specificity and effectiveness. *Medicine and Science in Sports and Exercise*, 27, 648-660.

Nadel, E.R. (ed.). (1977). *Problems with temperature regulation during exercise*. New York: Academic Press.

Nelson, M., Fiatarone, M., Morganti, C., Trice, I., Greengerg, R., & Evans, W. (1994). Effects of high-intensity strength training on multiple risk factors for osteoporotic fractures: A randomized controlled trial. *Journal of the American Medical Association*, 272, 1909-1914.

Newham, D. (1988). The consequences of eccentric contractions and their relationship to delayed onset muscle pain. *European Journal of Applied Physiology*, 57, 353-359.

Nikkila, E., Taskinen, M., Rehunen, S., & Harkonen, M. (1978). Lipoprotein lipase activity in adipose tissue and skeletal muscle of runners: Relationship to serum lipoproteins. *Metabolism*, 27, 1661-1667.

North, T., McCullagh, P., & Tran, Z.V. (1990). Effects of exercise on depression. *Exercise and Sport Science Reviews*, 18, 379-415.

Ornish, D. (1993). *Eat more, weigh less*. New York: Harper Collins.

Ornstein, R., & Sobel, D. (1989). *Healthy pleasures*. New York: Addison Wesley.

Oscai, L.B., & Holloszy, J.O. (1969). Effects of weight changes produced by exercise, food restriction or overeating on body composition. *Journal of Clinical Investigation*, 48, 2124-2128.

Paffenbarger, R. (1978). Physical activity as an index of heart disease risk in college alumni. *American Journal of Epidemiology*, 108, 161-172.

Paffenbarger, R. (1994). 40 years of progress: Physical activity, health and fitness. In American College of Sports Medicine, *40th Anniversary Lectures* (93-109). Indianapolis.

Paffenbarger, R., & Hale, W.E. (1975). Work activity and coronary heart mortality. *New England Journal of Medicine*, 292, 455-464.

Paffenbarger, R., Hyde, R., & Wing, A. (1986). Physical activity, all-cause mortality, and longevity of college alumni. *New England Journal of Medicine*, 314, 605-613.

Paffenbarger, R., Hyde, R., & Wing, A. (1990). Physical activity and physical fitness as determinants of health and longevity. In C. Bouchard, R.J. Shephard, T. Stephens, J.R. Sutton, & B.D. McPherson (eds.), *Exercise, fitness, and health*. Champaign, IL: Human Kinetics.

Passmore, R., & Durnin, J. (1955). Human energy expenditure. *Physiology Review*, 35, 801-824.

Pate, R., Pratt, M., Blair, S., Haskell, W., Macera, C., Bouchard, C., Buchner, D., Ettinger, W., Heath, G., King, A., Kriska, A., Leon, A., Marcus, B., Morris, J., Paffenbarger, R., Patrick, K., Pollock, M., Rippe, J., Sallis, J., & Wilmore, J. (1995). Physical activity and public health: A recommendation from the Centers for Disease Control and Prevention and the American College of Sports Medicine. *Journal of the American Medical Association*, 273, 402-407.

Pette, D. (1984). Activity induced fast to slow transitions in mammalian muscle. *Medicine and Science in Sports and Exercise*, 16, 517-528.

Pollock, M.L. (1973). The quantification of endurance training programs. In J.H. Wilmore (ed.), *Exercise and sports sciences reviews* (vol. 1). New York: Academic Press.

Pollock, M.L., Dimmick, J., Miller, H., Kendrick, Z., & Linnerud, A. (1975). Effects of mode of training on cardiovascular function and body composition of middle-aged men. *Medicine and Science in Sports and Exercise*, 7, 139-145.

Pollock, M. L., Wilmore, J., & Fox, S. (1984). *Exercise in health and disease*. Philadelphia: W.B. Saunders.

Pomerleau, O., Scherzer, H., Grunberg, N., Pomerleau, C., Judge, J., Fertig, J., & Burleson, J. (1987). The effects of acute exercise on subsequent cigarette smoking. *Journal of Behavioral Medicine*, 10 (2), 117-127.

Powel, K., & Paffenbarger, R. (1985). Workshop on epidemiologic and public health aspects of physical activity and exercise: A summary. *Public Health Reports*, 100, 118-126.

President's Council on Physical Fitness and Sport. (1973, May). National adult physical fitness survey. *PCPF&S Newsletter*, 1-27.

Pritikin, N. (1979). *The Pritikin program for diet and exercise*. New York: Bantam.

Raab, W. (1965). Prevention of ischaemic heart disease. *Medical Services Journal of Canada*, 21, 719-734.

Radcliffe, J., & Farentinos, R. (1985). *Plyometrics: Explosive power training*. Champaign, IL: Human Kinetics.

Rejeski, W., Neal, K., Wurst, M., et al. (1995). Walking, but not weight lifting, acutely reduces systolic blood pressure in older sedentary men and women. *Journal of Aging & Physical Activity*, 3, 163-177.

Rising, R., Harper, I., Fontvielle, A., Ferraro, R., Spraul, M., Ravussin, E. (1994). Determinants of total daily energy expenditure: Variability in physical activity. *American Journal of Clinical Nutrition*, 59, 800-804.

Ross, R., Pedwell, H., & Rissanen, J. (1995). Effects of energy restriction and exercise on skeletal muscle and adipose tissue in women as measured by magnetic resonance imaging. *American Journal of Clinical Nutrition*, 61, 1179-1185.

Roth, D., & Holmes, D. (1985). Influence of physical fitness in determining the impact of stressful life events on physical and psychological health. *Psychosomatic Medicine*, 47, 164-173.

Roth, E.M. (ed.). (1968). *Compendium of human responses to the aerospace environment III.* Washington, DC: National Aeronautics and Space Administration.

Ruby, B., & Robergs, R. (1994). Gender differences in substrate utilization during exercise. *Sports Medicine*, 17, 393-410.

Ryan, A., Pratley, R., Elahi, D., & Goldberg, A. (1995). Resistive training increases fat-free mass and maintains RMR despite weight loss in postmenopausal women. *Journal of Applied Physiology*, 79, 818-823.

Ryder, H.W., Carr, H.J., & Herget, R. (1976). Future performance in footracing. *Scientific American*, 234, 109-116.

Saltin, B. (1977). The interplay between peripheral and central factors in the adaptive response to exercise and training. In P. Milvy (ed.), *The marathon* (224-231). New York: New York Academy of Sciences.

Saltin, B., Blomqvist, G., Mitchell, J.H., Johnson, R.L., Jr., Wildenthal, K., & Chapman, C.B. (1968). Response to exercise after bed rest and after training. *Circulation*, 38 (suppl. 7), 1-78.

Seltzer, C.C., & Mayer, J. (1965). A simple criterion of obesity. *Postgraduate Medicine*, 38, A101-A106.

Selye, H. (1956). *The stress of life.* New York: McGraw-Hill.

Sharkey, B.J. (1970). Intensity and duration of training and the development of cardiorespiratory endurance. *Medicine and Science in Sports and Exercise*, 2, 197-202.

Sharkey, B.J. (1974). *Physiological fitness and weight control.* Missoula, MT: Mountain Press.

Sharkey, B.J. (1975). *Physiology and physical activity.* New York: Harper & Row.

Sharkey, B.J. (1977). *Fitness and work capacity.* Washington, DC: U.S. Government Printing Office.

Sharkey, B.J. (1979). *Heat stress.* Missoula, MT: U.S. Department of Agriculture/ Forest Service Equipment Development Center.

Sharkey, B.J. (1984). *Training for cross-country ski racing.* Champaign, IL: Human Kinetics.

Sharkey, B.J. (1986). *Coaches guide to sport physiology.* Champaign, IL: Human Kinetics.

Sharkey, B.J. (1987). Functional vs chronological age. *Medicine and Science in Sports and Exercise*, 19, 174-178.

Sharkey, B.J. (1991). *New dimensions in aerobic fitness.* Champaign, IL: Human Kinetics.

Sharkey, B.J., & Greatzer, D. (1993). Specificity of exercise, training and testing. In L. Durstine, A. King, P. Painter, & J. Roitman (eds.), *ACSM's resource manual for guidelines for exercise testing and prescription* (82-92). Philadelphia: Lea & Febiger.

Sharkey, B.J., & Holleman, J.P. (1967). Cardiorespiratory adaptations to training at specified intensities. *Research Quarterly*, 38, 398-404.

Sharkey, B.J., Jukkala, A., Putnam, T., & Tietz, J. (1978). *Fitness and work capacity: Wildland firefighting.* Missoula, MT: USDA Forest Service.

Sharkey, B.J., Simpson, C., Washburn, R., & Confessore, R. (1980). HDL cholesterol. *Running*, 5, 38-41.

Sharkey, B.J., Wilson, D., Whiddon, T., & Miller, K. (1978, Sept.). Fit to work? *Journal of Health, Physical Education and Recreation*, 18-21.

Sheehy, G. (1976). *Passages: Predictable crises of adult life*. New York: Bantam.

Simoes, E., Byers, T., Coates, R., Serdula, M., Mokdad, A., & Heath, G. (1995). The association between leisure-time physical activity and dietary fat in American adults. *American Journal of Public Health*, 85, 240-244.

Siscovick, D., LaPorte, R., & Newman, J. (1985). The disease-specific benefits and risks of physical activity and exercise. *Public Health Reports*, 100, 180-188.

Sleamaker, R. (1989). *Serious training for serious athletes*. Champaign, IL: Human Kinetics.

Smith, M., & Sharkey, B. (1984). Altitude training: Who benefits? *The Physician and Sportsmedicine*, 12, 48-62.

Smith, R., & Rutherford, O. (1995). The role of metabolites in strength training. 1. A comparison of eccentric and concentric contractions. *European Journal of Applied Physiology and Occupational Physiology*, 71, 332-336.

Spain, D.M. (1966). Atherosclerosis. *Scientific American*, 215, 48-56.

Stamler, J., Wentworth, D., & Neaton, J. (1986). Is relationship between serum cholesterol and risk of premature death from coronary heart disease continuous and graded? *Journal of the American Medical Association*, 256, 2823-2828.

Steed, J., Gaesser, G., & Weltman, A. (1994). Rating of perceived exertion and blood lactate concentration during submaximal running. *Medicine and Science in Sports and Exercise*, 26, 797-803.

Stephens, T. (1988). Physical activity and mental health in the United States and Canada: Evidence from four population surveys. *Preventive Medicine*, 17, 35-47.

Stephens, T., Jacobs, D., & White, C. (1985). A descriptive epidemiology of leisure-time physical activity. *Public Health Reports*, 100, 147-158.

Stevenson, J., Felek, V., Rechnitzer, P., & Beaton, J. (1964). Effect of exercise on coronary tree size in rats. *Circulation Research*, 15, 265-270.

Stray-Gunderson, J. (1986). The effect of pericardiectomy on maximal oxygen consumption and cardiac output in untrained dogs. *Circulation Research*, 58, 523-529.

Stunkard, A., Foch, T., & Hrubec, V. (1986). A twin study of human obesity. *Journal of the American Medical Association*, 256, 51-54.

Sundet, J., Magnus, P., & Tambs, K. (1994). The heritability of maximal aerobic power: A study of Norwegian twins. *Scandinavian Journal of Medical Science in Sports*, 4, 181-185.

Superko, R. (1988). The atherosclerotic process. In S. Blair, P. Painter, R. Pate, L.K. Smith, & C.B. Taylor (eds.), *Resource manual for guidelines for exercise testing and prescription* (101-110). Philadelphia: Lea & Febiger.

Suzuki, T. (1967). Effects of muscular exercise on adrenal 17-hydroxycorticosteroid secretion in the dog. *Endocrinology*, 80, 1148-1151.

Swinburn, B., & Ravussin, E. (1993). Energy balance or fat balance? *American Journal of Clinical Nutrition*, 57, 766S-771S.

Tarnopolsky, M., Atkinson, S., Phillips, S., & MacDougall, J. (1995). Carbohydrate loading and metabolism during exercise in men and women. *Journal of Applied Physiology*, 78, 1360-1368.

Taylor, C., & Miller, N. (1993). Principles of health behavior change. In L. Durstine, A. King, P. Painter, & J. Roitman (eds.), *ACSM's resource manual for guidelines for exercise testing and prescription*. Philadelphia: Lea & Febiger.

Taylor, D., Boyajian, J., James, N., Woods, D., Chiczdemet, A., Wilson, A., & Sandman, C. (1994). Acidosis stimulates Beta-endorphin release during exercise. *Journal of Applied Physiology*, 77, 1913-1918.

Tenebaum, G., & Singer, R. (1992). Physical activity and psychological benefits. Position statement of the International Society of Sport Psychology. *The Physician and Sportsmedicine*, 20, 179-184.

Tesch, P., Thorsson, A., & Kaiser, P. (1984). Muscle capillary supply and fiber type characteristics in weight and power lifters. *Journal of Applied Physiology*, 56, 35-38.

Tobin, J., Miller, K., Sharkey, B., & Coladarci, T. (1982). *Prediction of $\dot{V}O_2$max from a bicycle field test*. Missoula, MT: University of Montana Human Performance Lab.

Treuth, M., Hunter, G., Kezesszabo, T. (1995). Reduction in intraabdominal adipose tissue after strength training in older women. *Journal of Applied Physiology*, 78, 1425-1431.

Tutko, T., & Tosi, U. (1976). *Sports psyching*. New York: Hawthorn.

U.S. Department of Health and Human Services. (1980). *Promoting health/preventing disease: Objectives for the nation*. Washington, DC: U.S. Government Printing Office.

U.S. Department of Health and Human Services, Public Health Service. (1991). Healthy People 2000: National health promotion and disease prevention objectives (DHHS #91-50212). Washington, D.C.

U.S. Department of Labor. (1968). *Dictionary of occupational titles*. Washington, DC: U.S. Government Printing Office.

Van Aaken, E. (1976). *Van Aaken method*. Mountain View, CA: World Publications.

Van Linge, B. (1962). The response of muscle to strenuous exercise. *Journal of Bone and Joint Surgery*, 44, 711-721.

Vega deJesus, R., & Siconolfi, S. (1988). Fat mobilization and utilization during exercise at lactates of 2 and 4 mm. *Medicine and Science in Sports and Exercise*, 20, (suppl. 71).

Washburn, R., Sharkey, B., Narum, J., & Smith, M. (1982). Dryland training for cross-country skiers. *Ski Coach*, 5, 9-12.

Watson, P., Srivastava, A., & Booth, F. (1983). Cytochrome C synthesis rate is decreased in the 6th hour of hindlimb immobilization in the rat. In J. Knutgen, J. Vogel, & J. Poortmans (eds.), *Biochemistry of exercise* (vol. 13) (378-384). Champaign, IL: Human Kinetics.

Weltman, A. (1989). The lactate threshold and endurance performance. In W. Grana, J. Lombardo, B. Sharkey, & J. Stone (eds.), *Advances in sports medicine and fitness* (91-115). Chicago: Year Book Medical.

Weltman, A. (1995). *The blood lactate response to exercise*. Champaign, IL: Human Kinetics.

Wenger, C. (1988). Human heat acclimatization. In K. Pandolf, M. Sawka, & R. Gonzalez (eds.), *Human performance physiology and environmental medicine at terrestrial extremes*. Indianapolis: Benchmark.

Wenger, H., & Bell, G. (1986). The interaction of intensity, duration and frequency of exercise training in altering cardiorespiratory fitness. *Sports Medicine*, 3, 346-356.

Whiddon, T.R., Sharkey, B.J., & Steadman, R.J. (1969). Exercise, stress and blood clotting in men. *Research Quarterly*, 40, 431-434.

Williams, P. (1974). *Low back and neck pain*. Springfield, IL: Charles C. Thomas.

Willis, J., & Campbell, L. (1992). *Exercise psychology*. Champaign, IL: Human Kinetics.

Wilmore, J., & Costill, D. (1994). *Physiology of sport and exercise*. Champaign, IL: Human Kinetics.

Wilmore, J.H. (1983). *Athletic training and physical fitness*. Boston: Allyn & Bacon.

Wilson, P.K., Castelli, W., & Kannel, W. (1987). Coronary risk prediction in adults (The Framingham Study). *American Journal of Cardiology*, 59, 91-94.

Wood, P. (1975). Middle-aged joggers show healthy lipoprotein pattern. *Medical Tribune*, 38, 27.

Young, A. (1988). Human adaptation to cold. In K. Pandolf, M. Sawka, & R. Gonzalez, (eds.), *Human performance physiology and environmental medicine at terrestrial extremes*. Indianapolis: Benchmark.

Zauner, C.W., Burt, J.J., & Mapes, D.F. (1968). The effect of strenuous and mild premeal exercise on postprandial lipemia. *Research Quarterly, 39*, 395-401.

Zawadzki, K., Yaspelkis, B., & Ivy, J. (1992). Carbohydrate-protein complex increases the rate of muscle glycogen storage after exercise. *Journal of Applied Physiology, 72*

Zukel, W., Lewis, R.H., & Enterline, P. (1959). A short-term community study of the epidemiology of coronary heart disease. *American Journal of Public Health, 49*, 1630-1638.

Zuti, W.B., & Golding, L. (1976). Comparing diet and exercise as weight reduction tools. *The Physician and Sportsmedicine, 4*, 59-62.

Index

About the Author

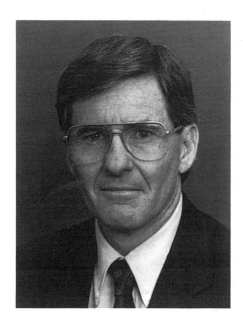

Brian Sharkey, past president of the American College of Sports Medicine, has more than 30 years' experience in the field of fitness as a teacher, researcher, consultant, and participant. A professor at the University of Montana (UM) since 1964, he also served as director of the school's Human Performance Laboratory. As professor emeritus, he remains associated with the university and the laboratory. Sharkey also works with the U.S. Forest Service as a consultant in the areas of fitness, health, and work capacity. He received the U.S. Department of Agriculture's Superior Service Award in 1977 and its Distinguished Service Award in 1993 for his contributions to the health, safety, and performance of wildland firefighters.

Known for his ability to translate complicated technical information into terms that the layperson can easily understand, Sharkey is the author of seven books on health and fitness, including three editions of *Physiology of Fitness*. From 1980 to 1986 he served as a consultant to the U.S. Nordic Ski Team, testing the limits of human performance in elite athletes. In his leisure time, Sharkey enjoys cross-country skiing, mountain biking, running, hiking, and canoeing.

More Books on
Improving Fitness and Health

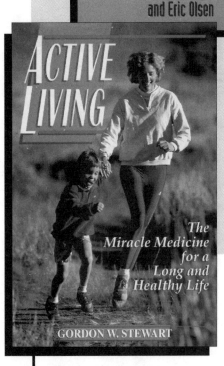

1996 • Paper • 432 pp
Item PPAF0429 • ISBN 0-87322-429-9
$16.95 ($24.95 Canadian)

Provides an easy-to-follow program for lengthening and improving the quality of your life. Dr. Ralph Paffenbarger presents this prescription based on more than three decades of studying the relations between physical activity, health, and fitness.

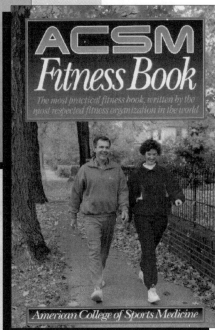

1992 • Paper • 128
Item PACS0460 • ISBN 0-88011-460-6
$13.95 ($19.95 Canadian)

This is the perfect beginner's guide for adults seeking a healthy exercise program. It's loaded with color photographs that show you how to perform over 45 stretching and strengthening exercises. The book contains an easy-to-use four-item fitness test, a walking program, and more!

1995 • Paper • 152 pp
Item PSTE0678 • ISBN 0-87322-678-X
$13.95 ($19.50 Canadian)

Shows how to attain better health through activities that are comfortable, meaningful, and right for you. You'll learn how to build physical activity into your daily routine, how to increase your activity level through various types of recreation—*and* how to stick to your program.

Prices subject to change.

Human Kinetics
The Premier Publisher for Sports & Fitness
http://www.humankinetics.com/
2335

To request more information or to place your order,
U.S. customers call **TOLL-FREE 1-800-747-4457**.
Customers outside the U.S. use appropriate telephone
number/address shown in the front of this book.